MICHAEL J. DALY, D.O.
MC, 497-62-9064

M Daly

D1762239

RENAL DISEASE
Classification and Atlas of Glomerular Diseases

Jacob Churg
Head, World Health Organization Collaborating Centre
for the Histological Classification of Renal Diseases,
Department of Pathology, Mount Sinai School of Medicine,
New York, N.Y., U.S.A.

in collaboration with

L. H. Sobin
Formerly Pathologist, World Health Organization
Geneva, Switzerland

and pathologists and nephrologists in 14 countries

IGAKU-SHOIN Tokyo · New York

Published and distributed by
IGAKU-SHOIN Ltd.,
　5-24-3 Hongo, Bunkyo-ku, Tokyo
IGAKU-SHOIN Medical Publishers, Inc.,
　1140 Avenue of the Americas, New York, N.Y. 10036

Library of Congress Cataloging in Publication Data

Churg, Jacob.
　Renal Disease.

　　Bibliography: p.
　　Includes index.
　　1. Kidneys—Diseases.　2. Glomerulonephritis.
I. Sobin, L. H.　II. Title. [DNLM: 1. Kidney diseases.
2. Kidney diseases—Classification WJ 300 C563r]
　RC903.9. C48　　　616.6'12　　81-13444
　ISBN 0-89640-066-2　　　　　AACR2

© First edition 1982 by IGAKU-SHOIN Ltd., Tokyo. All rights reserved. No part of this book may be translated or reproduced in any form by print, photoprint, microfilm or any other means without written permission from the publisher.

Printed and bound in Japan

World Health Organization

Collaborating Centre for the Histological Classification of Renal Diseases, Department of Pathology, Mount Sinai School of Medicine, New York, N.Y., USA.

Committee Members:

Dr. G. Avtandilov, Central Institute for Advanced Medical Studies. Moscow, USSR.
Dr. A. Bergstrand, Department of Pathlogy, Huddinge Hospital, Huddinge, Sweden.
Dr. A. Bohle, Department of Pathology, Faculty of Medicine, Tubingen, Federal Republic of Germany.
Dr. J. Churg (Chairman), Department of Pathology, Mount Sinai School of Medicine, New York, New York, USA.
Dr. R. Habib, Hospital des Enfants Malades, Paris, France.
Dr. F. Mota, Hospital Infantil de Mexico, Mexico, D.F., Mexico.
Dr. H. Sakaguchi, Department of Pathology, School of Medicine, Keio University, Tokyo, Japan.
Dr. A. E. Seymour, Department of Histopathology, The Queen Elizabeth Hospital, Woodville, South Australia.
Dr. L. H. Sobin, World Health Organization, Geneva, Switzerland.
Dr. D. R. Turner (Secretary), Department of Pathology, Guy's Hospital, London, England.

Consultants:

Dr. G. Andres, Department of Pathology, State University of New York at Buffalo, Buffalo, New York, USA.
Dr. E. L. Becker, Department of Medicine, Beth Israel Medical Center, New York, N.Y., USA.
Dr. J. Bernstein, Department of Anatomic Pathology, William Beaumont Hospital, Royal Oak, Michigan, USA.
Dr. J. S. Cameron, Renal Medicine, Guy's Hospital, London, England.
Dr. I. Greifer, Department of Pediatrics, Albert Einstein College of Medicine, Bronx, New York, USA.
Dr. P. Kincaid-Smith, Department of Medicine, Royal Melbourne Hospital, Melbourne, Australia.

Invited Participants:

Dr. G. Ditscherlein, Pathologisches Institut, Bereich Medizin (Charite) der Humboldt-Universitat zu Berlin, Berlin, German Democratic Republic.

Dr. S. Olsen, University Institute of Pathology, Aarhus Kommunehospital, Aarhus, Denmark.
Dr. R. Sinniah, Department of Pathology, University of Singapore, Singapore.
Dr. F. Skjorten, Patologisk anatomisk lab, Ulleval Sykehus, Oslo, Norway.
Dr. G. Tallqvist, Department of Pathology, Maria Hospital, Helsinki, Finland.

Ex-officio:

Dr. V. Khatchatourov, World Health Organization, Geneva, Switzerland.

Acknowledgment

Most of the illustrations in this monograph were supplied by members of the Committee, the consultants and other participants. Some illustrations came from friends and colleagues whose contributions are gratefully acknowledged: Doctors Roy N. Barnett, Samuel Dachs, Steven H. Dikman, R. S. Dobrin, John L. Duffy, Theodore Ehrenreich, Tullio Faraggiana, Burton Fine, Michael A. Gerber, Egil Gjone, Edith Grishman, Niilo Hallman, Gordon R. Henniger, Torstein Hovig, Hey-Chi Hsu, Jan Vincents Johannessen, David B. Jones, Edmund J. Lewis, Ching-Shen Lin, Jen H. Lin, A. F. Michael, Alfonso A. Madrazo, Willy Mautner, A. James McAdams, P.T. McEnery, Liliane Morel-Maroger, Takashi Morita, Mark Needle, William B. Ober, Bernard J. Panner, Conrad L. Pirani, Jerome G. Porush, Juhani Rapola, Mardoqueo Salomon, Melvin M. Schwartz, Raymond L. Sherman, Hidekazu Shigematsu, Richard K. Sibley, Fred G. Silva, K. Solling, Benjamin H. Spargo, Gerald S. Spear, Lotte Strauss, C. F. Strife, Yasunosuke Suzuki, R. L. Vernier, Brian H. Vitsky, Clark D. West and Richard H. R. White, and the International Study of Kidney Disease in Children. If any contributor's name has been inadvertently omitted, our gratitude is no less sincere.

Some of the illustrations are reproduced from books and journals with permission of the publishers and the authors:
Acta Medica Scandinavica: Fig. 3, Reference 148. *American Journal of Medicine*: Figs. 3, 4, 6, 8, Reference 104; Fig. 5, Reference 153. *American Journal of Pathology*: Fig. 7, Reference 121; Figs. 1, 8, 9, Reference 131. *Appleton-Century-Crofts*: Plate 2, Reference 44. *Dr. E. Lovell Becker*: Figs. 3-7, 3-11, Reference 2. *Clinical Nephrology*: Fig. 3, Reference 162; Figs. 3, 4, Reference 152. *Histopathology*: Fig. 8, Reference 87; Figs. 6, 11, Reference 191. *International Academy of Pathology, U.S.-Canadian Division*, and *Williams and Wilkins Co.*: Fig. 7, Chapter 2 and Fig. 7, Chapter 14, Reference 6. *International Academy of Pathology, U.S.-Canadian Division*, and *Laboratory Investigation*: Fig. 6, Reference 83. *Lancet*: Figs. 1, 2, Reference 108. *Little, Brown and Co.*: Fig. 13-11 and 13-20, Reference 8. *Springer-Verlag*: Figs. 21 and 23, Reference 22. *John Wiley & Sons*: Fig. 10, page 689, Reference 13; Fig. 21-11, Reference 14: Fig. 11, Reference 185. *Yearbook Medical Publishers, Inc.,* Chicago (© 1976): Figs. 7 and 9, Reference 109.

Appreciation is also expressed to all the technical personnel, especially Mr. Norman Katz, Mr. A. Prado and Miss Rosemary Lang.

Contents

	Page
Preface	ix
Introduction	x

Section I: Classification of Glomerular Diseases
- Glossary of Terms ... 3
- Basic Glomerular Alterations: Table I and Definitions ... 4
- Significant Qualifying Glomerular Changes: Table II and Definitions ... 5
- Clinical and Morphologic Correlations in Primary Glomerular Diseases (Glomerulonephritis and Related Conditions): Table III ... 7
- Clinical and Morphologic Correlations in Secondary Glomerular Diseases: Table IV ... 10
- Major Glomerular Syndromes and Associated Glomerular Lesions: Table V ... 18

Section II: Definitions, Descriptions and Illustrations of Glomerular Diseases
- Chapter 1. Normal Glomerulus ... 23

Primary Glomerular Diseases (Glomerulonephritis and Related Conditions)
- Chapter 2. Minor Glomerular Abnormalities (including Minimal Change Nephrotic Syndrome). Focal/Segmental Lesions (including Focal Segmental Glomerulosclerosis and Focal Glomerulonephritis) ... 35
- Chapter 3. Diffuse Membranous Glomerulonephritis ... 54
- Chapter 4. Diffuse Mesangial Proliferative Glomerulonephritis and Diffuse Endocapillary Proliferative Glomerulonephritis ... 67
- Chapter 5. Diffuse Mesangiocapillary Glomerulonephritis Types 1 and 3, and Dense Deposit Glomerulonephritis (Type 2) ... 83
- Chapter 6. Diffuse Crescentic Glomerulonephritis and Diffuse Sclerosing Glomerulonephritis ... 111

Glomerulonephritis of Systemic Diseases
- Chapter 7. Lupus Nephritis ... 127
- Chapter 8. Nephritis of Henoch-Schönlein Purpura, Berger's Disease, and Goodpasture's Syndrome ... 150

CONTENTS

Chapter 9. Glomerular Lesions in Systemic Infections
            (Septicemia, Infective Endocarditis, Shunt Nephritis,
            and Syphilis) 166
Chapter 10. Parasitic Nephropathies (Malaria, Schistosomiasis,
            and Strongyloidosis) 176

Glomerular Lesions in Vascular Diseases

Chapter 11. Periarteritis Nodosa and Wegener's Granulomatosis ... 188
Chapter 12. Hemolytic-Uremic Syndrome, Thrombotic Thrombo-
            cytopenic Purpura and Glomerular Thrombosis 198
Chapter 13. Benign Nephrosclerosis, Malignant Nephrosclerosis,
            and Scleroderma 211

Glomerular Lesions in Metabolic Diseases

Chapter 14. Diabetic Glomerulosclerosis 226
Chapter 15. Amyloidosis, Multiple Myeloma, Waldenstrom's
            Macroglobulinemia, and Cryoglobulinemia 240
Chapter 16. Nephropathies of Liver Disease, Sickle Cell Disease,
            and Cyanotic Congenital Heart Disease 262

Hereditary Nephropathies

Chapter 17. Alport's Syndrome, Thin Basement Membrane
            Syndrome, Nail-Patella Syndrome, Congenital
            Nephrotic Syndrome (Finnish Type) and Infantile
            Nephrotic Syndrome (French Type) 280
Chapter 18. Fabry's Disease, Familial Lecithin-Cholesterol Acyl
            Transferase Deviciency and I-Cell Disease 298

Miscellaneous Glomerular Diseases

Chapter 19. Nephropathy of Toxemia of Pregnancy and
            Radiation Nephritis 310
Chapter 20. *End Stage Kidney* 319
            Glomerular Lesions Following Transplantation 320

References 333

Appendix: Processing and Examination of Renal Biopsies 345

Index 351

Preface

Among the prerequisites for comparative studies on renal diseases are international agreement on criteria for diagnosis, a standardized nomenclature and a uniform system for classification. Without these ingredients, nephrologists, pathologists and epidemiologists, among others, would be uncertain whether studies carried out in one country were comparable to those from another.

Two notable recent efforts were made by international groups to bring order into this field.

The International Committee for Nomenclature and Nosology of Renal Disease working through subcommittees on anatomy, immunology, pathology, physiology, radiology and clinical medicine published "A Handbook of Kidney Nomenclature and Nosology" in 1975.

The International Collaborative Study of Kidney Disease in Children recognized the need to establish uniform criteria in this field owing to the special task they were undertaking. Their use of a panel of pathologists to review the material in the study helped pave the way towards developing acceptable terms and criteria for diagnosis.

Building on the experience of these groups, the World Health Organization in 1974 established a Collaborating Centre for the Histological Classification of Renal Diseases at the Department of Pathology, Mount Sinai School of Medicine, The City University of New York, in New York City, under the direction of Dr. J. Churg. The Centre worked with pathologists and nephrologists from fourteen countries to elaborate the material in this volume.

It is recognized that the classification reflects the present state of knowledge and modifications are almost certain to be needed as experience accumulates. Although some may wish to dissent from the views expressed, it is hoped that, in the interests of international cooperation, all will try to use the classification as put forward, particularly when international communication is intended.

Introduction

This monograph consists of two sections. The first provides a listing of glomerular lesions (Tables I and II) and gives their definitions. It also presents the main clinical and morphological features of glomerular processes in a tabular form (Tables III, IV and V). The second section describes in detail and illustrates the various glomerular processes. An Appendix contains information about some of the more useful histologic techniques and about examination of renal specimens.

Ideally, a classification of diseases should be based on etiology. However the current knowledge of etiology or even of pathogenesis of glomerular diseases is too limited to be of much value. As is well known, clinical classifications have proven unreliable because of considerable overlap in symptomatology. At the present time the most consistent classification is that based on morphology. This too has its limitations, because the pattern of glomerular change often lacks clinical specificity. It is to be understood that what is being classified here are histological patterns rather than diseases. Sometimes a pattern is sufficient to establish a specific diagnosis but in many cases it is necessary for that purpose to combine the morphological with the clinical data.

For some purposes the histological material has a further advantage over the clinical data: slides and photographs can be stored for a long period of time and retrieved for review whenever new clinical information in the individual cases, or a new way of classification becomes available. If need be, they can also be sent out for consultation over long distances.

The classification here presented harks back to Volhard and Fahr, but wears a modern dress. It is based primarily on light microscopy but also provides information about electron microscopic and immunofluorescent features. To avoid the increasing complexity of some of the current classifications, the glomerular lesions are divided into two categories: those representing the Basic Glomerular Patterns (Table I) and those considered to be the Qualifying Features (Table II). The lesions included in Table I are the constant changes, while those in Table II modify the appearance and sometimes even the evolution of the Basic lesion but do so inconstantly and only in some cases. For a complete definition of the histologic pattern in each individual case, the appropriate category from Table I should be supplemented by additional feature or features from Table II.

Perusing the Tables I and II makes it obvious that selection of the Basic Patterns is to a certain degree arbitrary. By combining sufficient number of Qualifying Features, it is feasible to define almost any entity in Table I, and if one so wishes, remove it from that Table. By this process one can reduce the number of Basic Patterns to very few, perhaps only two, in a manner reminiscent of Ellis' division of glomerulonephritis into Type 1 and

Type 2. For example, Table I could contain only Minor Changes and Mesangial Glomerulonephritis and all other entities would be defined by attaching appropriate qualifiers from Table II. However such classification would place under one heading entities with entirely different clinical behavior and would aggravate the problem of relating the clinical to the morphologic manifestations. The committee felt that the classification used in this monograph provides a reasonable compromise, which does not deviate too far from the current terminology and which offers a fairly consistent basis for clinicopathological correlation.

This monograph is meant not only for the specialist in renal diseases, but also for the general pathologist faced with examination of a renal biopsy or autopsy specimen. The first and most essential step of such examination is a careful study by light microscopy. This requires good tissue sections and proper stains (see Appendix). Information derived from such study, combined with the clinical and laboratory data and sometimes also with response to treatment, will be sufficient for diagnostic and prognostic purposes in a large majority of patients. In some cases the diagnosis should be considered provisional until it is further refined by electron microscopy and/or immunofluorescence microscopy, particularly in cases showing only minor changes by light microscopy, since clinically significant disease may occur with only slight glomerular changes. If only limited facilities are available, it is advisable to process and embed some of the renal biopsy tissue for electron microscopy (see Appendix for procedure). Such tissue can be examined at some future date, or be sent to an electron microscopy laboratory. A similar approach can be taken to immunofluorescence microscopy, though this may be somewhat more difficult to put into practice.

It is our sincere hope that pathologists and nephrologists will find this monograph useful as a basis for communication with their fellow workers throughout the world.

Key to Abbreviations

Am = amyloid
B = cytoplasmic bleb
BC = Bowman's capsule
BM, bm = basement membrane
BMM = basement membrane material
Br = break or defect of basement membrane
Cap = capillary
Col = collagen
Cr = crescent
Cr cell = cell of crescent
D = deposit
En = endothelial cell
Ep = epithelial cell
F = fibrin
FC = foam cell
FP = foot process or processes
Gr = granular material or granules
H = hyalin
I = interstitial tissue
JGC = juxtaglomerular cell
L = capillary lumen
l = lacuna or lucent area

LD = lamina densa
LRE = lamina rara externa
LRI = lamina rara interna
M = mesangium
MC = mesangial cell
MI = mesangial interposition in the capillary wall
MM = mesangial matrix
MN = mesangial nodule
Mon = mononuclear cell or monocyte
MV = microvillus or microvilli
P = podocyte
PAS = periodic acid-Schiff's reagent
PASM = periodic acid-silver methenamine
Pmn = polymorphonuclear leukocyte
PTA = phosphotungstic acid
PTAH = phosphotungstic acid-hematoxylin
RBC = red blood cell
S = spike or spikes
SM = smooth muscle
TBM = tubular basement membrane
TC = tubular cell
U = urinary space

Section I

Classification of Glomerular Diseases

GLOSSARY OF TERMS

Diffuse: A lesion involving all or nearly all glomeruli (i.e. $> 80\%$).

Focal: A lesion involving some but not all glomeruli ($< 80\%$).

Global: A lesion involving the whole glomerulus.

Segmental: A lesion involving a portion of the glomerulus (i.e. some capillary lumina remain uninvolved).

Hyalinosis: A lesion containing an acellular, structureless material (by light microscopy) consisting of glyco-proteins and sometimes incorporating lipids. The hyaline material stains intensely with eosin and PAS, red with Trichrome, and does not stain with periodic acid-silver methenamine (PASM).

Sclerosis: A lesion consisting of fibrillar material resulting from an increase in mesangial matrix and/or collapse and condensation of the basement membrane. The sclerotic material stains with eosin and PAS regent, blue/green with Trichrome stains and stains positively with PASM.

Fibrosis: A lesion consisting of collagen fibers which may be differentiated from sclerosis by *not* staining with PAS regent or PASM.

Necrosis (Glomerular): A lesion characterized by fragmentation of nuclei and/or disruption of the basement membrane, often associated with fibrin rich material.

Cellular Crescent: A lesion consisting of cellular proliferation (probably epithelial) which fills part or all of Bowman's space. Minimum requirement for this definition is the presence of at least two layers of cellular proliferation. Fibrin may often be associated with such lesions.

Fibro-cellular Crescent: A lesion which is similar to a cellular crescent but with the addition of a variable amount of fibrillar material. This fibrillar material may be either basement membrane-like material or collagen.

    N.B. This category includes those crescents with *almost* complete fibrous replacement.

Fibrous Crescent: A lesion within Bowman's space which is predominantly composed of fibrous tissue. This lesion may be the scarred remains of cellular and fibro-cellular crescents. However, it is important to note that identical lesions also occur in ischemic glomeruli where no evidence of glomerulonephritis can be obtained.

Note: Other terms in this monograph are used in a generally accepted sense as in standard textbooks of pathology and nephrology. A complete Glossary of terms can be found in a Handbook of Kidney Nomenclature and Nosology (see references). Histologic and clinical definitions follow Tables I, II and V in this monograph.

Table I BASIC GLOMERULAR ALTERATIONS.

1. **Primary Glomerular Diseases (Glomerulonephritis and Related Conditions)**
    A. Minor Glomerular Abnormalities
    B. Focal/Segmental Lesions (with only minor abnormalities in other glomeruli)
    C. Diffuse Glomerulonephritis
        a. Membranous Glomerulonephritis (Membranous Nephropathy)
        b. Proliferative Glomerulonephritis
            Mesangial Proliferative Glomerulonephritis
            Endocapillary Proliferative Glomerulonephritis
            Mesangiocapillary Glomerulonephritis (Membranoproliferative Glomerulonephritis Types 1 and 3)
            * Dense Deposit Glomerulonephritis (Dense Deposit Disease) (Membranoproliferative Glomerulonephritis Type 2)
            Crescentic (Extracapillary) Glomerulonephritis
        c. Sclerosing Glomerulonephritis
    D. Unclassified Glomerulonephritis
2. **Glomerulonephritis of Systemic Diseases**
    Lupus Nephritis
    Nephritis of Henoch-Schönlein Purpura (Anaphylactoid Purpura)
    Berger's Disease (IgA nephropathy)
    Goodpasture's Syndrome
    Glomerular Lesions in Systemic Infections
        Septicemia
        Infective Endocarditis
        Shunt Nephritis
        Syphilis
    Parasitic Nephropathies
        Malarial Nephropathy
        Schistosomal Nephropathy
        Strongyloides Nephropathy
3. **Glomerular lesions in Vascular Diseases**
    Periarteritis Nodosa
    Wegener's Granulomatosis
    Thrombotic Microangiopathy (Hemolytic-Uremic Syndrome and Thrombotic Thrombocytopenic Purpura)
    Glomerular Thrombosis (Intravascular Coagulation)
    Benign Nephrosclerosis
    Malignant Nephrosclerosis
    Scleroderma (Systemic Sclerosis)
4. **Glomerular Lesions in Metabolic Diseases**
    Diabetic Glomerulosclerosis
    Amyloidosis
    Nephropathy in Dysproteinemias
        Multiple Myeloma
        Waldenstrom's Macroglobulinemia
        Cryoglobulinemia

---

* May belong in a different category — Metabolic Disease?

Nephropathy of Liver Disease
Nephropathy of Sickle Cell Disease
Nephropathy of Cyanotic Congenital Heart Disease and in Pulmonary Hypertension

5. Hereditary Nephropathies
Alport's Syndrome
Benign Recurrent Hematuria
   Thin Basement Membrane Syndrome
Nail-Patella Syndrome (Osteo-onychodysplasia)
Congenital Nephrotic Syndrome (Finnish Type)
Infantile Nephrotic Syndrome (French Type) (Diffuse Mesangial Sclerosis)
Fabry's Disease and Other Lipidoses

6. Miscellaneous Glomerular Diseases
Nephropathy of Toxemia of Pregnancy (Pre-eclamptic Nephropathy)
Radiation Nephritis

7. End Stage Kidney

8. Glomerular Lesions Following Transplantation

Definitions to Table I will be found in Section II of this monograph together with clinical and morphological descriptions and illustrations of each entity.

Table II SIGNIFICANT QUALIFYING GLOMERULAR CHANGES.

The lesions may be diffuse or focal. If focal, then give percentage of glomeruli affected.
   (a) Segmental Mesangial/Endocapillary Proliferation
   (b) Segmental Hyalinosis
   (c) Segmental Sclerosis
   (d) Segmental Necrosis
   (e) Segmental Capillary Wall Abnormality
   (f) Capillary Thrombosis
   (g) Adhesions
   (h) Cellular and/or Fibrocellular Crescents
   (j) Global Sclerosis
   (k) Leukocytic Infiltration
   (l) Subepithelial Deposits
   (m) Transmembranous and Intramembranous Deposits
   (n) Subendothelial Deposits
   (p) Mesangial Deposits
Additional Non-Glomerular Lesions: Specify Type and Extent.
   Vacular
   Tubular
   Interstitial

DEFINITIONS TO TABLE II

(a) Segmental Mesangial/Endocapillary Proliferation
Focal involvement of glomeruli by segmental increase in mesangial cells and matrix (more than four cells/mesangial area), which may encroach upon capillary lumina. Proliferation of endothelial cells may also occur.

(b) Segmental Hyalinosis
Focal involvement of glomeruli by segmental hyalinosis.

(c) Segmental Sclerosis
Focal involvement of glomeruli by segmental sclerosis.

(d) Segmental Necrosis
Focal involvement of glomeruli by segmental necrosis.

(e) Segmental Capilary Wall Abnormality
Focal involvement of glomeruli by occasional splitting, wrinkling or thickening of the glomerular capillary wall.

(f) Capillary Thrombosis
Capillary lumina occluded by either protein, fibrin, platelet or mixed thrombi. Thrombi should be differentiated from emboli where possible.

(g) Adhesions
The attachment of part or all of the circumference of the glomerular tuft to Bowman's capsule. Adhesions may be either fibrinous or fibrous.

(h) Cellular and/or Fibrocellular Crescents
Focal involvement of glomeruli by either cellular or fibrocellular crescents.

(j) Global Sclerosis
Focal involvement of glomeruli by global sclerosis.

(k) Leukocytic Infiltration
The presence of five or more leukocytes per glomerulus.

(l) Subepithelial Deposits
Small accumulations of homogeneous eosinophilic material situated on the external aspect of the basement membrane. They may be relatively large and scattered (i.e., "humps") or small, frequent and closely applied to the basement membrane as seen in membranous glomerulonephritis.

(m) Transmembranous and Intramembranous Deposits
Accumulations of homogeneous eosinophilic material on both sides and within the basement membrane.

(n) Subdendothelial Deposits
Accumulation of homogeneous eosinophilic material in the subendothelial zone affecting occasional capillary walls.

(p) Mesangial Deposits
Rounded accumulations of homogenous eosinophilic material within the mesangial areas.

Table III CLINICAL AND MORPHOLOGICAL CORRELATIONS IN PRIMARY GLOMERULAR DISEASES (GLOMERULONEPHRITIS AND RELATED CONDITIONS)

GLOMERULAR CLASSIFICATION	CLINICAL MANIFESTATIONS	LIGHT MICROSCOPY	ELECTRON MICROSCOPY	IMMUNOFLUORES-CENCE MICROSCOPY
Minor Glomerular Abnormalities	Nephrotic syndrome steroid sensitive	Minor changes of epithelial cells, sometimes slight mesangial thickening or minimal increase in cells.	Foot process effacement	Nil (rarely, minor deposits of immunoglobulins or complement)
	Nephrotic syndrome steroid resistant	(Should be differentiated from very early membranous glomerulonephritis, early amyloidosis, early hereditary nephritis. See under appropriate headings)	Foot process effacement ± irregularities basement membrane	0 or IgM ± IgG
	Isolated proteinuria and/or microscopic hematuria		0 or minor changes of basement membrane, or mesangial changes. ± mesangial deposits	0 or IgM or IgA, IgG, C3 or IgA – C3 (predominantly mesangial)
	Macroscopic or microscopic hematuria, persistent or recurrent		Mesangial deposits or 0	IgA and/or IgG, C3, ± fibrin (predominantly mesangial); or IgM or 0
Focal and Segmental Hyalinosis and Sclerosis	Nephrotic syndrome Steroid resistant, sometimes steroid sensitive	Focal segmental hyalinosis and sclerosis Sometimes mild to moderate mesangial widening and cellularity	Diffuse foot process effacement, focal segmental collapse, increase in mesangial matrix (basement membrane-like material) and sometimes cells, occasional homogeneous electron dense deposits, lipid droplets	± IgM, ± C3, C1q (segmental, occasionally diffuse mesangial)
	Isolated proteinuria and/or macroscopic or microscopic hematuria	Focal segmental hyalinosis and sclerosis Sometimes mild to moderate mesangial widening and cellularity	No or only segmental foot process effacement, rest as above	As above

NOTE: ± This sign is used throughout Table III and Table IV to mean: present or absent.

GLOMERULAR CLASSIFICATION	CLINICAL MANIFESTATIONS	LIGHT MICROSCOPY	ELECTRON MICROSCOPY	IMMUNOFLUORESCENCE MICROSCOPY
Focal Glomerulonephritis	Macroscopic hematuria Proteinuria and/or microscopic hematuria Nephrotic syndrome Acute nephritic syndrome	Focal/segmental or focal/global lesions (exudative, proliferative, necrotizing, sclerosing) involving only some glomeruli (usually less than 50%)	Mesangial cellularity and increased amount of mesangial matrix. Mesangial (paramesangial) deposits. Capillary thrombosis and necrosis. Fibrin and crescents progressing to collagenous fibrosis. Subendothelial widening with translucent deposits.	IgA, ± IgG, C3, fibrin-segmental or diffuse mesangial. Diffuse mesangial IgG or 0 Fibrin Linear IgG, C3
Diffuse Membranous Glomerulonephritis	Nephrotic syndrome Isolated proteinuria ± Microscopic hematuria	Diffuse thickening of capillary walls due to subepithelial deposits (red with Trichrome stain) and projections of basement membrane (blue or green with Trichrome, black with silver)	Diffuse discrete regular subepithelial deposits, with intervening projections of basement membrane (spikes). Deposits may become intramembranous.	Uniform granular peripheral deposits of IgG and C3, less frequently IgM, rarely IgA, C1q, C4, fibrin.
Diffuse Mesangial Proliferative Glomerulonephritis	Isolated proteinuria and/or microscopic hematuria Nephrotic syndrome Massive proteinuria Macroscopic hematuria	Mesangial hypercellularity ± Increase mesangial matrix ± Mesangial deposits	Increased mesangial cells and matrix. ± Mesangial deposits As above and foot process effacement Increased mesangial cells and matrix ± Mesangial deposits	IgA ± IgG, ± C3 or 0 or IgM ± C3 Diffuse mesangial IgM ± C3 or 0 IgA ± IgG or 0
Diffuse Endocapillary Glomerulonephritis	Acute nephritic syndrome Acute nephritic syndrome with renal failure Acute nephritic syndrome with massive proteinuria (Other presentations rare)	Mesangial and endothelial cell hypercellularity Mesangial monocytes ± Polymorphonuclear leukocytes Capillary lumen reduced May show capillary thrombi and crescents	Subepithelial deposits ("humps") (not always present) Subendothelial deposits, mesangial deposits	Granular C3, early, along capillary wall IgG, early, sometimes IgM, IgA Occasional C1q, C4, properdin Fibrin

GLOMERULAR CLASSIFICATION	CLINICAL MANIFESTATIONS	LIGHT MICROSCOPY	ELECTRON MICROSCOPY	IMMUNOFLUORESCENCE MICROSCOPY
Diffuse Mesangiocapillary Glomerulonephritis (Membranoproliferative Type I)	Nephrotic syndrome or massive proteinuria Acute nephritic syndrome Macroscopic hematuria Rapidly progressive renal failure Isolated proteinuria (minimal or moderate) ± hematuria	Double contours or outlines (mesangial interposition), increased mesangial matrix and cells ± Enlargement of glomeruli ± Lobularity ± Crescents	Mesangial matrix increase, Mesangial cellularity "subendothelial" deposits mesangial interposition with double outlines. Mesangial, intramembranous and sometimes subepithelial deposits. Foot process effacement Crescents	Coarse irregular confluent deposits of C3, mainly peripheral, also mesangial. Less constant – IgG, IgM, IgA, C1q, C4, properdin, fibrin
Diffuse Mesangiocapillary Glomerulonephritis (Membranoproliferative Type III)	Same as Type I	Similar to Type I but thickening and irregularity of the basement membrane and poor staining with PASM	Similar to Type I but disruption of the lamina densa with intramembranous deposits. "Subendothelial" deposits rare. Subepithelial deposits more common.	Similar to Type I.
Dense Deposit Glomerulonephritis	Nephrotic syndrome Rapidly progressing renal failure Macroscopic hematuria Isolated proteinuria and/or microscopic hematuria	Silver negative layer in basement membrane. Basement membrane stains strongly with PAS, eosin, light green of Masson stain and thioflavin T. Crescents in about one-third of cases.	Electron dense "deposits" in the lamina densa and ± in mesangial matrix; also in tubular basement membranes and Bowman's capsules.	Coarse granular C3 in the mesangium, sometimes along basement membranes; usually no immunoglobulins. Occasionally no deposits.
Diffuse Crescentic Glomerulonephritis	Rapidly progressive glomerulonephritis Occasionally nephrotic syndrome	Large occluding crescents (cellular, fibrocellular, fibrous) in at least 50% and usually over 80% of glomeruli. (If endocapillary proliferation present, see endocapillary glomerulonephritis, also Henoch-Schönlein purpura, systemic lupus erythematosus) (Vasculitis – see also periarteritis nodosa, Wegener's granulomatosis, cryoglobulinemia)	Frequent breaks in the basement membrane. Sometimes electron dense or translucent subendothelial deposits. ("Humps" – see endocapillary glomerulonephritis).	Fibrin in crescents and capillary lumina. Linear IgG and C3 or 0 (In secondary crescentic glomerulonephritis, immunofluorescence reflects the basic lesion)

GLOMERULAR CLASSIFICATION	CLINICAL MANIFESTATIONS	LIGHT MICROSCOPY	ELECTRON MICROSCOPY	IMMUNOFLUORES-CENCE MICROSCOPY
Diffuse Sclerosing Glomerulonephritis	Chronic renal failure	Extensive glomerular sclerosis, mostly global in type. Thickening of Bowman's capsule. Capsular adhesions. Tubular atrophy and interstitial fibrosis.	Reflects original lesions	Immunofluorescence microscopy reflects original lesion, but non-specific deposits may be present (IgG, IgM, C3)

Table IV CLINICAL AND MORPHOLOGICAL CORRELATIONS IN SECONDARY GLOMERULAR DISEASES (SYSTEMIC, VASCULAR, METABOLIC, HEREDITARY AND OTHER NEPHROPATHIES)

GLOMERULAR CLASSIFICATION	CLINICAL MANIFESTATIONS	LIGHT MICROSCOPY	ELECTRON MICROSCOPY	IMMUNOFLUORES-CENCE MICROSCOPY
Lupus Nephritis	Proteinuria, mild to massive Nephrotic syndrome Hematuria "Telescoped" sediment Reduced glomerular filtration rate Decreased complement Anti-nuclear anti-bodies	Minor abnormalities Mesangial proliferative Focal segmental proliferative and necrotizing Diffuse proliferative (hematoxylin bodies, crescents, wire loops) Mesangiocapillary Membranous	Mesangial, subendothelial, intramembranous and subepithelial deposits. "Fingerprint" deposits Tubulo-reticular bodies	IgG + (all immunoglobulins) C3, Clq, C4, fibrin, DNA in glomeruli, especially in the mesangium and also along capillary walls. Deposits along tubular basement membranes and in the walls of blood vessels.
Henoch-Schönlein Purpura Nephritis	Hematuria Proteinuria Occasionally nephrotic syndrome	Minor abnormalities Mesangial proliferative Focal segmental necrotizing and proliferative Mesangiocapillary Crescentic	Mesangial and subendothelial deposits, also subepithelial "humps"	IgA, IgG, C3 and fibrin in the mesangium. Fibrin in capillary lumen and wall and in urinary space
Berger's Disease (IgA Nephropathy)	Persistent or recurrent hematuria, proteinuria, occasionally nephrotic syndrome. Slow progression to renal failure.	Mild diffuse or segmental mesangial widening with increase of cells and matrix and deposits. Occasionally diffuse cellularity or crescents.	Mesangial deposits, occasionally also subendothelial and subepithelial deposits.	Predominantly mesangial deposits of IgA and C3, often also IgG, occasionally IgM.

GLOMERULAR CLASSIFICATION	CLINICAL MANIFESTATIONS	LIGHT MICROSCOPY	ELECTRON MICROSCOPY	IMMUNOFLUORES-CENCE MICROSCOPY
Goodpasture's Syndrome	Lung hemorrhage and nephritis (Similar syndrome occasionally occurs in Henoch-Schönlein purpura, Wegener's granulomatosis, periarteritis nodosa, systemic lupus erythematosus. Differentiation by additional symptoms and by immunofluorescence microscopy).	Focal necrotizing glomerulonephritis Diffuse crescentic glomerulonephritis (see under this heading) Hemorrhagic pneumonia	Often no deposits Sometimes subendothelial, translucent or electron dense deposits Crescents	Linear deposits of IgG, C3 (on occasion, may be granular) Fibrin
Glomerulonephritis in Infective Endocarditis	Symptoms of acute or subacute endocarditis Hematuria and proteinuria Acute nephritic syndrome Rapidly progressive glomerulonephritis	Focal necrotizing and crescentic glomerulonephritis Mesangial proliferative glomerulonephritis Glomerular scars	Mesangial proliferation Mesangial subendothelial and subepithelial deposits Crescents	Granular deposits of IgG and C3, sometimes also IgM, IgA Fibrin
Shunt Nephritis	Nephrotic syndrome Microscopic hematuria Azotemia Positive blood culture (Staphylococcus albus)	Diffuse mesangiocapillary glomerulonephritis Rarely crescentic glomerulonephritis	Double outline of capillary walls Subendothelial deposits	Granular deposits of IgG, IgM, C3 along capillary walls, also bacterial antigens
Malarial Nephropathy	Acute form: hematuria and proteinuria Chronic form: nephrotic syndrome progressing to renal failure	Acute: Mild proliferative glomerulonephritis, segmental or mesangial Chronic: Capillary wall thickening with or without cellular proliferation	Mesangial proliferation with electron dense deposits. Basement membrane thickening, sometimes "plexiform" Subepithelial intramembranous, occasionally subendothelial deposits	IgM, IgG, C3, occasionally C1q, C4. Sometimes malarial antigens
Schistosomal Nephropathy	Hepatosplenic schistosomiasis Nephrotic syndrome or proteinuria Microscopic hematuria Slowly progressive renal failure	Mesangial proliferative glomerulonephritis Diffuse proliferative glomerulonephritis Mesangiocapillary glomerulonephritis Focal segmental sclerosis	Mesangial cellularity and matrix deposition. Deposits under the epithelium, in the basement membrane, under the endothelium and in the mesangium.	IgG, IgM, occasionally IgA and IgE, and also C3 in the mesangium and along capillary walls. Schistosomal antigens.

Table IV (Continued) CLINICAL AND MORPHOLOGICAL CORRELATIONS IN SECONDARY GLOMERULAR DISEASES (SYSTEMIC, VASCULAR, METABOLIC, HEREDITARY AND OTHER NEPHROPATHIES) GLOMERULAR LESIONS IN VASCULAR DISEASES

GLOMERULAR CLASSIFICATION	CLINICAL MANIFESTATIONS	LIGHT MICROSCOPY	ELECTRON MICROSCOPY	IMMUNOFLUORESCENCE MICROSCOPY
Periarteritis Nodosa and Wegener's Granulomatosis	Hematuria Proteinuria Acute renal failure Hypertension	Focal and segmental necrotizing glomerulonephritis Diffuse proliferative glomerulonephritis Mesangiocapillary glomerulonephritis Crescents	Capillary thrombosis Variable mesangial proliferation Occasional deposits Breaks in basement membrane Crescents	Fibrin ± Immunoglobulins, C3 ±
Thrombotic Microangiopathy	Hemolytic uremic syndrome Thrombotic thrombocytopenic purpura Postpartum renal failure	"Double outline" of capillary walls Translucent deposits Wrinkling (ischemic) Subendothelial deposits Thrombi Fragmented RBCs	Translucent subendothelial deposits ± Fibrin. Wrinkling of basement membranes Mesangial edema, mesangiolysis	Fibrinogen ± Occasionally IgG, C3
Glomerular Thrombosis (Intravascular Coagulation)	May be associated with gram-negative sepsis, shock, renal failure	Fibrin thrombi in glomerular capillaries, as well as arterioles, arteries and occasionally veins	Pure fibrin or fibrin mixed with structureless protein precipitate in the capillary lumina and occasionally under the endothelium	Fibrin, occasionally other proteins
Benign Nephrosclerosis	Hypertension (diastolic pressure 90–120 mm Hg) Microscopic hematuria Slight proteinuria	Hyaline sclerosis of arterioles Glomerular capillary wrinkling Mesangial widening Fibrous crescents	Increase in mesangial matrix Occasional small mesangial deposits	No data
Malignant Nephrosclerosis	Hypertension, severe Hematuria, proteinuria Renal failure	Ischemic wrinkling, segmental and hilar necrosis, crescents	Wrinkling of basement membranes Translucent subendothelial zone Occasional mesangiolysis	Fibrin in glomeruli and arteries Occasionally immunoglobulins and complement

GLOMERULAR CLASSIFICATION	CLINICAL MANIFESTATIONS	LIGHT MICROSCOPY	ELECTRON MICROSCOPY	IMMUNOFLUORES-CENCE MICROSCOPY
Scleroderma (Systemic Sclerosis)	Cutaneous and systemic manifestations Proteinuria Occasional nephrotic syndrome Azotemia Malignant hypertension	Vascular lesions, mild or severe Glomerular capillary wrinkling Thrombosis, necrosis Infarction	Capillary wrinkling Segmental basement membrane thickening Increased mesangial matrix	Fibrin, immunoglobulins, complement in areas of necrosis

Table IV (Continued) CLINICAL AND MORPHOLOGICAL CORRELATIONS IN SECONDARY GLOMERULAR DISEASES (SYSTEMIC, VASCULAR, METABOLIC, HEREDITARY AND OTHER NEPHROPATHIES) GLOMERULAR LESIONS IN METABOLIC DISEASES

GLOMERULAR CLASSIFICATION	CLINICAL MANIFESTATIONS	LIGHT MICROSCOPY	ELECTRON MICROSCOPY	IMMUNOFLUORES-CENCE MICROSCOPY
Diabetic Glomerulosclerosis	Proteinuria Occasional nephrotic syndrome Moderate hypertension Late renal failure	Basement membrane thickening, mesangial matrix increase Nodular form Capillary microaneurysms Hyaline or insudative lesions Thickening of tubular basement membranes Arteriolar hyalin at the hilus (afferent and efferent arterioles)	Basement membrane thickening Mesangial matrix increase Occasional deposits in the basement membranes and in the mesangium	Linear IgG, usually faint, also in the tubular basement membranes Occasionally IgM and C3 in the mesangium
Amyloidosis	Proteinuria Nephrotic syndrome Occasional renal vein thrombosis Acute renal failure Chronic renal failure	Deposits of amyloid in capillary wall and mesangium, stainable with Thioflavin T, crystal violet, Congo red (polarized)	Characteristic fibrillar deposits Subepithelial "spikes" composed of amyloid fibrils	IgG, C3, variable, generally weak (Specific antiserum available for light chain proteins)
Multiple Myeloma	Bence Jones proteinuria Chronic renal failure Acute renal failure Rarely nephrotic syndrome	Plugging of capillaries (rare) Mesangial nodules (similar to those in diabetes) 5–15% have amyloid with proteinuria Atrophy of tubules, dense lamellated casts, multinucleated giant cells	Mesangial widening Mesangial nodules Subendothelial deposits (kappa chain) Peritubular deposits (kappa chain)	Casts may show bright immunofluorescence but may be positive for kappa chain May be positive for kappa or lambda chain

GLOMERULAR CLASSIFICATION	CLINICAL MANIFESTATIONS	LIGHT MICROSCOPY	ELECTRON MICROSCOPY	IMMUNOFLUORES-CENCE MICROSCOPY
Waldrenstrom's Macroglobulinemia	Proteinuria, rarely nephrotic syndrome Bence-Jones proteinuria Acute renal failure	Plugging of capillaries Mesangial nodules (related to "light chain" production)	Mesangial widening Mesangial nodules Subendothelial deposits (kappa chain) Peritubular deposits (kappa chain) Plugging of capillaries by finely granular material	IgM of the same type as in serum
Mixed Cryoglobulinemia	Proteinuria Nephrotic syndrome Hematuria Acute renal failure	Plugging of capillaries Mesangiocapillary glomerulonephritis with large deposits	Hyaline deposits in capillaries; subendothelial deposits which show crystalline pattern (tubular or fibrillar)	Variable, concordant with circulating globulins: IgM, IgG, rarely IgA
Nephropathy of Sickle Cell Disease	Proteinuria Nephrotic syndrome Hematuria	Minor changes Focal segmental glomerulosclerosis "Mesangiocapillary" glomerulonephritis	Cellular proliferation Mesangial interposition Deposits in the mesangium, under the endothelium and in the basement membrane	Granular deposits of IgG and C3 in capillary walls and mesangium or 0
Nephropathy of Liver Disease	None or proteinuria and hematuria Functional renal failure	Minor changes Mesangial widening Mesangiocapillary glomerulonephritis Membranous glomerulonephritis	Occasional deposits in the mesangium, under endothelium or epithelium. Dark particles surrounded by clear zones in the mesangium and under the endothelium	IgA, IgG, IgM, C3, Hbs antigen
Nephropathy of Cyanotic Congenital Heart Disease	None or mild proteinuria, rarely hematuria, hypertension and azotemia	Glomeruli are large and congested Mesangium considerably widened with occasional nodular formations	Mesangial cell and matrix increase, fine collagen fibrils	IgM, inconstant

Table IV (Continued) CLINICAL AND MORPHOLOGICAL CORRELATIONS IN SECONDARY GLOMERULAR DISEASES (SYSTEMIC, VASCULAR, METABOLIC, HEREDITARY AND OTHER NEPHROPATHIES)

HEREDITARY NEPHROPATHIES

GLOMERULAR CLASSIFICATION	CLINICAL MANIFESTATIONS	LIGHT MICROSCOPY	ELECTRON MICROSCOPY	IMMUNOFLUORESCENCE MICROSCOPY
Alport's Syndrome	Hematuria, proteinuria, ear and eye manifestations, chronic renal failure	Minor changes Slight mesangial proliferation Focal segmental glomerulosclerosis Diffuse sclerosing glomerulonephritis Interstitial "foam" cells	Thickening and splitting of lamina densa with granular inclusions Focal thinning of lamina densa (early in the disease?)	C3 occasionally
Benign Recurrent Hematuria	Hematuria Chronic renal failure?	Minor changes or mild mesangial proliferation	Thinning of basement membrane	Negative
Nail-Patella Syndrome	Proteinuria Hematuria Occasional chronic renal failure Bone and nail changes	Minor changes Focal and segmental sclerosis Diffuse sclerosing glomerulonephritis	Thickening of basement membrane Collagen in basement membrane and in the mesangial matrix	Negative
Congenital Nephrotic Syndrome (Finnish Type)	Proteinuria, nephrotic syndrome Renal failure in first year of life	Microcysts Glomerular sclerosis	Foot process loss	IgG, C3 – occasionally
Infantile Nephrotic Syndrome (French Type)	Proteinuria, nephrotic syndrome Chronic renal failure	Mesangial sclerosis Global sclerosis	Foot process loss Irregular thickening or basement membranes	Negative
Fabry's Disease	Hematuria, proteinuria Chronic renal failure, especially in males Skin and mucous membrane lesions	Vacuolated epithelial cells in glomeruli and in tubules Similar cells in the interstitium and arteriole walls Progressive vascular and glomerular sclerosis	Dense myelin-like structures in the cytoplasm	Negative
Familial Lecithin-Cholesterol Acyltransferase Deficiency	Proteinuria Late renal failure Corneal opacities High serum lipids but low cholesterol esters	Foam cells in glomeruli and interstitium Thickening of glomerular basement membranes and widening of mesangium Progressive glomerular sclerosis	Widening of lamina rara interna and mesangium with accumulation of dark particles lying in clear zones	No data

Table IV (Continued) CLINICAL AND MORPHOLOGICAL CORRELATIONS IN SECONDARY GLOMERULAR DISEASES
(SYSTEMIC, VASCULAR, METABOLIC, HEREDITARY AND OTHER NEPHROPATHIES)
MISCELLANEOUS GLOMERULAR DISEASES

GLOMERULAR CLASSSIFICATION	CLINICAL MANIFESTATIONS	LIGHT MICROSCOPY	ELECTRON MICROSCOPY	IMMUNOFLUORESCENCE MICROSCOPY
Toxemia of Pregnancy (Pre-eclampsia)	Proteinuria Hypertension Occasionally microscopic hematuria	Mesangial and endothelial cell swelling with capillary narrowing	Mesangial and endothelial swelling. Subendothelial and mesangial deposits	Fibrin + IgM, IgG, C3 ±
Radiation Nephritis	Proteinuria Hypertension Renal failure	Thickening and wrinkling of capillary walls Segmental necrosis and cell proliferation Segmental or diffuse sclerosis Capsular adhesions	Endothelial detachment Translucent subendothelial deposits Foot process loss Mesangiolysis Mesangial sclerosis	0 or segmental IgM

Table IV (Continued) CLINICAL AND MORPHOLOGICAL CORRELATIONS IN SECONDARY GLOMERULAR DISEASES
(SYSTEMIC, VASCULAR, METABOLIC, HEREDITARY AND OTHER NEPHROPATHIES)
END STAGE KIDNEY

GLOMERULAR CLASSSIFICATION	CLINICAL MANIFESTATIONS	LIGHT MICROSCOPY	ELECTRON MICROSCOPY	IMMUNOFLUORESCENCE MICROSCOPY
End Stage Kidney	Terminal renal failure	Sclerosis of almost all glomeruli Extensive tubular atrophy Prominent vascular sclerosis	Capillary collapse Extensive sclerosis	Inconstant deposits of immune globulins and C3

Table IV (Continued) CLINICAL AND MORPHOLOGICAL CORRELATIONS IN SECONDARY GLOMERULAR DISEASES (SYSTEMIC, VASCULAR, METABOLIC, HEREDITARY AND OTHER NEPHROPATHIES) GLOMERULAR LESIONS OCCURRING IN TRANSPLANTED KIDNEYS

GLOMERULAR CLASSSIFICATION	CLINICAL MANIFESTATIONS	LIGHT MICROSCOPY	ELECTRON MICROSCOPY	IMMUNOFLUORESCENCE MICROSCOPY
Glomerular Lesions Occurring in Transplanted Kidneys	Deteriorating glomerular filtration rate. Proteinuria, occasionally nephrotic syndrome. Hemolytic-uremic syndrome may be seen. Note: Almost all case have vascular involvement	Almost any lesion in Tables I and II may be present and may be recurrent or *de novo*. Only some can be identified as recurrent, such as Dense Deposit Disease, mesangial IgA, diffuse crescents with linear IgG (anti-GBM), focal and segmental hyalinosis or sclerosis (with immediate nephrotic syndrome), hemolytic-uremic syndrome. Systemic diseases, e.g. diabetes may have recurrent lesions. Others may not be recurrent but arise *de novo*. Among *de novo* lesions irregular double contour without proliferation is the most frequent change.	Translucent subendothelial zone with some mesangial cell interposition (as distinct from electron dense subendothelial deposits in recurrent MCGN Type I)	Variable IgM, C3 Fibrin, early

Table V CLINICAL SYNDROMES AND GLOMERULAR HISTOPATHOLOGY

Acute Nephritic Syndrome
Definition: A syndrome characterized by abrupt onset of hematuria, proteinuria, hypertension, decreased glomerular filtration and retention of sodium and water.
Common Histopathologic Patterns or Diseases:
    Diffuse endocapillary proliferative glomerulonephritis
    Diffuse crescentic glomerulonephritis
    Diffuse mesangiocapillary glomerulonephritis
    Dense deposit glomerulonephritis
    Diffuse sclerosing glomerulonephritis (acute exacerbation)
    Focal proliferative or necrotizing glomerulonephritis
    Lupus nephritis
    Henoch-Schönlein purpura
    Berger's disease (IgA nephropathy)
    Hereditary nephritis (Alport's syndrome)
    Periarteritis nodosa
    Wegener's granulomatosis

Rapidly Progressive Nephritic Syndrome (Rapidly Progressive Glomerulonephritis)
Definition: An abrupt or insidious onset of hematuria, proteinuria, anemia and rapidly progressing renal failure.
Common Histopathologic Patterns or Diseases:
    Diffuse crescentic glomerulonephritis
    Goodpasture's syndrome
    Diffuse endocapillary proliferative glomerulonephritis
    Diffuse mesangiocapillary glomerulonephritis with crescents
    Dense deposit glomerulonephritis with crescents
    Henoch-Schönlein purpura
    Lupus nephritis
    Periarteritis nodosa
    Wegener's granulomatosis
    Infective endocarditis
    Diffuse membranous glomerulonephritis with crescents
    Mixed essential cryoglobulinemia
    Hemolytic-uremic syndrome

Recurrent or Persistent Hematuria
Definition: Insidious or abrupt onset of gross or microscopic hematuria with little or no proteinuria and no evidence of other features of nephritic syndrome.
Common Histopathologic Patterns or Diseases:
    Focal proliferative or necrotizing glomerulonephritis
    Berger's disease (IgA nephropathy)
    IgM nephropathy
    Diffuse mesangial proliferative glomerulonephritis
    Diffuse mesangiocapillary glomerulonephritis

Focal segmental glomerulosclerosis
Diffuse sclerosing glomerulonephritis
Alport's syndrome
Lupus nephritis
Sickle cell disease
Thin basement membrane syndrome
No glomerular abnormalities

Chronic Nephritic Syndrome
Definition: Slowly developing renal failure accompanied by proteinuria, hematuria and hypertension
Common Histopathologic Patterns or Diseases:
Diffuse mesangial proliferative and sclerosing glomerulonephritis
Diffuse mesangiocapillary glomerulonephritis
Diffuse mesangial glomerulonephritis including Berger's disease (IgA nephropathy)
Diffuse membranous glomerulonephritis
Focal segmental glomerulosclerosis
Lupus nephritis
Diabetic glomerulosclerosis
Renal amyloidosis
Hereditary nephritis: Alport's syndrome, nail patella syndrome

Nephrotic Syndrome
Definition: A syndrome of massive proteinuria, edema, hypoalbuminemia and frequently, hypercholesteremia. Associated with a great variety of glomerular lesions.
Common Histopathologic Patterns or Diseases:
Lipoid nephrosis (Minimal change)
Focal segmental glomerulosclerosis
Diffuse membranous glomerulonephritis
Diffuse mesangial proliferative glomerulonephritis
Diffuse mesangiocapillary glomerulonephritis
Dense deposit glomerulonephritis
Berger's disease (IgA nephropathy)
IgM nephropathy
Mixed essential cryoglobulinemia
Lupus nephritis
Henoch-Schönlein purpura
Diabetes mellitus
Amyloidosis
Hereditary nephritis: Alport's syndrome, nail patella syndrome
Congenital nephrotic syndrome
Infantile nephrotic syndrome
Transplant rejection

Section II

Definitions, Descriptions and Illustrations of Glomerular Diseases

CHAPTER 1

Normal Glomerulus
(Figs. 1-1 to 1-11)

Normal Glomerulus

The renal glomerulus consists of a bundle of capillaries (capillary tuft) invaginated into the modified and dilated end of the proximal tubule, so-called urinary or Bowman's space. Some authors reserve the name glomerulus for the capillary tuft alone, and use the term "renal corpuscle" to denote the capillaries together with the urinary space and its capsule (Bowman's capsule). Others, including ourselves, use glomerulus in a broader sense, identifying it with the entire renal corpuscle. So conceived, the glomerulus is seen to consist of three structural elements: the Bowman's capsule, the capillary walls and the mesangium, the latter being a slender branching stalk of specialized connective tissue which holds together and supports the capillaries. These structural elements delineate two spaces: the urinary space and the capillary lumina.

The glomerular capillaries arise by subdivision of the afferent arteriole. The latter gives rise to several primary branches which form glomerular lobes and which give off anastomosing secondary branches. The latter curl around the terminal portions of the mesangial stalk and form glomerular lobules. The capillaries reunite into the efferent arteriole which leaves the glomerulus at the hilus, close to the entrances of afferent arteriole. However occasionally the arterioles lie at a distance even as far as the opposite poles. The efferent arteriole after leaving the glomerulus tends to curve along the outside aspect of the Bowman's capsule.

The Bowman's capsule consists of a thick, occasionally multilayered basement membrane which supports a single layer of flattened epithelial cells (parietal epithelial cells). At the vascular pole, the parietal cell layer is continuous with the visceral cells, so-called podocytes.

The capillary wall consists of a basement membrane covered by a thin sheet of endothelial cytoplasm on its inner aspect and by epithelial podocytes on its outer aspect, facing the urinary space. The attenuated endothelial cytoplasm is studded with rounded pores measuring about 70 nm in diameter, and covered by very thin diaphragms. The nuclei and the bodies of the endothelial cells are usually located in the part of the capillary closest to the mesangium. The podocytes have relatively small bodies which give rise to long trabeculae bearing numerous foot processes which rest upon and are attached to the basement membrane. The surface of the podocytes facing the urinary space is covered by a fairly thick coat of mucous substances, mainly mucopolysaccharides. Similar cell coat also covered the surfaces of the foot processes. Where foot processes are attached to the basement membrane, a similar but much thinner coat is present. The basement membrane consists of three layers: the middle, lamina densa; the outer, lamina rara externa and the inner, lamina rara interna. The thickness of the basement membrane varies with the species and with age. In adult humans, it measures 200–400 nm, with an average around 300 nm; in children under three years of age, it is probably half that thickness.

The mesangium arises at the glomerular hilus, where it appears to be continuous with the lacis cells of the juxtaglomerular apparatus, and follows the branching capillaries as far as the centers of individual glomerular lobules. It consists of cells (mesangial cells) and intercellular material (mesangial matrix). The cells have irregular bodies with numerous cytoplasmic processes and contain bundles of fine fibrils arranged perpendicularly to the plasma membrane. The cells are probably analogous to capillary pericytes elsewhere in the body. They have contractile properties, phagocytic properties and probably also the potential ability to produce inner secretion (renin). The mesangial matrix forms a branching meshwork surrounding the cells and separating them, though incompletely from the endothelial cells. The matrix resembles the basement membranes in its staining characteristics and electron microscopic appearance, but is coarser and looser in texture and probably somewhat different in chemical composition, and in its immunological reactions. Where the mesangium does not abut upon the endothelial cells, it is covered by the capillary basement membrane and by the epithelial foot processes. Thus both the capillary endothelium and the mesangium lie on the "inside" of the basement membrane ("intracapillary"). The region of the mesangium directly under the basement membrane is often referred to as the paramesangial area. This area extends slightly into the capillary wall, lying between the endothelium and the basement membrane.

NORMAL GLOMERULUS

NORMAL GLOMERULUS

Fig. 1-1 Normal glomerulus cut through the hilus. The branching mesangial stalk is clearly seen. The capillaries are attached to the stalk, forming peripheral lobules.
2 mu. section, PAS stain.   x 260.

Fig. 1-2 Normal glomerulus cut through the hilus. The mesangial stalk is visible but somewhat obscured by the stained nuclei and cytoplasm of the glomerular cells.
Trichrome stain.   x 260.

Fig. 1-3 Normal glomerulus showing fine mesangial stalk and the glomerular capillaries.
PASM stain with counterstain.   x 260.

Fig. 1-4 Normal glomerulus stained with colloidal iron. The cell coat of the podocytes is clearly outlined.   x 410.

Fig. 1-5 Normal glomerulus in a new born infant (age 11 days). The mesangium is relatively wide. The nuclei of the podocytes are prominent.
PAS stain.   x 410.

Fig. 1-6 Part of a normal glomerulus showing peripheral lobules with their mesangial stalks and attached capillaries.
1 mu. section, PAS stain.   x 1,000.

NORMAL GLOMERULUS

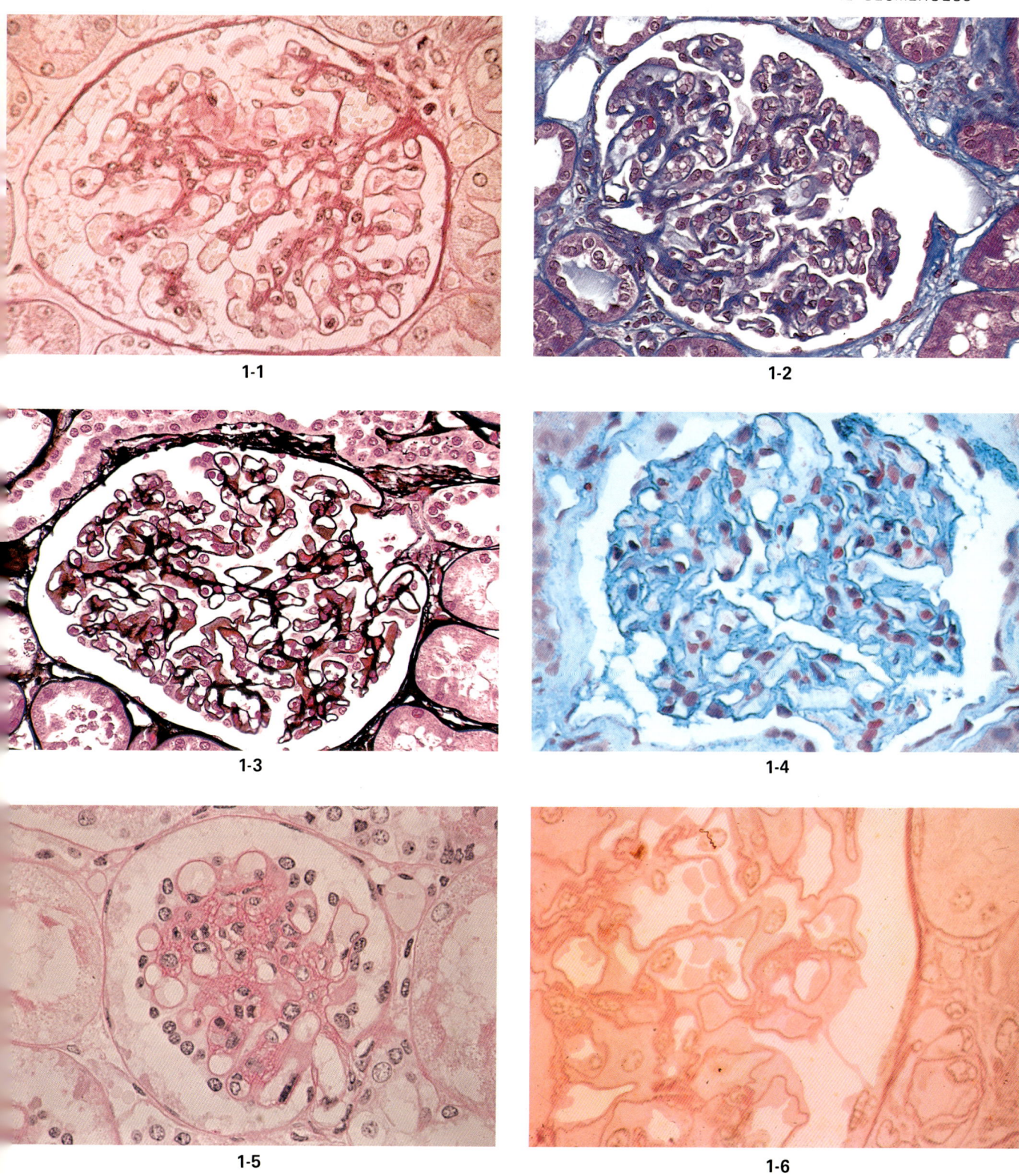

1-1

1-2

1-3

1-4

1-5

1-6

NORMAL GLOMERULUS

NORMAL GLOMERULUS

Fig. 1-7 A single glomerular lobule under high magnification. The mesangial stalk is in the center. Two nuclei of mesangial cells (MC) are visible as well as small strands of mesangial matrix. The matrix (MM) forms thin discontinuous lines separating the mesangium from the capillary lumina. Endothelial cells (En) are seen in two of the capillaries. Epithelial cells (podocytes) (P) are attached to the basement membrane (BM). Bowman's capsule (BC) is present in the left upper corner.
0.5 mu. section, PAS stain. x 2,000.

Fig. 1-8 Electron micrograph of the mesangial stalk. Two mesangial cells (MC) are present together with strands of mesangial matrix (MM). An extension of one cell, so-called "bleb" (B), is seen in the capillary lumen (left upper corner). The basement membrane covering the mesangium is somewhat wrinkled and is covered by foot processes of the podocytes (P). x 12,000.

U: urinary space, L: capillary lumen, En: endothelial cell.

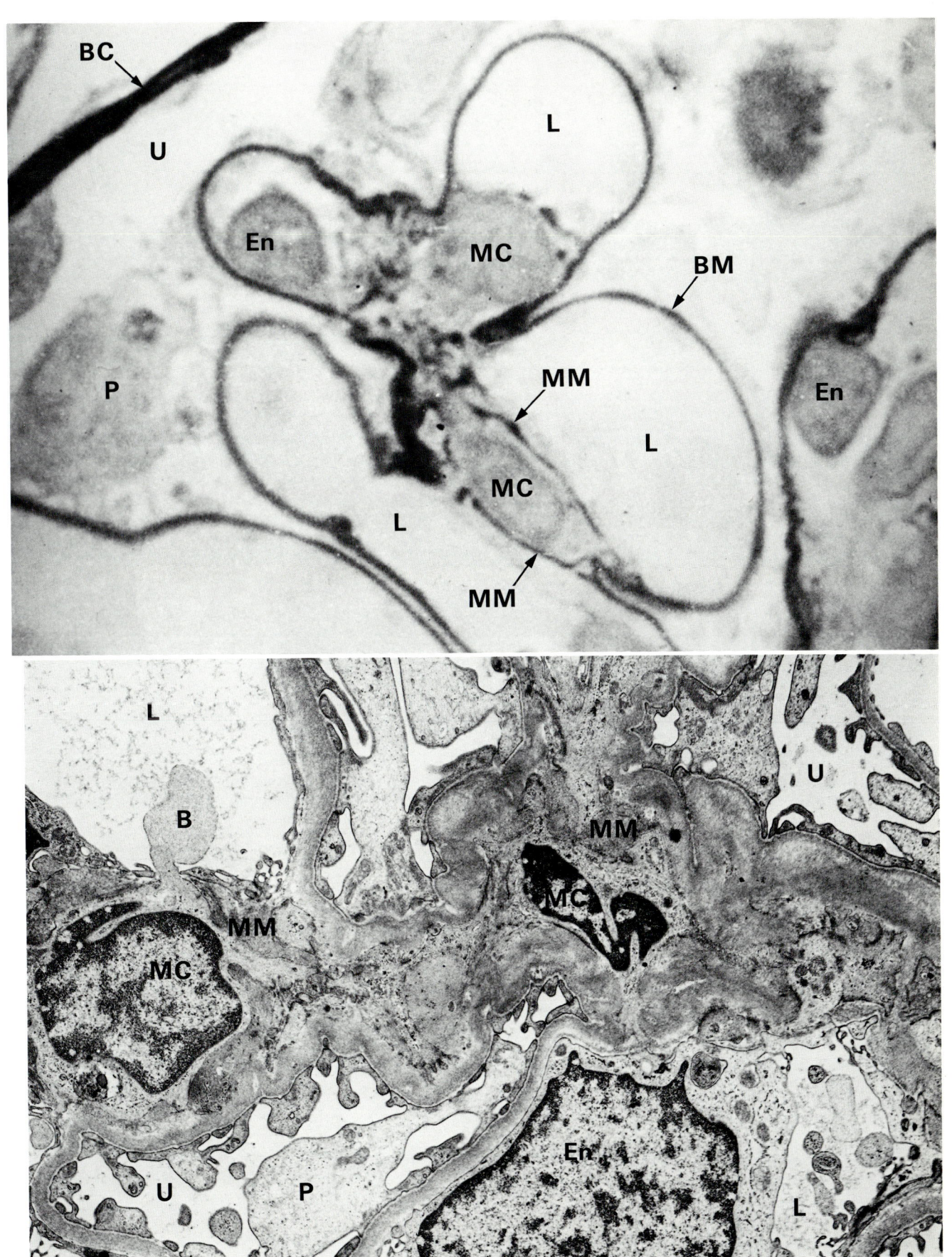

NORMAL GLOMERULUS

Fig. 1-9 Electron micrograph. Part of a glomerular capillary showing the endothelial lining, the basement membrane (BM) and foot processes, some of which are attached to the cytoplasm of the podocytes (P). Bowman's capsule (BC) with its basement membrane and the parietal epithelial cells is also visible.
x 12,000.

Fig. 1-10 Electron micrograph. Part of a glomerular capillary wall under higher magnification. Endothelial pores are visible in places. The basement membrane shows three layers: lamina rara interna (LRI), lamina densa (LD) and lamina rara externa (LRE) x 18,000.

U: urinary space, L: capillary lumen, FP: foot process of processes.

NORMAL GLOMERULUS

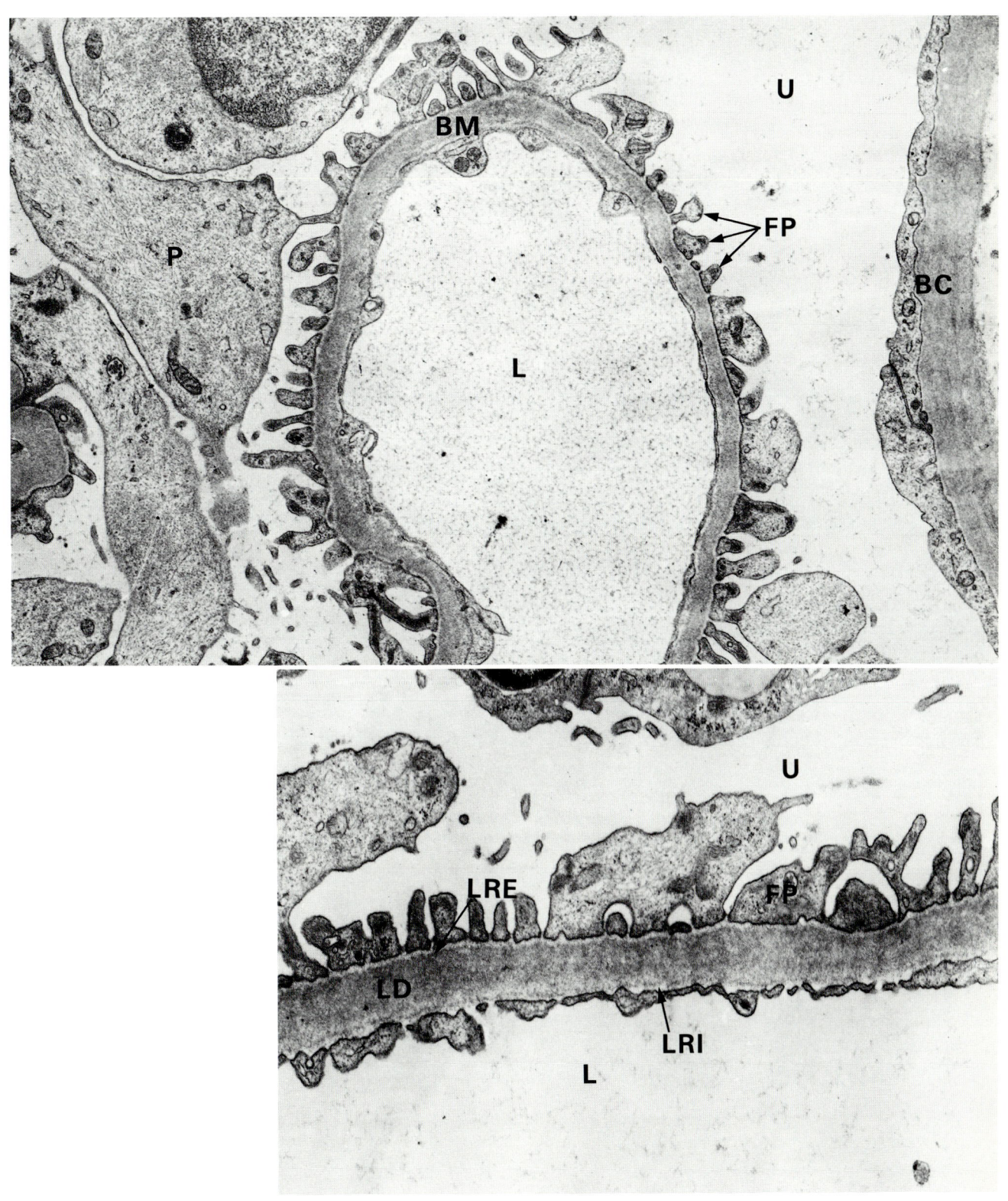

NORMAL GLOMERULUS

Fig. 1-11 Normal glomerulus under scanning electron microscope. Cell body of a podocyte (P) gives rise to numerous trabeculae and secondary foot processes. x 9,900.

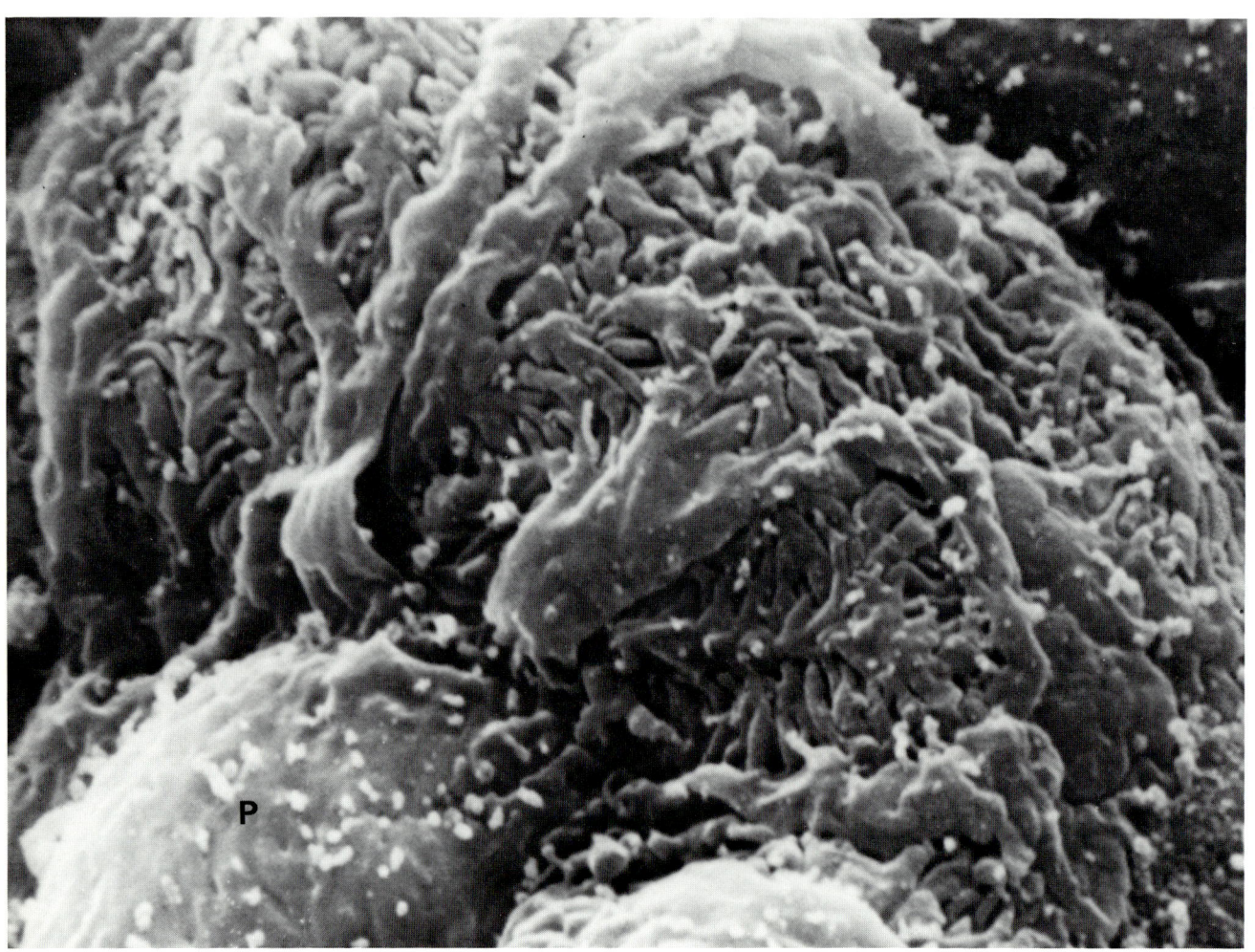

Primary Glomerular Diseases
(Glomerulonephritis and Related Conditions)

CHAPTER 2

Minor Glomerular Abnormalities
  Minimal Change Nephrotic Syndrome
    (Figs. 2-1 to 2-5 and Figs. 2-19 to 2-20)
Focal/Segmental Lesions
  Focal Segmental Hyalinosis and Sclerosis
    (Figs. 2-6 to 2-14 and Figs. 2-21 to 2-24)
  Focal Glomerulonephritis
    (Figs. 2-15 to 2-18 and Figs 2-25)

Minor Glomerular Abnormalities

Definition: This category includes glomeruli which are apparently normal by light microscopy or show minor changes such as: — (i) increased cellularity of some peripheral mesangial areas (groups of up to 3 cells/area), (ii) widening of the mesangium (up to twice normal), (iii) occasional capillary wall abnormalities, i.e. splitting, wrinkling or thickening, (iv) generalized increase in thickness of glomerular capillary basement membranes (up to twice normal for age). This category includes what has previously been called minimal change disease and excludes cases with focal/segmental lesions.

Additional features other than focal/segmental lesions should be recorded according to Table II; e.g. minor changes with mesangial deposits (see Section I).

Clinical Manifestations: Renal tissue in several different clinical syndromes may show only minor glomerular abnormalities. The most important of these is an entity known as *minimal change nephrotic syndrome*, lipoid nephrosis or nil disease; the term idiopathic nephrotic syndrome is sometimes used as a synonym, but others apply this name also to membranous glomerulonephritis. The disease occurs at any age but is seen more frequently in young children between the ages of one and five. In this age group, minimal change nephrotic syndrome (MCNS) accounts for at least three-quarters of all cases of nephrotic syndrome while in adults it constitutes 10–15% and in some series up to 30% of cases of nephrotic syndrome. In children, but not in adults, males are affected more frequently than females by a ratio of about 1.5 to 1 or 2 to 1. The nephrotic syndrome often develops without any prodromes though a minor infection or immunization may precede it by a few days. Some patients have a history of allergy and others a family history of diabetes. The disease develops rapidly, edema being often the first clue. Urine examination reveals heavy proteinuria sometimes as high as 20g/24hours. Serum albumin is decreased, often below 2g/100ml and cholesterol is usually elevated. The proteinuria is of the selective type, in that smaller molecules, approximately the size of albumin and smaller are excreted. Microscopic hematuria is not uncommon and mild to moderate elevation of blood pressure is seen on occasion. If renal insufficiency is present, it is usually the result of hypovolemia due to rapid loss of fluids into the tissues. However, sometimes true acute renal failure develops.

The disease responds very well to steroid therapy. Adults fare as well as children, in whom the initial response rate is greater than 90%. Relapses at all ages are common but respond to re-treatment. The ultimate cure rate in children approaches 90% though in adults it is probably lower. Steroid resistant nephrotic syndrome is almost always associated with other categories of glomerular disease, e.g. focal segmental glomerulosclerosis, although the microscopic features of these categories are sometimes inconspicuous in the first biopsy.

Isolated proteinuria, that is, proteinuria below the nephrotic range (usually less than 2 g/24 hours) may also be associated with minor glomerular abnormalities. Other symptoms are rare though microscopic hematuria may be observed on occasion. Isolated proteinuria is rather infrequent in children but more common in adults. In some cases it is probably of the same origin as the nephrotic syndrome except that the proteinuria is less severe. Other cases probably have a different basis such as asymptomatic essential hypertension or early diabetes. Orthostatic proteinuria may also fall into this category.

Minor glomerular changes may also constitute the histologic finding in *"pure" hematuria*, either gross or microscopic, recurrent or persistent. It is, of course, understood that hematuria from the lower urinary tract had been excluded. Some of these patients may have focal lesions in other glomeruli (not included in the biopsy); some have hereditary nephritis without electron microscopic changes in the examined glomeruli. Gross hematuria after exercise is typically associated with apparently normal glomeruli, and a syndrome of loin pain and gross hematuria has been described with minor glomerular changes but significant vascular abnormalities on renal angiography. Cases where immunofluorescence microscopy demonstrates deposits of IgA usually represent Berger's disease. Very early stages of lupus nephritis may show no deposits or only small deposits of various immunoglobulins.

Light Microscopy: On light microscopy the glomeruli appear normal or show only minor changes. In cases of hematuria, Bowman's space and tubules may contain red blood cells. In patients with nephrotic syndrome or proteinuria, close examination may reveal enlargement of podocytes and protein precipitate in the Bowman's space. Mesangium may be slightly widened containing more mesangial matrix and perhaps a few extra cells. Careful counts have demonstrated increase in the number of mesangial cells on the order of up to 30%. Occasionally a completely sclerosed glomerulus is noted. The tubules may exhibit the usual findings of nephrotic syndrome, that is hyaline casts, hyaline droplets in the cytoplasm and occasionally small areas of calcification. The presence of lipid can be demonstrated by special procedures. Tubular atrophy, particularly in young people, casts doubt on the diagnosis of minimal change nephrotic syndrome and indicates a thorough search for another lesion, especially focal segmental glomerulosclerosis. It must be remembered that in principle the diagnosis of minimal change nephrotic syndrome is established by exclusion.

Electron Microscopy: The most characteristic feature in patients with the nephrotic syndrome is the loss or effacement of foot processes of the epithelial cells so that the surface of the cell is in direct contact with the basement membrane. The cell cytoplasm is often edematous with focal loss or focal increase of organelles. The zone adjacent to the basement membrane often contains a layer of dark fibrillar material. Vacuoles, lipid droplets and hyaline droplets may be present. The surfaces of the podocytes facing the urinary space show numerous fine microvilli. The lamina rara interna is sometimes widened and the lamina densa may be finely "mottled". The capillary lumen may on occasion contain fibrin and platelet aggregates. Sometimes small, moderately dense deposits are present in the mesangium or under the endothelium but such deposits do not necessarily contain immune globulins or complement. When the patient goes into remission, the foot processes promptly reappear though they may show some distortion. The microvilli persist for some time. Patients with isolated proteinuria usually have less severe alteration of foot processes. Patients with recurrent hematuria may have no ultrastructural alterations.

Immunofluorescence Microscopy: In Minimal Change Nephrotic Syndrome immunofluorescence studies are usually completely negative. Flecks of C3 and rarely C1q occur in 20–30% of patients either in the mesangium or along the periphery. On occasion small amount of immune globulins, such as IgM or IgG, may be found in the mesangium.

Focal/Segmental Lesions
(With only Minor Abnormalities in Other Glomeruli)

Definition: This category is reserved for those cases where the basic lesion is focal and segmental, that is involving only some glomeruli and only parts (segments) of the glomeruli, while the remaining glomeruli show no more than minor changes described under Minor Glomerular Abnormalities.

Focal/segmental lesions are a heterogeneous category which includes several types of glomerular lesions and several clinical syndromes or manifestations. The nomenclature is somewhat confused since many authors distinguish sharply between "focal segmental hyalinosis and sclerosis" and "focal glomerulonephritis" while others do not separate them, applying the last name to the whole group. While the histological lesions cannot always be clearly recognized, they occur with rather distinct clinical settings and generally have different prognostic significance. For this reason they will be described separately.

Focal/segmental lesions may be further qualified by additional features according to Table II: Example – focal segmental *hyalinosis* and *sclerosis* (see Section I).

Clinical Manifestations: The main manifestation of *focal segmental hyalinosis and sclerosis (FSHS)* (focal segmental glomerulosclerosis-FSGS) is massive proteinuria which in children is almost invariably accompanied by other features of nephrotic syndrome. Microscopic hematuria is not infrequent, the proteinuria is usually non-selective and hypertension is often present. In adults a certain proportion of cases do not have a nephrotic syndrome but merely isolated proteinuria with or without hematuria and hypertension. An occasional patient will have isolated or recurrent hematuria. The feature that distinguishes this process from minimal change nephrotic syndrome is resistance to steroid therapy in the majority of patients. Some respond to steroid therapy either temporarily or permanently; some become steroid dependent and eventually steroid resistant. Those patients who do not improve tend to progress to renal failure over a period as short as 2–3 years or as long as 15 years or more. On the other hand, those who respond to steroids usually have a benign course. Transplantation in patients with FSHS is usually complicated by the rapid recurrence of massive proteinuria, sometimes with the reappearance of the lesion in the graft, but proteinuria often resolves to allow good graft survival.

FSHS is considered by some to be an independent disease entity and by others a more severe or more advanced form of minimal change nephrotic syndrome. The histologic changes of FSHS are not specific, and are seen in other glomerular diseases, such as membranous glomerulonephritis, Alport's syndrome, nail-patella syndrome, hypertension and pyelonephritis.

Light Microscopy: The characteristic lesion on light microscopy is a segmental area of glomerular "solidification". The juxtamedullary glomeruli are more often affected than the subcapsular glomeruli. The "solidity" is caused by mesangial expansion and collapse of the capillaries. The expanded mesangium contains an increased amount of mesangial matrix and a variable number of cells. In addition, hyaline deposits may be present in the mesangium or in the lumina of the capillaries. Sometimes the order is reversed and hyalin precedes the sclerosis. The lesion is frequently seen at the glomerular hilus, but may first appear in one of the peripheral lobules. The endothelial cells often contain lipid vacuoles. Lipid can also be found in the interstitial cells (so-called "foam cells"). The glomerular lesions are frequently overlain by prominent epithelial cells (podocytes) which may form small crescents not attached to the Bowman's capsule. A narrow clear space may be seen between epithelial cell layer and the underlying basement membrane. More commonly adhesions develop between the area of sclerosis and Bowman's capsule, which are unrelated to crescents.

With progression of the disease more lobules become affected and more glomeruli are involved gradually affecting the function of the kidney. In the advanced stage the appearance is that of "chronic" that is diffuse sclerosing glomerulonephritis. Tubular atrophy is one of the early signs and is an indication for a thorough search for FSHS in an otherwise minimal change nephrotic syndrome. In addition to atrophy, tubules exhibit the usual findings of nephrotic syndrome. The amount of interstitial fibrosis and inflammatory infiltration is proportional to the degree of tubular damage. In more advanced cases vascular sclerosis often supervenes.

In a fair proportion of cases of FSHS there is diffuse increase in the number of mesangial cells, similar to that seen in mesangial glomerulonephritis. In patients with mesangial glomerulonephritis and nephrotic syndrome a search should be made for segmental lesions.

Electron Microscopy: On electron microscopy diffuse as well as segmental lesions are found in the glomeruli. The diffuse lesions are similar to those seen in minimal change nephrotic syndrome, that is changes in the podocytes, loss of foot processes, formation of microvilli and rather prominent widening of the lamina rara interna. There may be obvious mesangial cellularity. The segmental lesions are in essence the same as in light microscopy, that is mesangial expansion, capillary collapse and deposits, which when present may be mesangial, subendothelial or intraluminal. Areas of epithelial detachment, with the formation of subepithelial zones containing lucent fibrillar material, are common over sclerotic segments and may occur elsewhere.

Immunofluorescence Microscopy: This often shows no immune deposits. However, localized deposits of immune globulins and complement may be noted in the sclerotic areas and sometimes more diffusely in the mesangium of the affected glomeruli. The most common constituents are IgM and C3, occasionally also IgG, C1q and fibrin.

The second major subdivision in the category of Focal/Segmental Lesions is *Focal Glomerulonephritis*. This is more often a manifestation of a systemic disease rather than idiopathic. It is seen in systemic lupus erythematosus, Henoch-Schönlein purpura, Wegener's granulomatosis and periateritis nodosa, in endocarditis, and in rheumatic fever. Most of these systemic diseases are discussed under appropriate headings.

Clinical Manifestations: The main clinical manifestation is hematuria either gross or microscopic. There may be an accompanying proteinuria which on rare occasion reaches the nephrotic levels. Hypertension and renal insufficiency are absent as a rule, but if a large number of glomeruli is involved, acute nephritic syndrome may ensue. Hematuria is often accompanied by red cell casts testifying to its renal origin. With successful treatment of the primary disease, the renal manifestations abate. Spontaneous healing occurs in the idiopathic form. The latter has a tendency to recur after minor intercurrent infections or other forms of stress. After repeated attacks sufficient number of glomeruli may become damaged to cause renal insufficiency.

Light Microscopy: Focal glomerulonephritis can be subdivided into several histological types: proliferative, necrotizing, crescentic, and sclerosing. This subdivision is similar to what is seen in diffuse glomerulonephritis and indeed some cases of focal glomerulonephritis progress to diffuse disease and on the other hand, resolving diffuse disease at some point of its evolution may resemble focal glomerulonephritis.

Focal proliferative glomerulonephritis is a rather mild disease which usually resolves, though it sometimes leads to a segmental scar. Necrotizing lesions often begin as segmental thrombosis of capillaries, perhaps due to endothelial damage, and usually lead to rupture of the capillaries and spilling of the material into the Bowman's space. This in turn provokes proliferative reaction with formation of crescents. Healing of necrotizing and crescentic glomerulonephritis is by segmental scarring and adhesion to Bowman's capsule with preservation of the remainder of the tuft. Such sclerotic lesions are non-progressive and will affect the renal function only if their number is large.

Electron Microscopy: In some cases of focal glomerulonephritis mesangial cellularity and sclerosis may be accompanied by small mesangial deposits. In cases with necrosis and crescent formation, fibrin may be seen in the capillaries and in the Bowman's space. Occasionally subendothelial deposits occur, either of the usual dense variety or on the contrary quite lucent. Subepithelial deposits are rare.

Immunofluorescence Microscopy: Immunofluorescence microscopy helps to identify one type of focal proliferative glomerulonephritis as a specific entity, so-called Berger's or IgA disease (see under appropriate heading). This is characterized by the presence of IgA immunoglobulins in the mesangium usually in association with C3 and variable amounts of IgG. In some patients with crescent formation linear IgG and C3 may be found. Such patients usually represent an early stage of Goodpasture's syndrome (see there).

In addition to the two categories discussed above, that is FSHS and focal glomerulonephritis, various lesions listed in Table II may occur in a pattern of focal segmental distribution with only minor changes in other glomeruli. This is also true of some of the entities in Table I, such as those listed in the category of Diffuse Glomerulonephritis. In an occasional case the histologic changes remain limited to only some glomeruli, or to segments of some glomeruli. Such cases should be classified as Focal Glomerulonephritis of the appropriate type (membranous, mesangial proliferative, endocapillary proliferative, mesangiocapillary, crescentic).

PRIMARY GLOMERULAR DISEASES

MINIMAL CHANGE NEPHROTIC SYNDROME

Fig. 2-1 Essentially a normal glomerulus as seen by light microscopy. (In some cases slight mesangial widening may be noted.)
PAS stain. x 410.

Fig. 2-2 Immunofluorescence microscopy showing small granular deposits of complement (C3), mainly in the glomerular mesangium. Such deposits occur in a minority of cases of minimal change nephrotic syndrome (MCNS). x 260.

Fig. 2-3 Proximal tubules showing numerous hyaline (protein) droplets.
PAS stain. x 410.

Fig. 2-4 Proximal tubules showing lipid droplets. Sudan stain on frozen section. x 260.

Fig. 2-5 Interstitial "foam" cells. These cells contain lipid which has been washed out in the process of paraffin embedding.
H&E stain. x 410.

FOCAL SEGMENTAL HYALINOSIS AND SCLEROSIS (FOCAL SEGMENTAL GLOMERULOSCLEROSIS)

Fig. 2-6 Early focal segmental glomerulosclerosis showing a small, almost completely sclerosed lobule attached to the capsule and surrounded by prominent epithelial cells.
PAS stain. x 410.

MINOR GLOMERULAR ABNORMALITIES

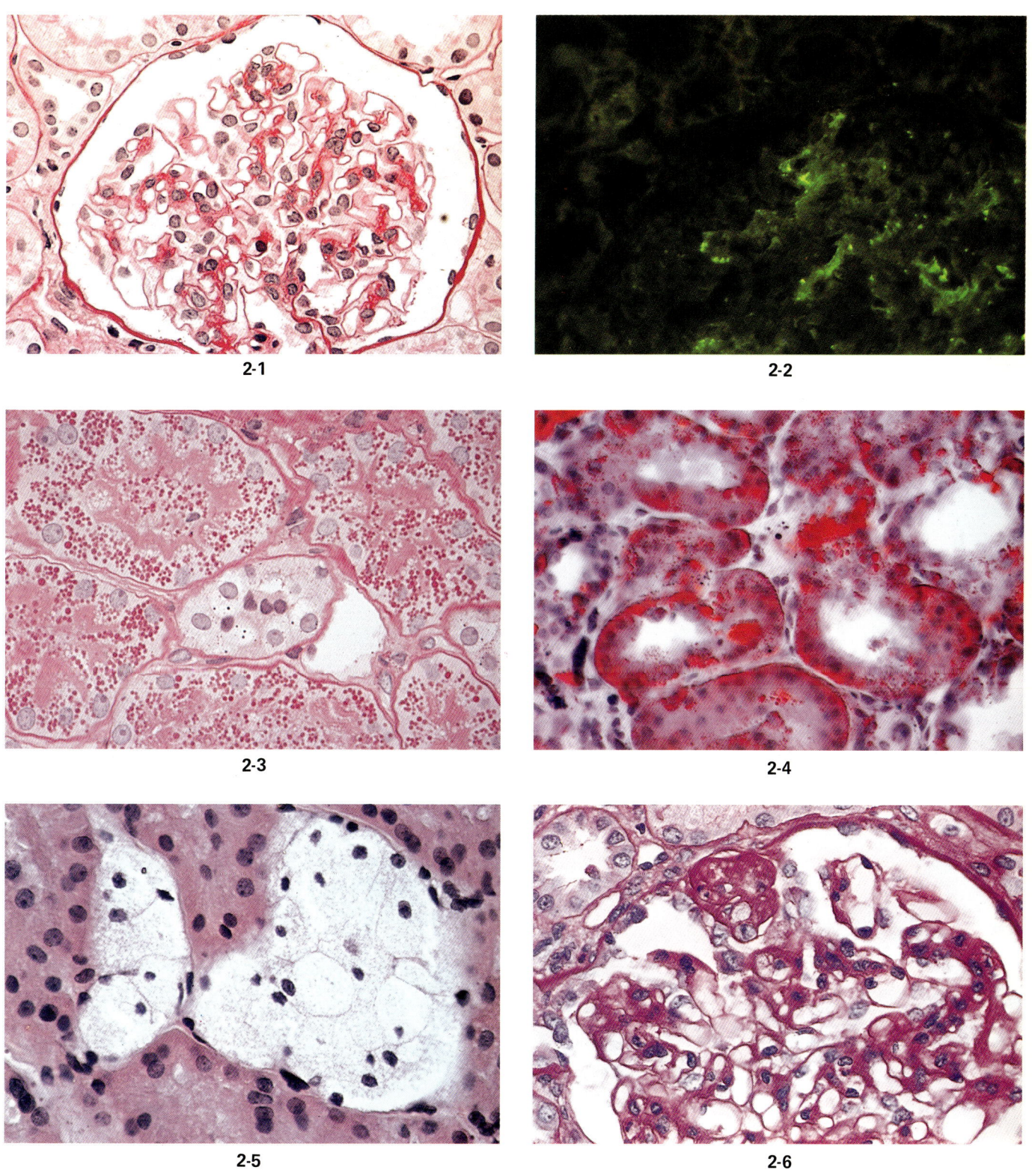

PRIMARY GLOMERULAR DISEASES

FOCAL SEGMENTAL HYAC/NOSIS AND SCLEROSIS (FOCAL SEGMENTAL GLOMERULOSCLEROSIS)

Fig. 2-7 A more advanced stage with sclerosis in the hilar region and hyaline deposits in the involved area. The wall of the adjacent arteriole is slightly thickened. PAS stain. x 260.

Fig. 2-8 Part of a glomerulus showing striking proliferation of podocytes. Some cells contain hyaline droplets. PAS stain. x 1,000.

Fig. 2-9 Immunofluorescence microscopy showing segmental deposits of IgM. x 260.

Fig. 2-10 Immunofluorescence microscopy showing segmental deposits of complement (C3). x 410.

Fig. 2-11 Focal segmental glomerulosclerosis in a heroin addict. Rather extensive sclerosis involving most of the glomerular lobules. PAS stain. x 260.

Fig. 2-12 Immunofluorescence microscopy. Heroin addict. Fairly extensive deposits of IgM. x 260.

FOCAL/SEGMENTAL LESIONS

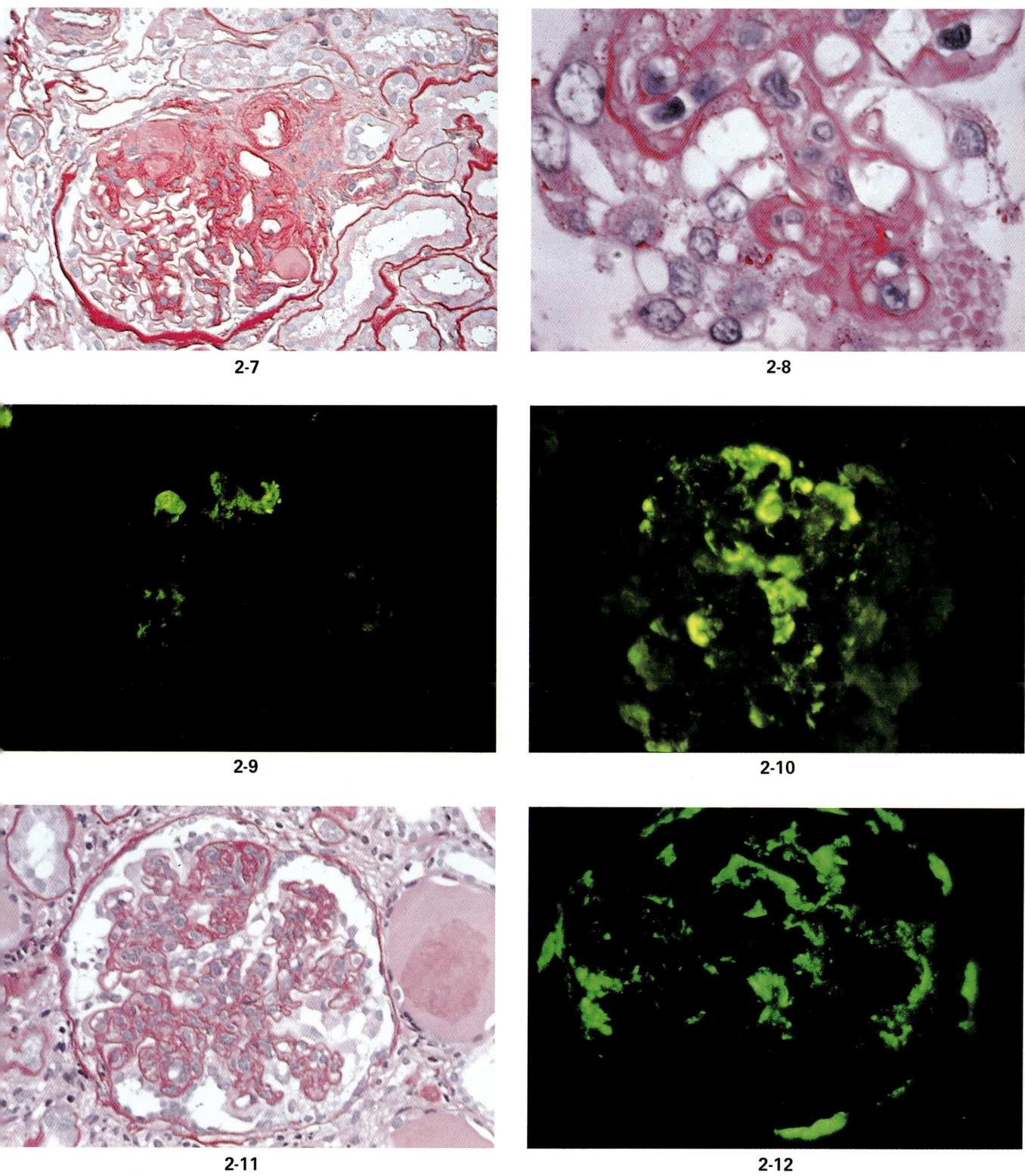

2-7

2-8

2-9

2-10

2-11

2-12

43

PRIMARY GLOMERULAR DISEASES

FOCAL SEGMENTAL GLOMERULOSCLEROSIS

Fig. 2-13   Focal tubular atrophy in a case of focal segmental glomerulosclerosis. The glomerulus shows no significant changes.
PAS stain. × 100.

Fig. 2-14   Advanced stage of focal segmental glomerulosclerosis with sclerosis of most of the glomeruli and tubular atrophy.
PAS stain. × 100.

FOCAL GLOMERULONEPHRITIS

Fig. 2-15   Focal proliferative glomerulonephritis. Mild proliferation best seen in a lobule at eleven o'clock.
H&E stain. × 260.

Fig. 2-16   Focal proliferative glomerulonephritis.   Segmental proliferation in a lobule at seven o'clock.
PAS stain. × 260.

Fig. 2-17   More extensive focal proliferative glomerulonephritis accompanied by some diffuse mesangial proliferation.
PAS stain. × 260.

Fig. 2-18   Focal crescentic glomerulonephritis showing slight proliferation in the tuft and a crescent in the left lower half of the Bowman's space.
PAS stain. × 260.

FOCAL/SEGMENTAL LESIONS

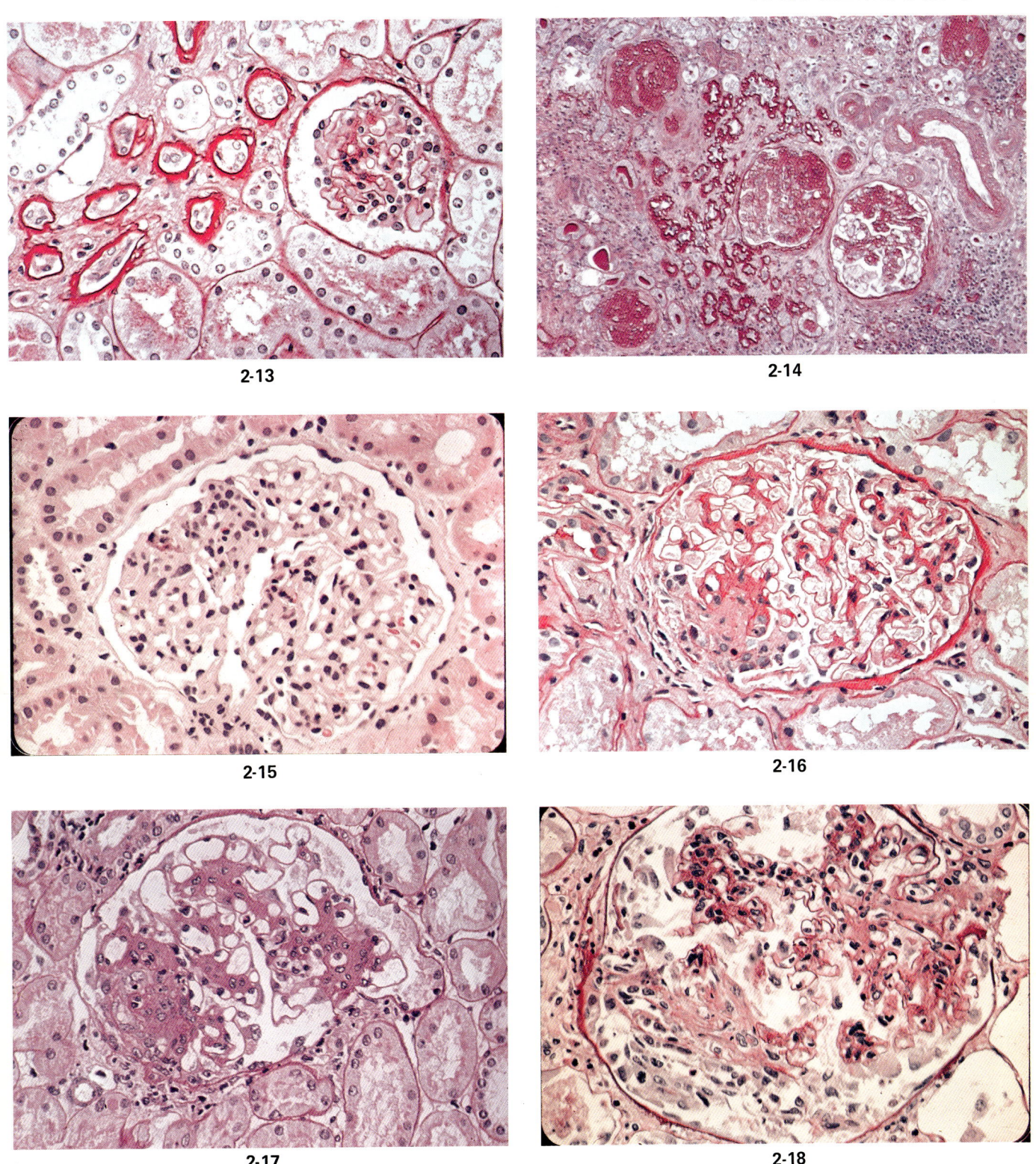

PRIMARY GLOMERULAR DISEASES

MINIMAL CHANGE NEPHROTIC SYNDROME

Fig. 2-19 A glomerular capillary loop showing typical changes of nephrotic syndrome. There is extensive effacement of the epithelial foot processes (FP), microvilli (MV) in the urinary space (U) (right lower corner) and edema of the podocytes (P). There is also some edema of the endothelial cells (En).
Electron Micrograph × 17,000.

Fig. 2-20 Glomerulus in MCNS under the scanning electron microscope. The foot processes are mainly effaced. The microvilli are prominent.
× 7,000.
BM: basement membrane, L: capillary lumen, P: podocyte, Cap: capillary.

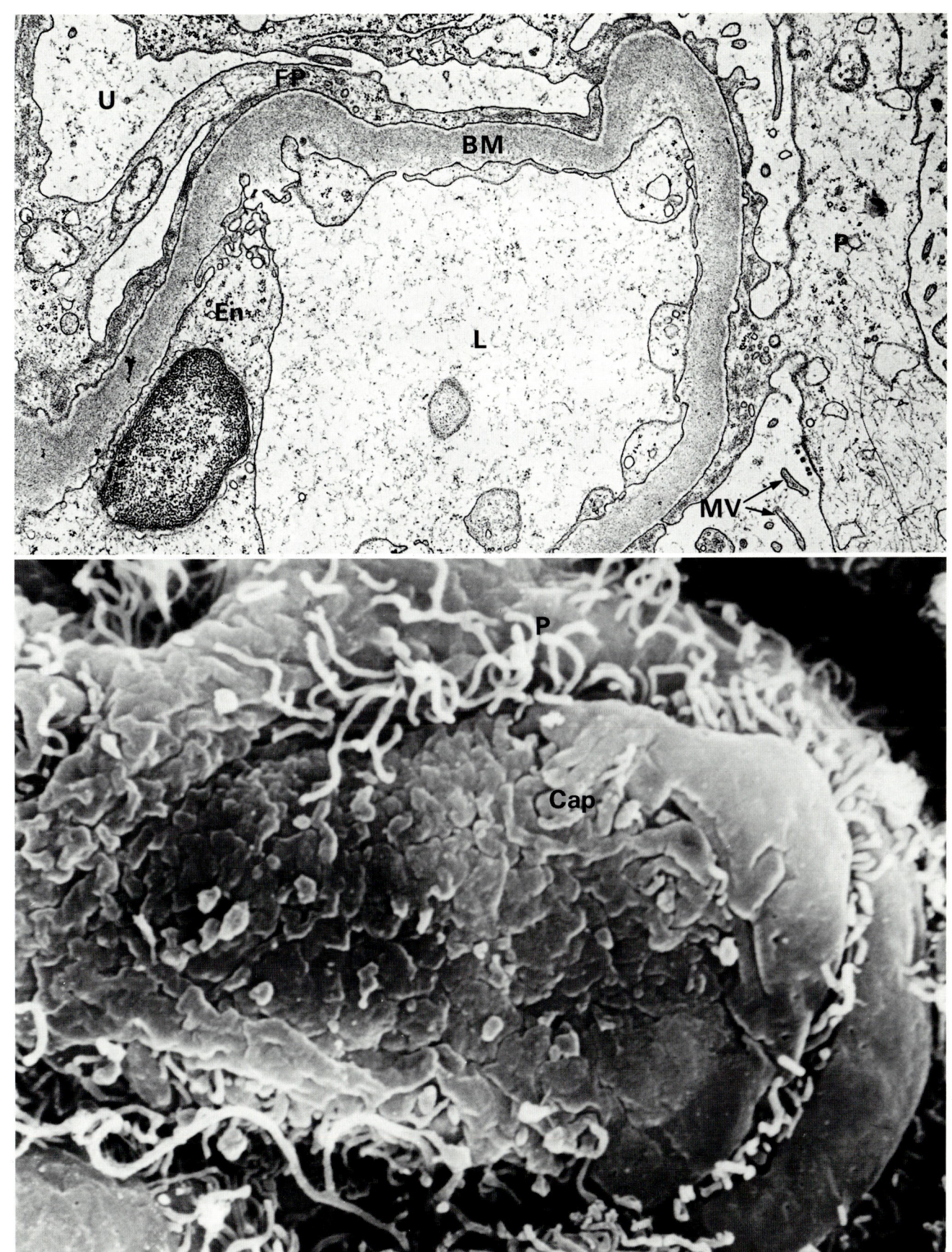

PRIMARY GLOMERULAR DISEASES

FOCAL SEGMENTAL HYALINOSIS AND SCLEROSIS (FOCAL SEGMENTAL GLOMERULOSCLEROSIS)

Fig. 2-21   Electron micrograph. Part of a glomerulus showing capillary collapse, mesangial sclerosis and small electron dense subendothelial deposits (D). The podocyte (P) is detached from the basement membrane (BM) and the space is filled with layers of new basement membrane material (BMM).
x 3,300.

Fig. 2-22   Electron micrograph. Completely collapsed glomerular lobule surrounded by hypertrophied epithelial cells. As in the previous picture, the podocytes (P) are detached in some areas.
x 1,700.

MM: mesangial matrix

FOCAL/SEGMENTAL LESIONS

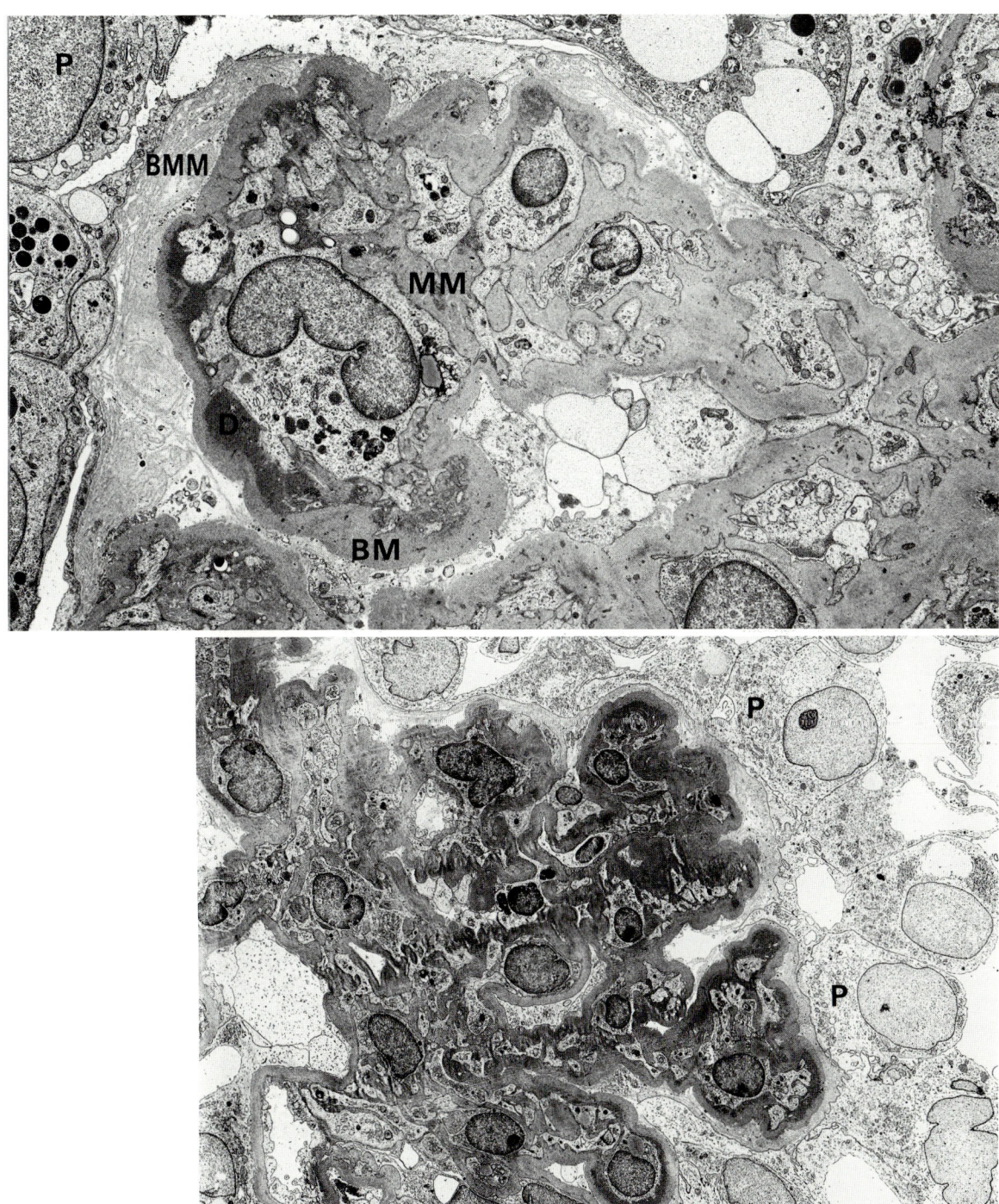

PRIMARY GLOMERULAR DISEASES

FOCAL SEGMENTAL GLOMERULOSCLEROSIS

Fig. 2-23 Electron micrograph. Early stage of podocyte (P) detachment creating an empty space between the cell cytoplasm and the basement membrane (BM). × 8,900.

Fig. 2-24 Electron micrograph. Later stage of podocyte (P) detachment. The space between the basement membrane (BM) and the epithelial cytoplasm contains finely fibrillar layers and remnants of cytoplasm(*). × 13,000.

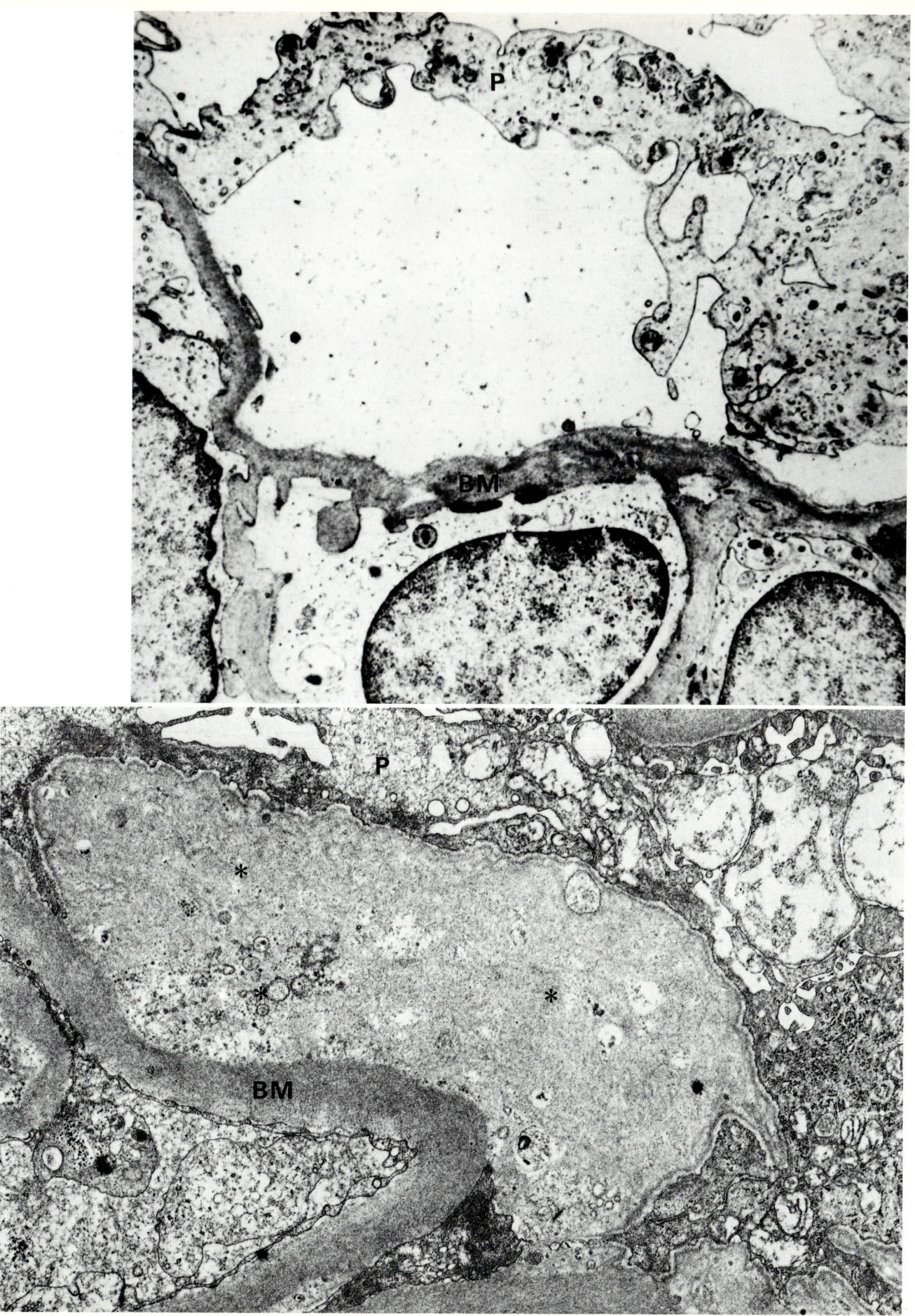

PRIMARY GLOMERULAR DISEASES

FOCAL GLOMERULONEPHRITIS

Fig. 2-25 Electron micrograph. Focal crescentic glomerulonephritis showing fibrin (F), and cell proliferation in the urinary space and partial collapse of glomerular capillaries. × 4,000.

Ep: epithelial cell, BM: basement membrane, En: endothelial cell.

FOCAL/SEGMENTAL LESIONS

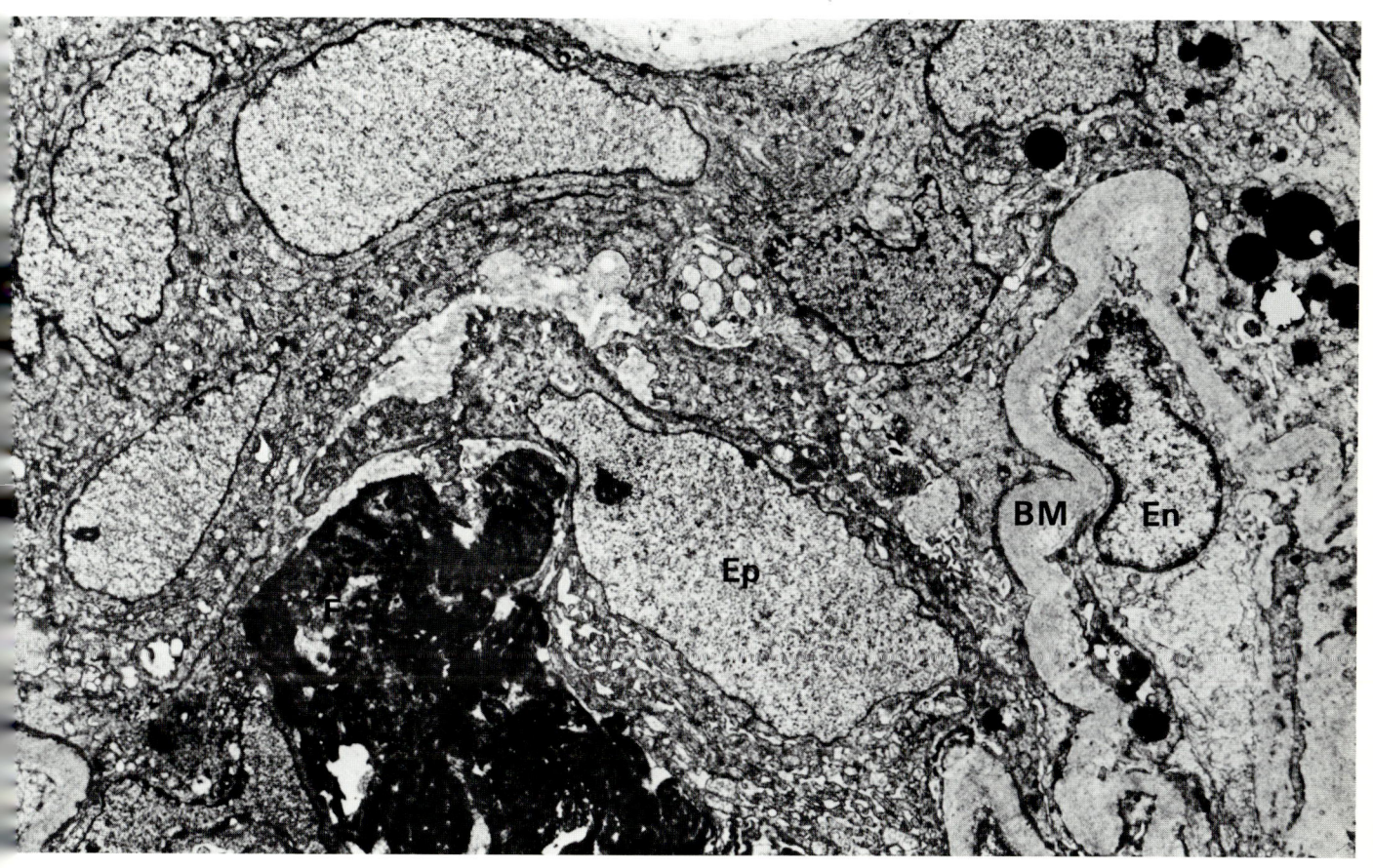

CHAPTER 3

Diffuse Membranous Glomerulonephritis
(Figs. 3-1 to 3-17)

Diffuse Membranous Glomerulonephritis

Definition: All or nearly all glomeruli are affected by a diffuse thickening of capillary walls. This derives from the presence of subepithelial deposits which may sometimes be demonstrable by light microscopy (red with Trichrome stain). Silver impregnation typically reveals the presence of basement membrane projections (spikes) between the deposits. In the early stages spikes are small or absent; in the late stages spikes join up to form a greatly thickened basement membrane with the appearance of a twisted rope or linked chain. The mesangium shows only minor changes but appreciable proliferation may be noted in some cases. Although the lesions of membranous glomerulonephritis are usually diffuse, in a small percentage of cases they are focally distributed.

Example of additional features from Table II: diffuse membranous glomerulonephritis with segmental sclerosis (see Section I).

Clinical Manifestations: The disease occurs at any age, but is rare in children. The majority of patients are over the age of 40 with the peak incidence in the fourth to sixth decades. A small secondary peak is seen in the second or third decade. Males are affected more often than females. The onset is insidious with the main manifestation being the nephrotic syndrome. In a minority the disease begins as asymptomatic proteinuria, which almost invariably progresses to nephrotic syndrome. Proteinuria is non-selective. Microscopic hematuria is not uncommon, but gross hematuria is rare. Hypertension is sometimes seen at the onset but more often develops late in the course of the disease, together with renal insufficiency.

In about 70% of cases the disease is "idiopathic", that is, has no known cause. A variety of systemic diseases is seen in the remaining 30%: systemic lupus erythematosus (see there); sarcoidosis; infections — secondary or congenital syphilis (see there), filariasis, schistosomiasis; malignant tumors; drugs and chemicals — penicillamine, gold, mercury. With appropriate and early treatment of the systemic diseases, the symptoms and morphological changes of membranous glomerulonephritis abate. The idiopathic form runs a slowly progressive course, though in some patients (5–25%) the disease remits spontaneously; one-quarter develop renal failure in 5–10 years, and the remainder may last 10–20 years or longer. The rate of recovery with reversion of glomerular abnormalities is the highest in children under five years. It has been suggested that therapy with steroids accelerates clinical remission in a proportion of patients and may also delay the development of renal insufficiency.

Renal vein thrombosis often occurs in association with membranous glomerulonephritis. It was believed at one time that thrombosis induces the glomerular disease but nowadays it is considered that more often thrombosis is a secondary phenomenon, perhaps due to increased coagulability of blood in patients with a nephrotic syndrome.

Light Microscopy: The characteristic finding is thickening of the capillary walls in the glomeruli. In the early stages this thickening is slight and distinction from minimal change nephrotic syndrome may be difficult. In typical cases special stains (PAS, PASM, Trichrome) clearly demonstrate that thickening is caused by changes on the epithelial side of the basement membrane — deposition of proteinaceous material which stains red with Trichrome stains, and formation of "spikes", that is extension of basement membrane between the deposits. In more advanced stages the "spikes", that is extensions of basement membrane is transformed into a thick rope-like or chain-like structure. The capillary lumina are proportionally narrowed. However in some cases there is complete or almost complete restoration to normal.

The mesangial areas are unaffected as a rule but in a small percentage of patients mild or moderate cellular proliferation and sclerosis occur. Progression of the disease is quite often accompanied by development of segmental and focal areas of sclerosis, somewhat similar to those described in idiopathic focal segmental glomerulosclerosis. Such areas may be seen even in the first biopsy. Eventually most of the glomeruli become sclerotic leading to the histological picture of sclerosing glomerulonephritis. This process may be slow (15–20 years or longer) or, on the contrary, quite rapid (2–3 years). In a few cases crescents develop in the glomeruli and may be accompanied by the clinical picture of rapidly progressive glomerulonephritis and linear deposits of immunoglobulins.

Electron Microscopy: The changes in the capillary walls develop in four stages: Stage I is characterized by the presence of small scattered subepithelial electron dense deposits along the capillary walls. The foot processes first become effaced over the deposits and later over the entire circumference of the capillary. In Stage II the deposits are numerous and evenly distributed and are separated by projections ("spikes") which arise from and have the appearance similar to that of the lamina densa. In Stage III the "spikes" fuse over the deposits incorporating them into a markedly thickened basement membrane, while some of the deposits became rarified. In Stage IV most of the deposits disappear leaving an irregularly thickened lamina densa. Quite often more than one stage is seen at the same time.

In a few cases small deposits are also found in the mesangium. Most of these cases turn out to be examples of systemic lupus erythematosus, hepatitis B or syphilis, but a few are genuinely idiopathic. In cases in which the disease resolves, the basement membrane is partially or completely reconstructed and may approach the normal appearance.

Immunofluorescence Microscopy: In typical cases numerous, evenly distributed granular deposits of IgG and usually also of C3 are seen along the glomerular capillary walls. Sometimes these deposits may be recognized before they become visible on electron microscopy. When the granules are small and very numerous a "pseudolinear" appearance may result. In rare cases IgM, IgA or early components of complement are also present. Fibrin is rather infrequent. In the advanced stages of disease, the deposits become scantier and less regular. In secondary types of membranous glomerulonephritis the relevant antigen can sometimes be demonstrated, such as tumor protein or hepatitis B derivatives.

PRIMARY GLOMERULAR DISEASES

MEMBRANOUS GLOMERULONEPHRITIS

Fig. 3-1   Early membranous glomerulonephritis. At this magnification only minimal changes can be recognized.
PAS stain.   x 320.

Fig. 3-2   Same case as Fig. 3-1 under oil immersion. A row of small pink deposits can be recognized along the capillary on the left. Chromotrope-silver methenamine stain (CSM)   x 1,000.

Fig. 3-3   Fully developed membranous glomerulonephritis showing marked thickening of capillary walls and little or no cellular proliferation.
PAS stain.   x 320.

Fig. 3-4   Same case as Fig. 3-3. Capillary loops of glomerulus showing numerous pink subepithelial deposits and black "spikes".
CSM stain.   x 1,000.

Fig. 3-5   Immunofluorescence microscopy. Diffuse granular deposits of IgG along the capillary walls.   x 260.

Fig. 3-6   Immunofluorescence microscopy. Another case of membranous glomerulonephritis showing extensive deposits of IgG along the capillary walls. The deposits are so closely packed as to create the impression of pseudolinear staining.   x 260.

DIFFUSE MEMBRANOUS GLOMERULONEPHRITIS

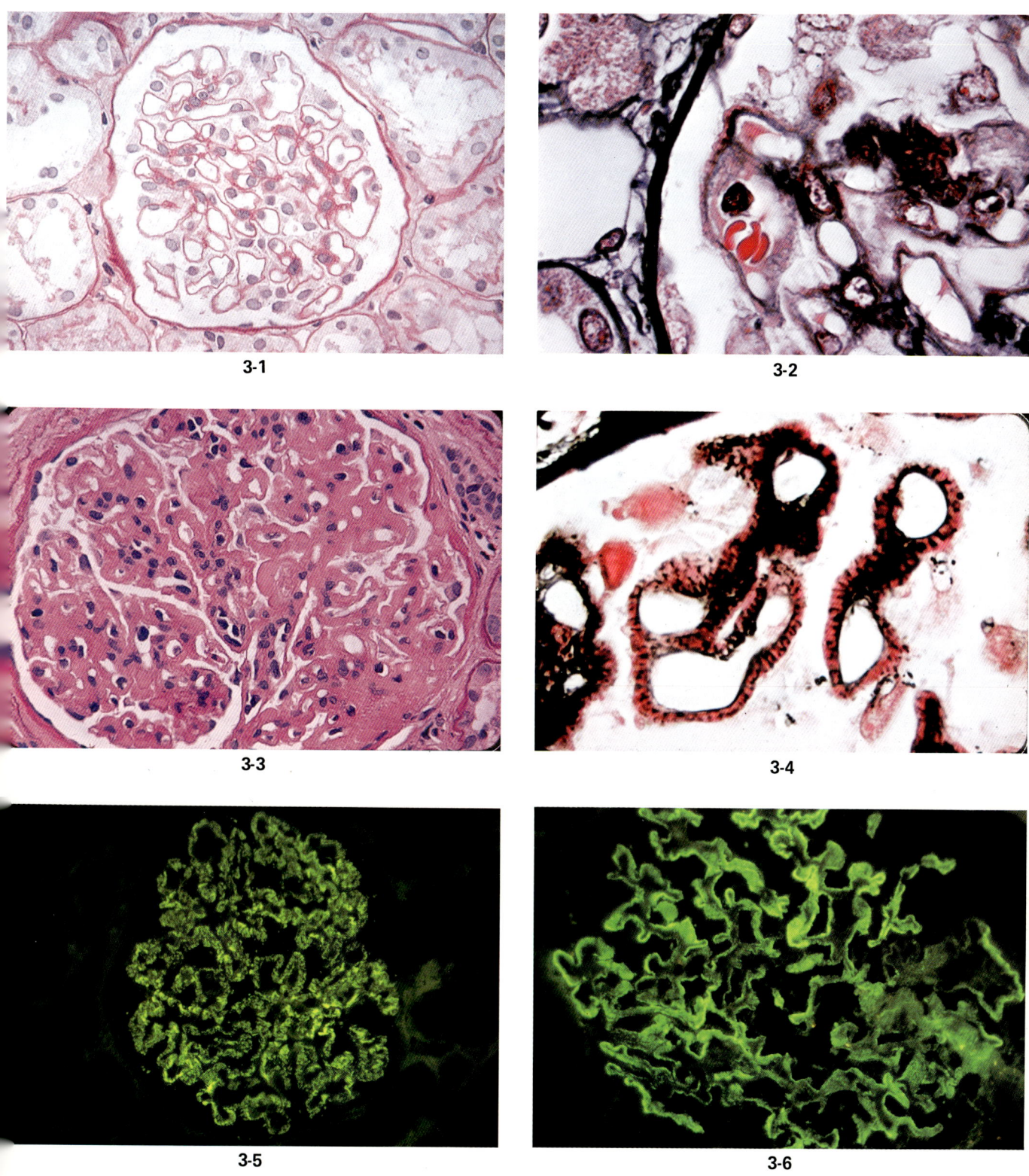

PRIMARY GLOMERULAR DISEASES

MEMBRANOUS GLOMERULONEPHRITIS

Fig. 3-7   Schematic representation of four stages of membranous glomerulonephritis. In stage 1 only scattered deposits (red) are located on the epithelial side of basement membrane (blue) and are overlaid by the podocytes (yellow). Stage 2: numerous deposits completely encircle the capillary wall. They are separated from each other by "spikes" arising from the basement membrane. Stage 3: the spikes encircle and fuse over the deposits. Some of the deposits begin to dissolve. Stage 4: irregularly thickened basement mebrane incoporating remnants of deposits.

Fig. 3-8   Membranous glomerulonephritis showing an area of segmental sclerosis at four o'clock.
PAS stain.   x 260.

Fig. 3-9   Membranous glomerulonephritis showing mesangial proliferation and matrix deposition in the lower half of the glomerulus. Periodic acid-silver methenamine counterstained with H&E.   x 410.

Fig. 3-10   Membranous glomerulonephritis showing an epithelial crescent at the top of the glomerulus.
PAS stain.   x 260.

Fig. 3-11   Advanced membranous glomerulonephritis showing extensive glomerular sclerosis. Same case as Fig. 3-1 three years later.
PAS stain.   x 40.

DIFFUSE MEMBRANOUS GLOMERULONEPHRITIS

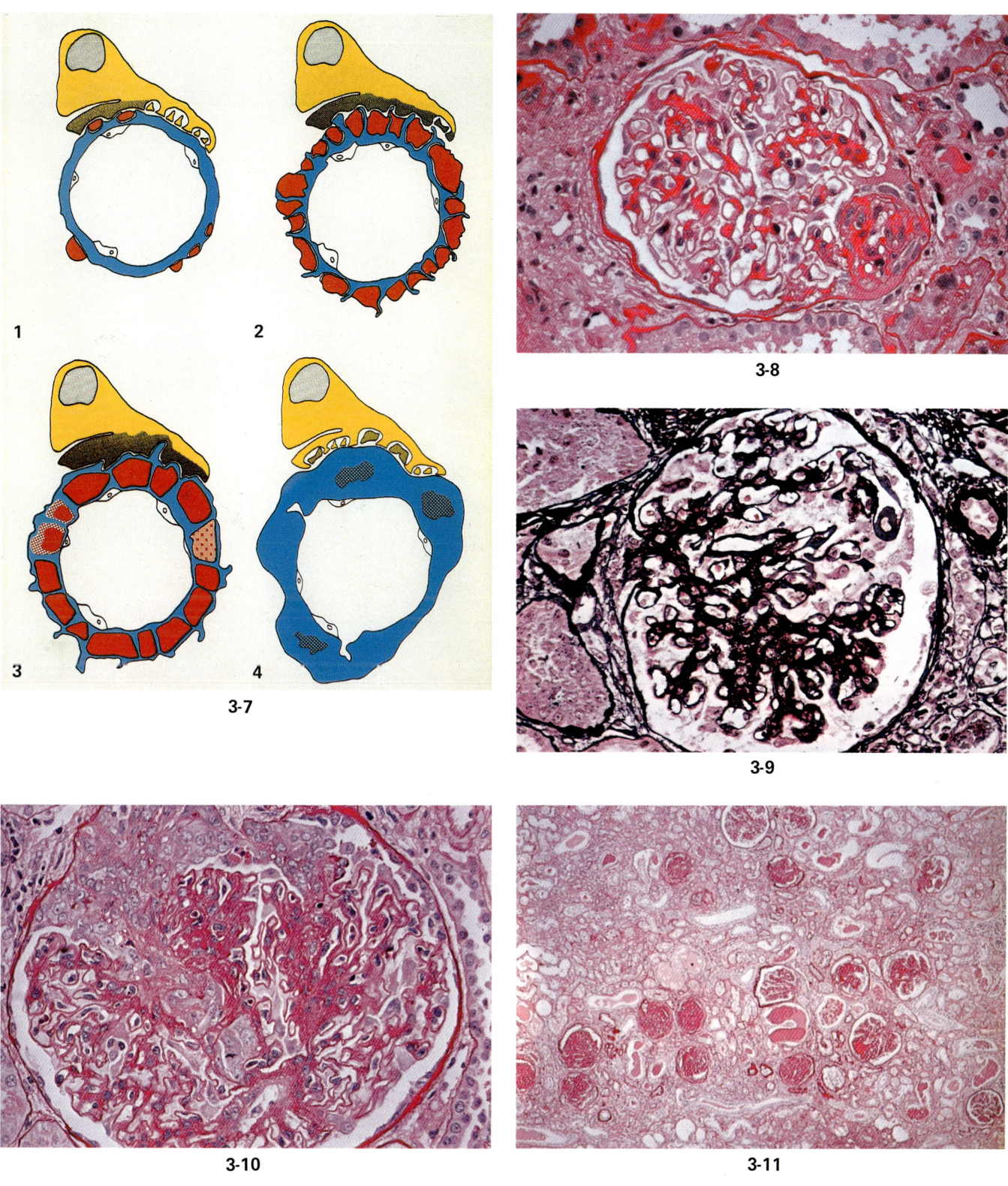

3-7

3-8

3-9

3-10

3-11

59

PRIMARY GLOMERULAR DISEASES

MEMBRANOUS GLOMERULONEPHRITIS

Fig. 3-12 Electron micrograph. Membranous glomerulonephritis Stage 1. Small deposits (D) are located between the basement membrane (BM) and the cytoplasm of the podocyte (P). The outlines of the basement membrane are slightly irregular. The podocytes have been completly effaced.   x 23,000.

Fig. 3-13 Electron micrograph. Membranous glomerulonephritis Stage 1-2. Glomerular capillary loop showing deposits (D) and small spikes (S) along its subepithelial surface. The foot processes (FP) are completely effaced. The cell cytoplasm is edematous. There are many microvilli (MV) in the urinary space (U).
x 16,000.

L: capillary lumen.

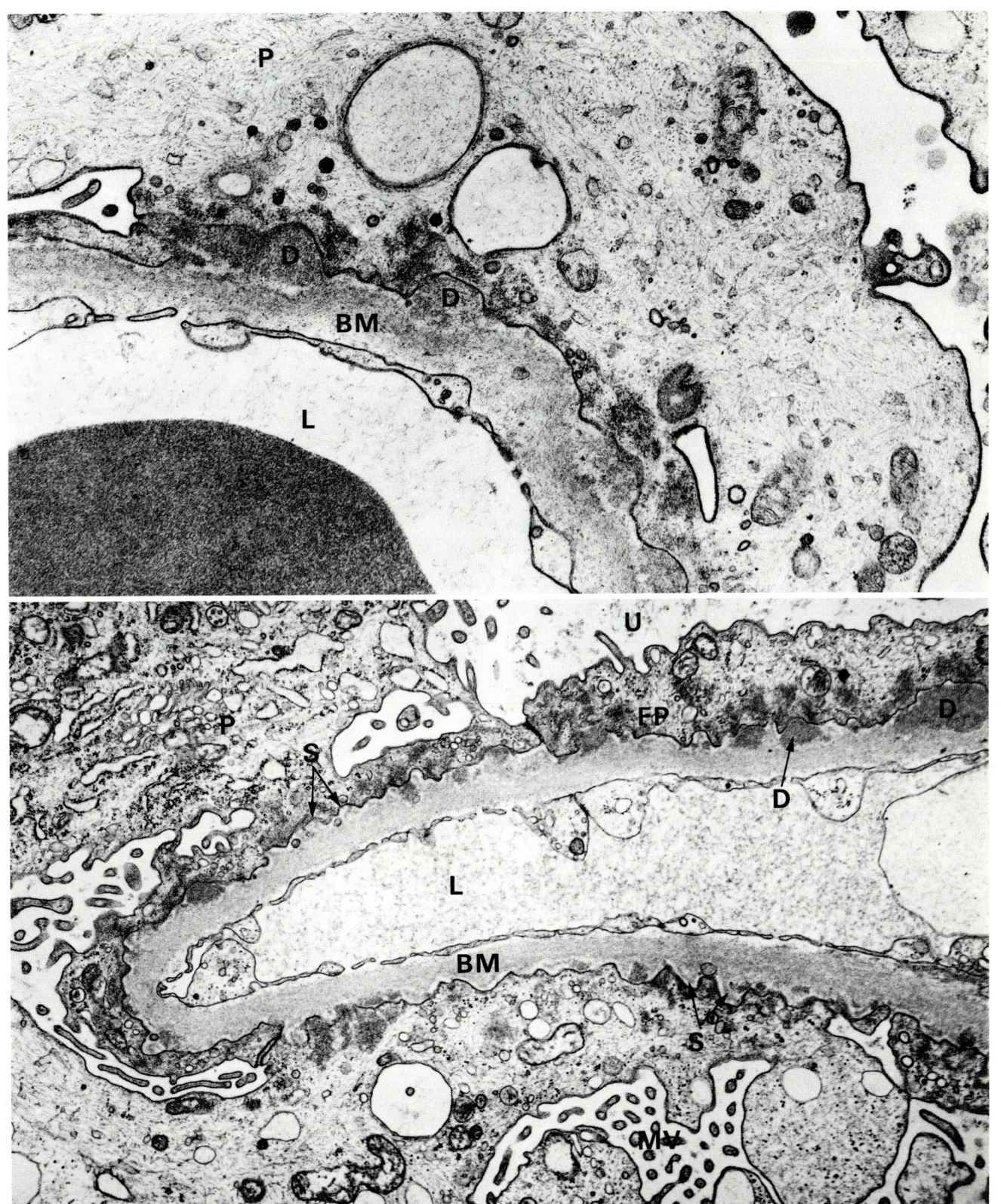

PRIMARY GLOMERULAR DISEASES

MEMBRANOUS GLOMERULONEPHRITIS

Fig. 3-14 Electron micrograph. Membranous glomerulonephritis Stage 2. Large deposits (D) and spikes (S) along the basement membrane. The foot processes (Fp) are effaced. The cell cytoplasm is edematous.   x 16,000.

Fig. 3-15 Electron micrograph. Membranous glomerulonephritis Stage 2. The basement membrane and the spikes (S) are intensely black. The deposits (D) are less intensely stained.
PASM stain.   x 25,000.

U: urinary space, P: podocyte, L: capillary lumen.

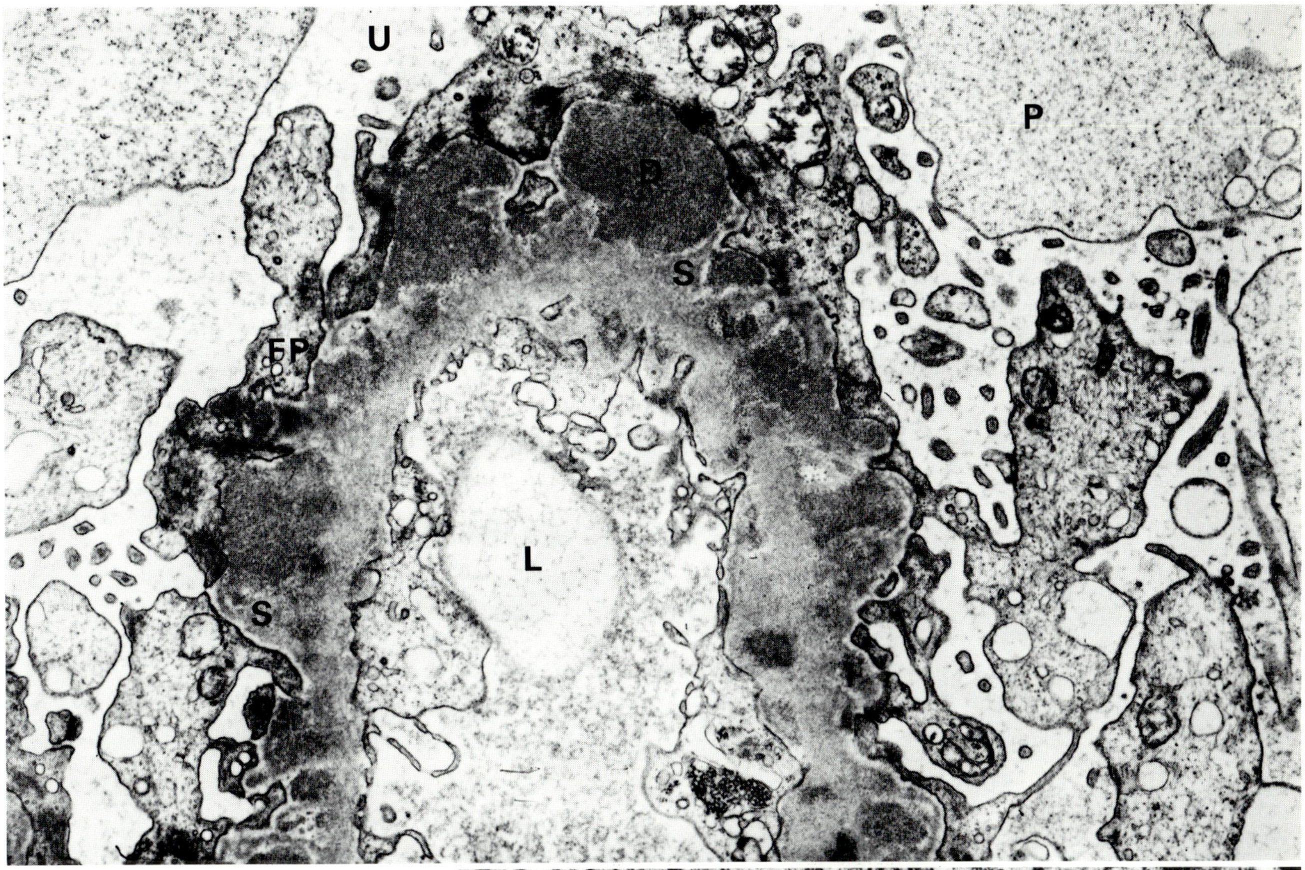

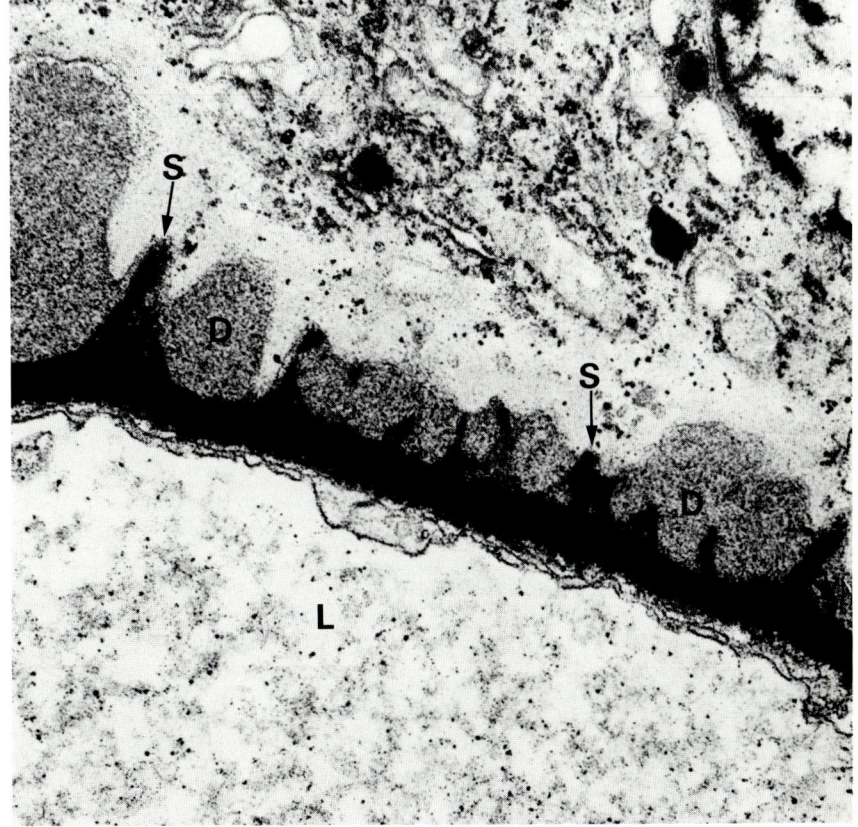

PRIMARY GLOMERULAR DISEASES

MEMBRANOUS GLOMERULONEPHRITIS

Fig. 3-16 Electron micrograph. Membranous glomerulonephritis Stage 3. Deposits (D) of varying density, washed out areas and thin spikes (S), some covering the deposits, along the subepithelial surface of the basement membrane.
x 8,400.

Fig. 3-17 Electron micrograph. Membranous glomerulonephritis Stage 4. Markedly thickened basement membrane incorporating vaguely outlined deposits.
x 12,000.

U: urinary space, L: capillary lumen.

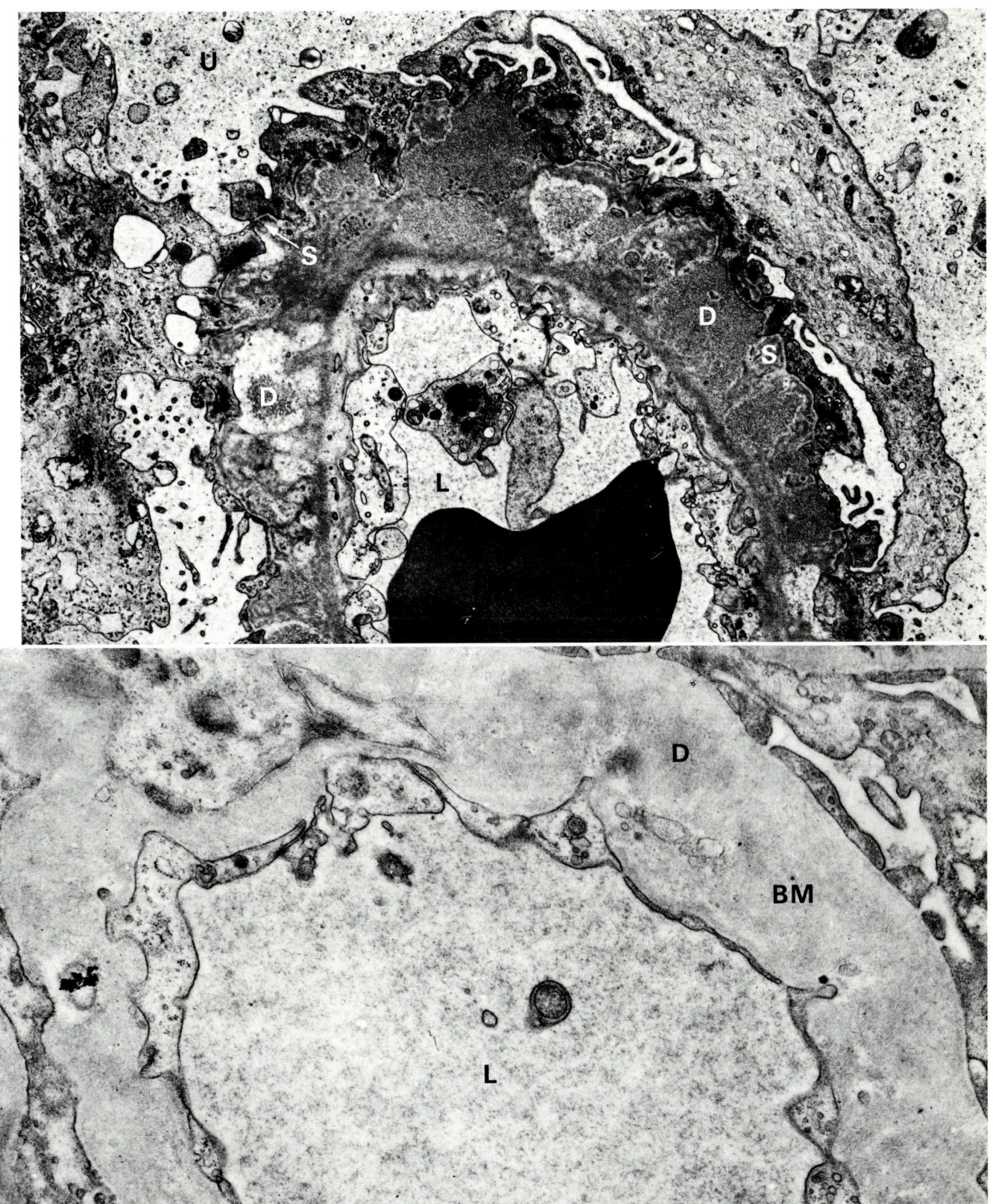

CHAPTER 4

Diffuse Mesangial Proliferative Glomerulonephritis
(Figs. 4-1 to 4-7 and Figs. 4-19 to 4-21)
Diffuse Endocapillary Proliferative Glomelonephritis
(Figs. 4-8 to 4-18 and Figs. 4-22 to 4-26)

Diffuse Mesangial Proliferative Glomerulonephritis

Definition: This is characterized by an essentially uniform increase in mesangial cells (with clusters of four cells or more per mesangial area) in all or nearly all glomeruli (over 80%). Cell proliferation may be accompanied by an increase in mesangial matrix. The capillary lumina remain patent. In advanced cases mesangial sclerosis may predominate. Although the lesions of mesangial proliferative glomerulonephritis are usually diffuse, in a small percentage of cases they are focally distributed.

Example of additional features from Table II: mesangial proliferative glomerulonephritis with capsular adhesions in 30% of glomeruli (see Section I).

Clinical Manifestations: Mesangial proliferation may occur in systemic conditions such as systemic lupus erythematosus, Henoch-Schönlein purpura and infective endocarditis — which are discussed elsewhere — or may be a component of focal segmental hyalinosis and sclerosis, membranous nephropathy, IgA nephropathy and mild or resolving postinfectious glomerulonephritis. A small proportion of cases have no associated glomerular or systemic disorder and may present with gross or microscopic hematuria, proteinuria, combined proteinuria and hematuria or the nephrotic syndrome. The prognosis of these idiopathic forms is uncertain but some cases progress to chronic renal failure.

Light Microscopy: Light microscopy shows expansion of the mesangium with little or no involvement of capillary lumina. The expanded mesangium contains mononuclear cells, presumably of mesangial origin, with clusters of four cells or more per mesangial area. This cell increase is essentially uniform and involves all or nearly all glomeruli (over 80%). Cell proliferation may be accompanied by an increase in mesangial matrix and in advanced cases by mesangial sclerosis.

Electron Microscopy: Electron microscopy generally confirms the light microscopic observations including the presence of any deposits.

Immunofluorescence Microscopy: Immunofluorescence microscopy correlates more closely with the clinical picture. Thus patients with nephrotic syndrome often have deposits of IgM with or without C3, while patients with hematuria more often have deposits of IgA with IgG and C3 which places them in the category of Berger's disease (see there). It has been also suggested that patients with only IgG and C3 represent cases of resolving endocapillary glomerulonephritis. However this has not been definitely confirmed.

Diffuse Endocapillary Proliferative Glomelonephritis

Definition: All or nearly all glomeruli show an essentially uniform increase in cellularity, affecting both mesangial areas and the capillary lumina. The latter are narrowed or occluded due in part to endothelial cell swelling and in part to mesangial cell proliferation. Additional features may be present such as leukocytic infiltration on light microscopy and subepithelial deposits ("humps") on electron microscopy. Although the lesions of endocapillary glomerulonephritis are usually diffuse, in a small percentage of cases they are focally distributed.

Example of additional features from Table II: diffuse endocapillary proliferative glomerulonephritis with focal capillary thrombosis and crescents in 10% of glomeruli (see Section I).

Clinical Manifestations: The disease usually follows an infection (post-infectious glomerulonephritis), though similar histological picture occurs in systemic affections, such as systemic lupus erythematosus, Henoch-Schönlein purpura, polyarteritis nodosa, infective endocarditis and necrotizing arteritis (see under appropriate headings). Among the infective agents, the most common is beta hemolytic Streptococcus but Staphylococcus, Pneumococcus, other bacteria, viruses and parasites account for a proportion of cases. In temperate and cold climates Streptococcal infection is usually in the upper respiratory passages (Streptococcal sore throat); in warm and tropical climates, skin infection (pyoderma) predominates. Only certain serological types (nephritogenic Streptococci) cause glomerulonephritis. The disease occurs more often in children but is more severe in adults. Males are more frequently affected.

A characteristic feature is a latent period, particularly in post-streptococcal disease, where it usually lasts 1–2 weeks. This latent period is less noticeable with other infections.

The main manifestation is the *acute nephritic syndrome*, that is, hematuria, proteinuria, edema, hypertension and renal insufficiency. There is, however, a wide range of severity from a transient illness, manifest only as microscopic hematuria, to fulminant renal failure. Hematuria may either be gross, with reddish or brownish (coca-cola colored) urine, or microscopic. The presence of red cell casts in the sediment testifies to its renal origin. Proteinuria is usually mild or moderate, though on occasion it is severe enogh to lead to nephrotic syndrome. Edema is mild and differs from the nephrotic edema by its tendency to occur on the face and upper extremities rather than lower extremities. It is probably due to salt and water retention, but possibly also to diffuse capillary damage similar to that seen in the glomeruli. Hypertension is mild or moderate and tends to subside with the resolution of the disease. Renal insufficiency is evidenced by decreased glomerular filtration rate, and in more severe cases by oliguria or even anuria.

In many cases clinical symptoms are very mild and the diagnosis may be missed or established only after routine examination of urine. Severe disease with prolonged renal failure is uncommon in children, but more common in adults. Even in relatively mild cases recovery is often gradual, with mild proteinuria and hematuria persisting for months or years. A small percentage of children, but perhaps a larger percentage of adults develop diffuse sclerosing glomerulonephritis.

Laboratory findings also include elevation of anti-streptolysin titer (in post-streptococcal glomerulonephritis), presence of Streptococci in the throat or skin eruptions, positive blood culture in staphylococcal infections, cryoglobulins in the serum, and depression of complement including some of its early components (C4, C2) and C3.

Light Microscopy: The glomeruli are large and cellular often filling the whole Bowman's space. The capillary walls are thickened, the lumina reduced in size and sometimes completely compressed. In the early stages appreciable numbers of polymorphonuclear leukocytes may be seen. Otherwise the predominant cells are mononuclear probably representing blood monocytes and the native mesangial cells. Capillary thrombi and crescents may be seen in severe cases. Occasionally small deposits which stain red with Trichrome stain may be recognized under the epithelium of the capillary wall. They correspond to the "humps" seen on electron microscopy. Resolution of the disease is characterized by rapid clearing of the capillaries, but much slower restoration to normal in the mesangial areas with resulting picture of mesangial glomerulonephritis.

Electron Microscopy: The characteristic feature is marked enlargement of the mesangium due to cell proliferation and also some increase of the mesangial matrix. Polymorphonuclear leukocytes may be found in the mesangium and adherent to the capillary wall. Deposits, so-called humps, are usually seen on the epithelial side of the capillary basement membrane. The humps vary in size and number and are often inhomogeneous. The foot processes overlying the humps are effaced but are preserved elsewhere unless the patient has the nephrotic syndrome. Small deposits may also be found in the subendothelial location and rarely in the mesangium. All deposits tend to disappear in a matter of a few weeks even if other changes persist. However in some patients deposits persist or recur and are accompanied by formation of "spikes", thus producing a picture of focal or diffuse membranous glomerulonephritis. Occasionally breaks or discontinuities are found in the capillary basement membrane. Mild mesangial cellularity, focal or diffuse, may persist for some time in patients who continue to excrete small amounts of protein and red blood cells, or even after apparent clinical recovery.

Immunofluorescence Microscopy: The most constant finding is granular deposition of C3 along the capillary walls. It is not quite certain whether these deposits always correspond to the humps seen by electron microscopy. C3 is usually accompanied by IgG, sometimes also IgM and IgA. Fibrin is more often seen in the mesangium or in the Bowman's space. The mesangium may also contain deposits of C3 and IgG and sometimes IgM and these tend to persist in cases with incomplete resolution. In post-streptococcal disease Streptococcal antigens can sometimes be demonstrated, more often in the mesangium than in the subepithelial humps.

PRIMARY GLOMERULAR DISEASES

MESANGIAL PROLIFERATIVE GLOMERULONEPHRITIS

Fig. 4-1 Mesangial widening with slightly increased number of cells and mesangial matrix. An adhesion to the capsule is seen at eight o'clock. Note: This is the same case as Figs. 4-13 and 4-14 — Endocapillary Glomerulonephritis, six months after onset of illness. It is meant to show that resolving endocapillary glomerulonephritis may have the appearance of mesangial glomerulonephritis.
PAS stain. X 260.

Fig. 4-2 and 4-3 Mesangial proliferative glomerulonephritis in a six-year-old boy. Acute onset with nephritic syndrome accompanied by nephrotic syndrome. Spontaneous resolution after two months. No streptococcal etiology demonstrated.
Fig. 4-2 — PAS stain. X 410.
Fig. 4-3 — H&E stain. X 410.

Fig. 4-4 Mesangial proliferative glomerulonephritis. Insidious onset of nephrotic syndrome with poor response to therapy.
PAS stain. X 260.

Fig. 4-5 Mesangial glomerulonephritis with considerable mesangial involvement. Insidious onset. No specific etiology.
PAS stain. X 260.

Fig. 4-6 Immunofluorescence microscopy. Mesangial glomerulonephritis with nephrotic syndrome. Mesangial deposits of IgM. X 260.

MESANGIAL PROLIFERATIVE GLOMERULONEPHRITIS

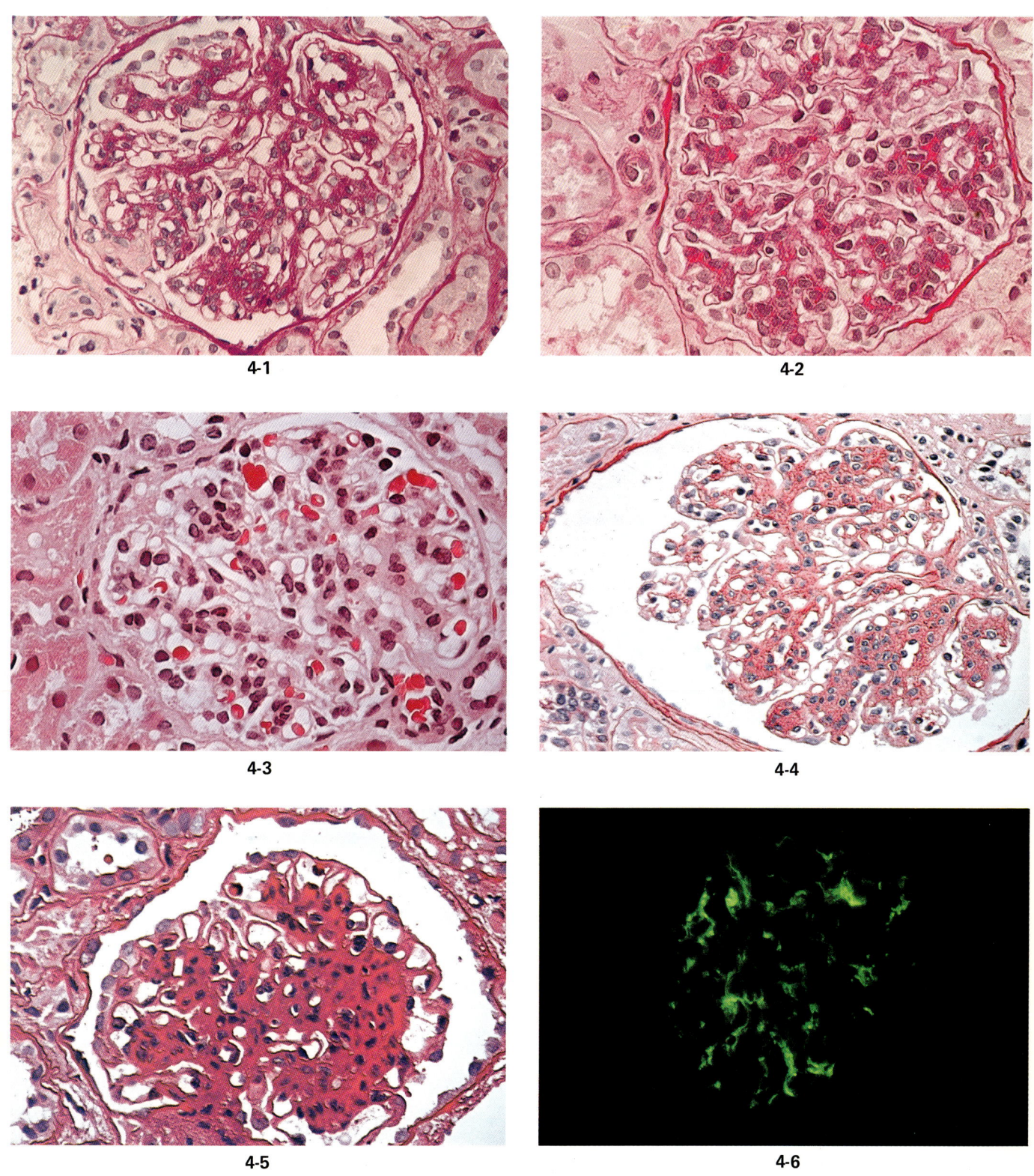

PRIMARY GLOMERULAR DISEASES

MESANGIAL PROLIFERATIVE GLOMERULONEPHRITIS

Fig. 4-7   Progression of mesangial glomerulonephritis to glomerular sclerosis.
PAS stain.   x 260.

ENDOCAPILLARY PROLIFERATIVE GLOMERULONEPHRITS

Fig. 4-8   Endocapillary proliferative glomerulonephritis. Diffuse proliferative changes with sparing of some capillary loops. Periglomerular inflammatory infiltrate is seen.
H&E stain.   x 260.

Fig. 4-9   One micron section of a glomerular lobule showing a large number of mononuclear cells filling the mesangium and the capillary lumina, and a few polymorphonuclear leukocytes. Note fine dark blue granules along the right border of the lobule, representing deposits ("humps").
Toluidine blue stain.   x 1,000.

Fig. 4-10   Immunofluorescence microscopy. Numerous larger and smaller granules of IgG along the capillary loops.   x 260.

Fig. 4-11   Immunofluorescence microscopy. Same case as in Fig. 4-10 stained for C3.   x 260.

Fig. 4-12   Diffuse proliferation with lobular accentuation. A crescent is seen in the right lower corner.
PAS stain.   x 260.

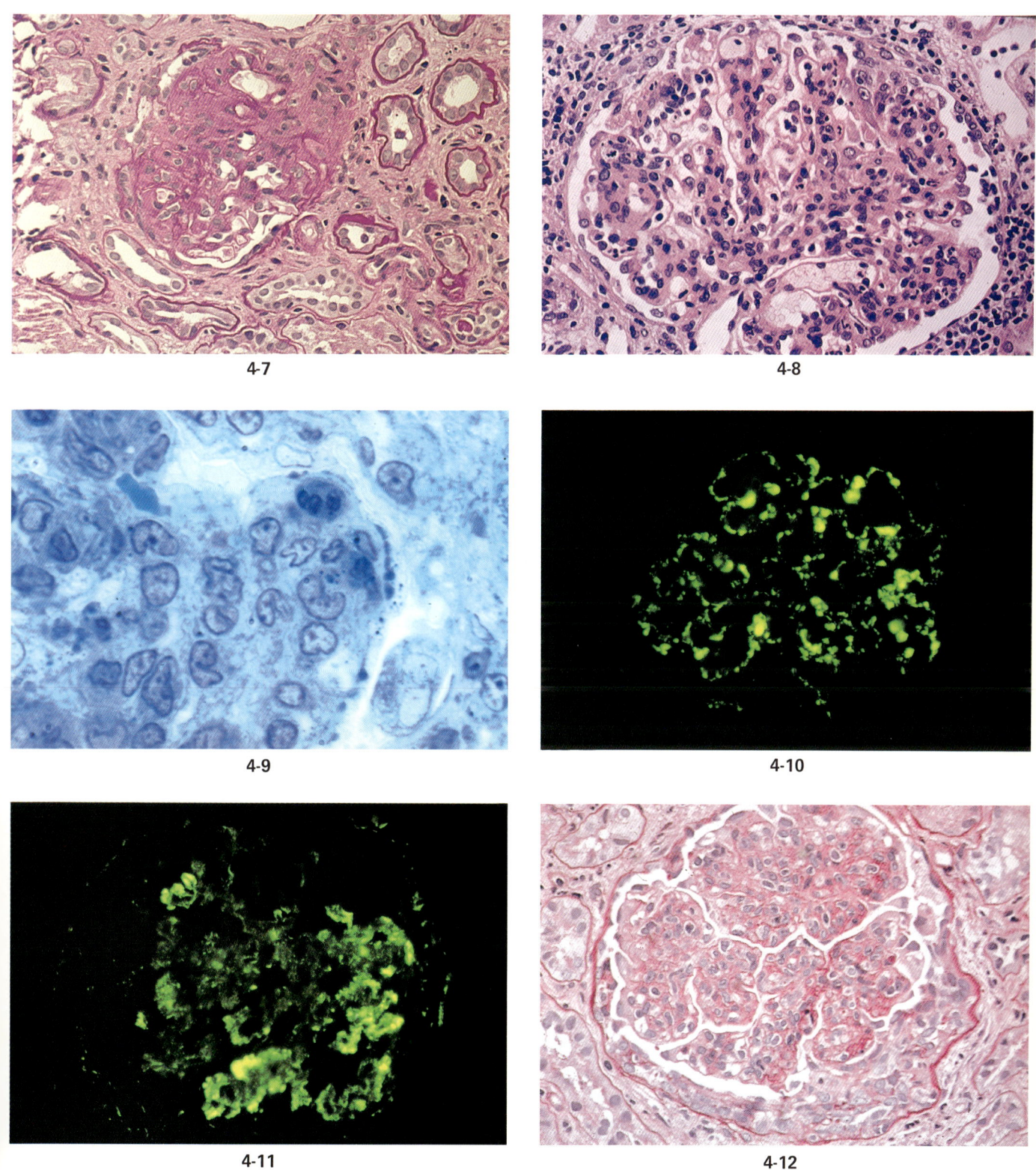

PRIMARY GLOMERULAR DISEASES

ENDOCAPILLARY PROLIFERATIVE GLOMERULONEPHRITIS

Fig. 4-13   Typical diffuse proliferative endocapillary glomerulonephritis in an adult. There is marked cellularity caused by both mononuclear cells and polymorphonuclear leukocytes.
H&E stain.   x 260.

Fig. 4-14   Same case as Fig. 4-13 six months later showing partial resolution of the proliferative process. (Compare also with Fig. 4-8 — Mesangial Proliferative Glomerulonephritis, which shows another glomerulus from the same biopsy but with a more advanced resolution).
H&E stain.   x 260.

Fig. 4-15   Same case as Figs. 4-13 and 4-14 two years later. There is almost complete resolution of the proliferative process with slight segmental mesangial thickening and small capsular adhesions. There is also pericapsular fibrosis.
PAS stain.   x 260.

Fig. 4-16   Typical endocapillary proliferative glomerulonephritis in a child showing distinct lobulation.
H&E stain.   x 410.

Fig. 4-17 and 4-18   Same case as Fig. 4-16 two years later. Complete resolution of the disease process in most of the glomeruli and sclerosis of some of the glomeruli.
Fig. 4-17 H&E stain.   x 100.
Fig. 4-18 PAS stain.   x 410.

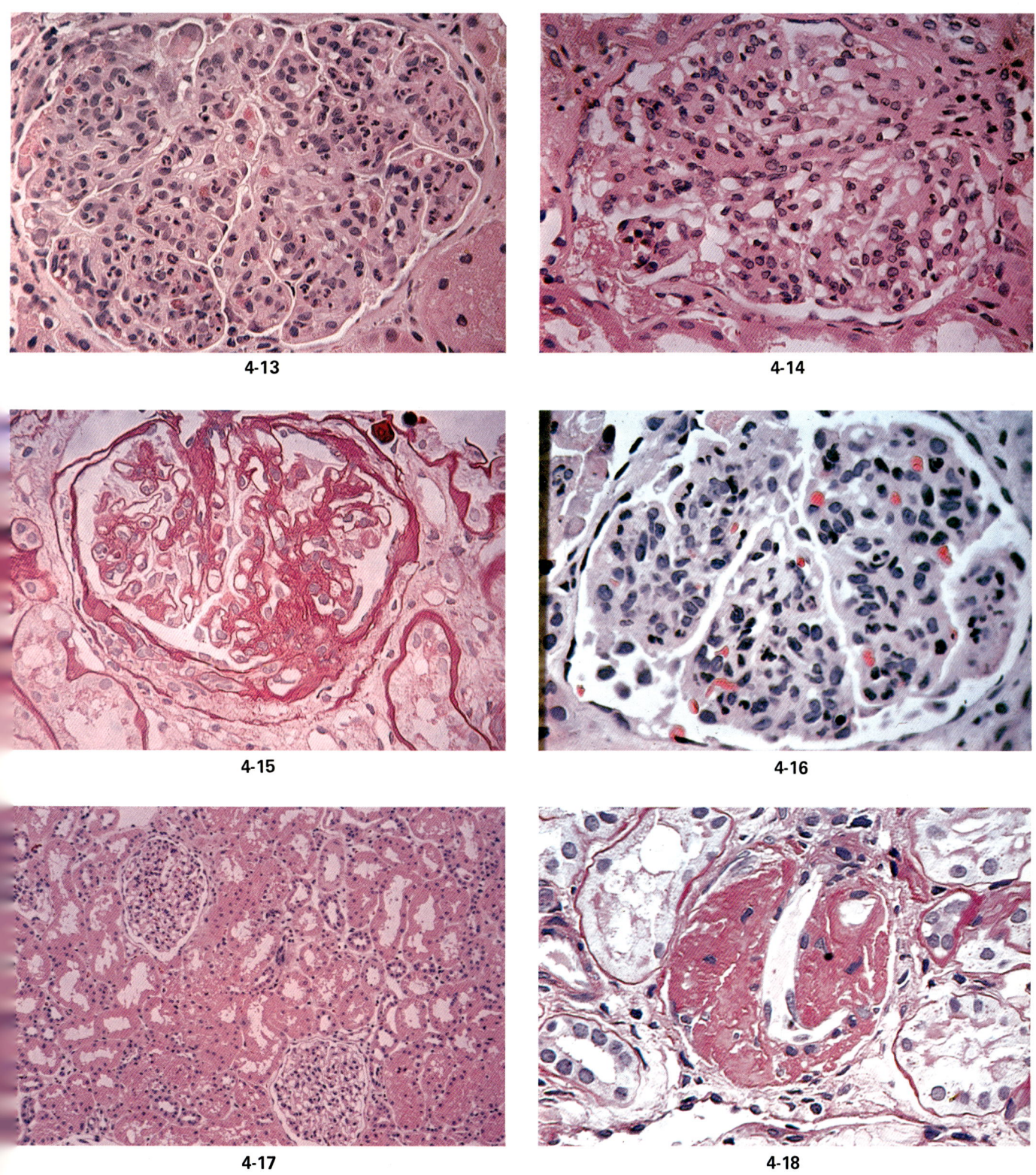

MESANGIAL PROLIFERATIVE GLOMERULONEPHRITIS

Fig. 4-19, 4-20 and 4-21   Electron micrographs. Same case as Fig. 4-5.
   Fig. 4-19 — Mesangial proliferation and scattered deposits (D).   x 7,000.
   Fig. 4-20 — Paramesangial deposit.   x 20,000.
   Fig. 4-21 — Subepithelial deposit.   x 20,000.
   These deposits contain only IgG on immunofluorescence microscopy. The case may represent a milder or partly resolved stage of endocapillary glomerulonephritis.

   BM: basement membrane, En: endothelial cell, MC: mesangial cell, MM: mesangial matrix, FP: foot process, L: capillary lumen.

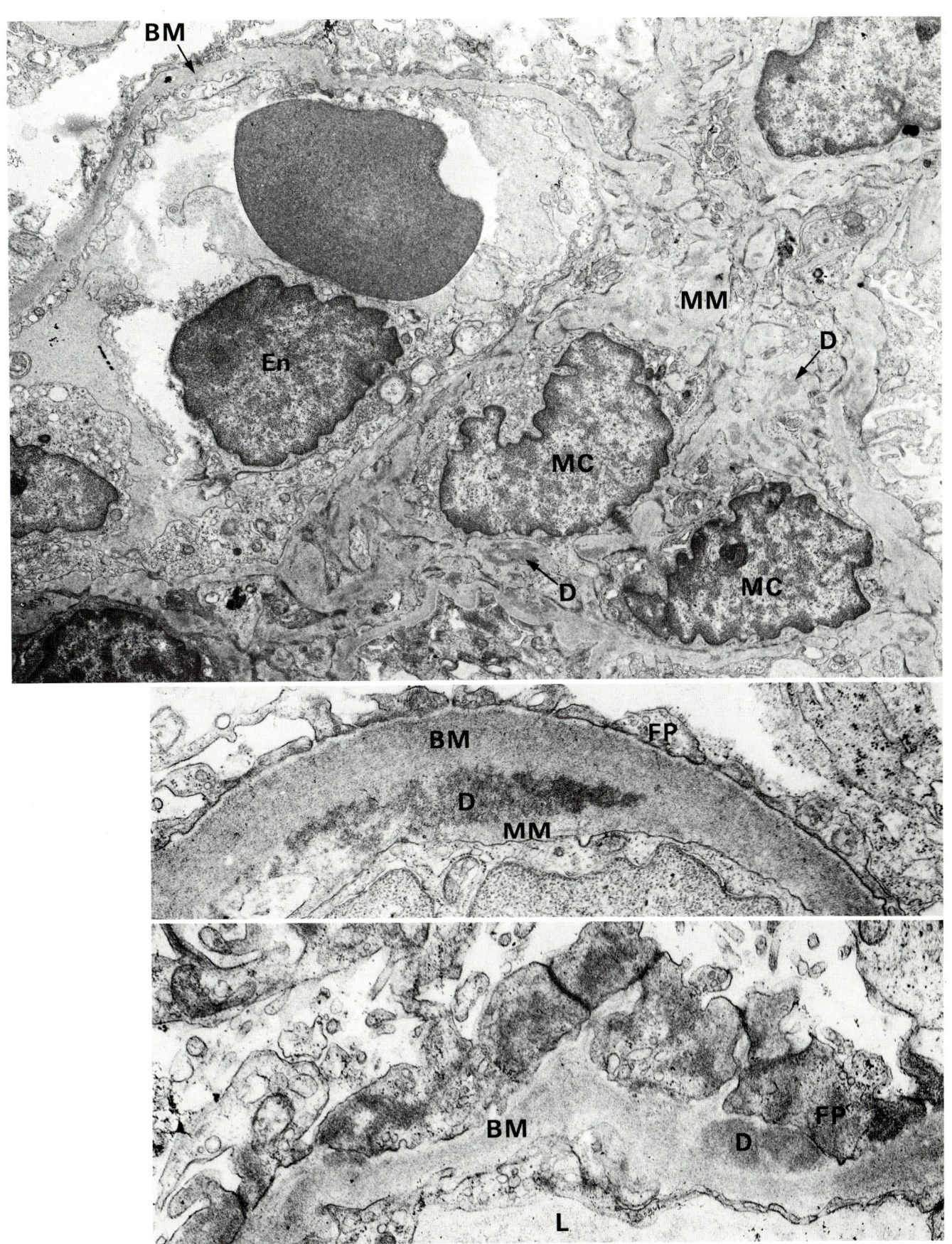

PRIMARY GLOMERULAR DISEASES

ENDOCAPILLARY PROLIFERATIVE GLOMERULONEPHRITIS

Fig. 4-22 Electron micrograph. Part of a glomerular lobule in an early stage of endocapillary proliferative glomerulonephritis. There is a large number of mononuclear cells in the mesangium compressig the capillary lumina. Strands of mesangial matrix (MM), are also present. Polymorphonuclear leukocytes (Pmn) are seen, some attached to the capillary wall. Many deposits ("humps") (D) of various sizes are present along the epithelial aspect of the capillary basement membrane.   x 2,900.

Fig. 4-23 Electron micrograph. Part of a glomerular capillary showing large, partly fused humps (D).   x 15,000.

P: podocyte, En: endothelial cell, MC: mesangial cell, BM: basement membrane.

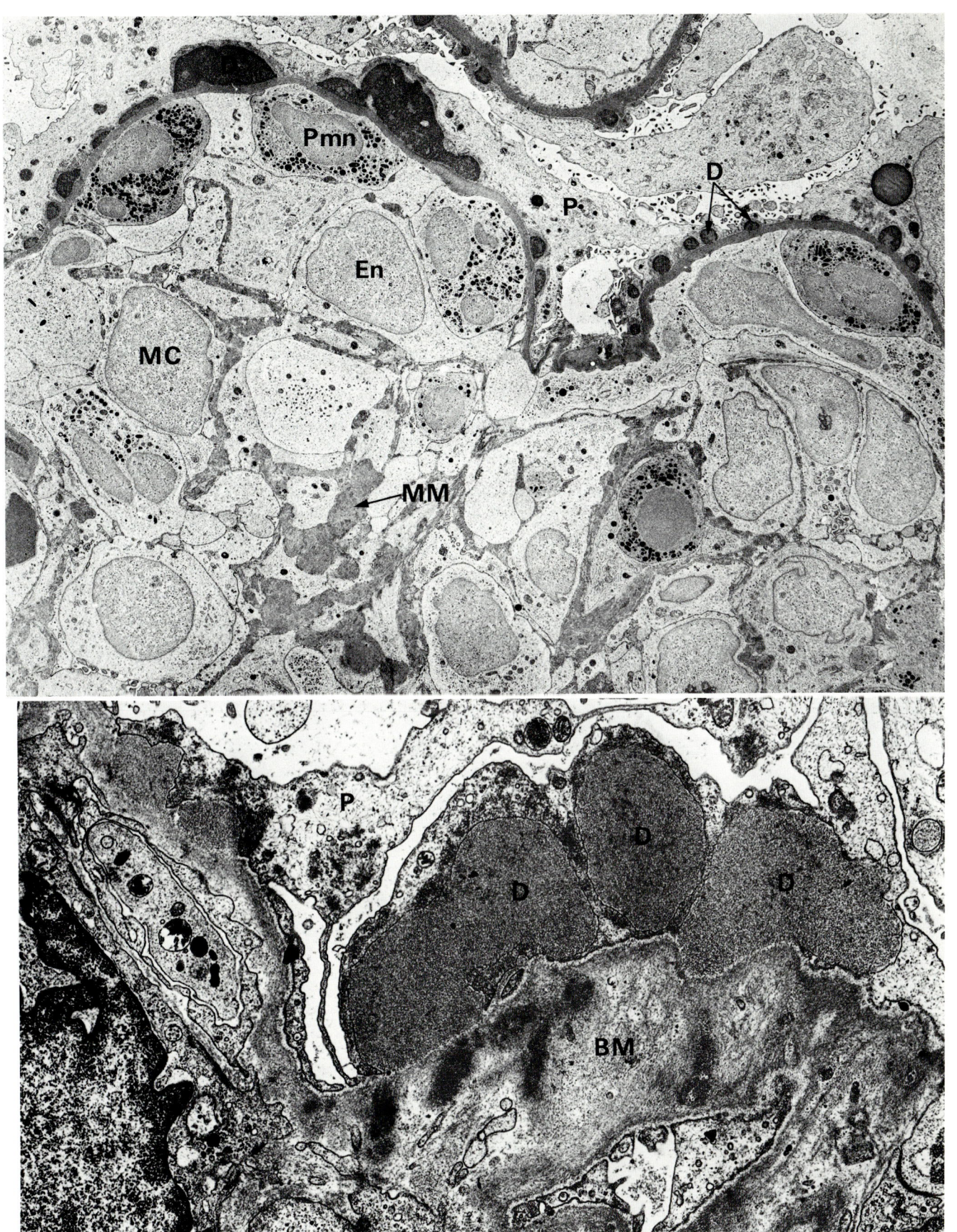

ENDOCAPILLARY PROLIFERATIVE GLOMERULONEPHRITIS

Fig. 4-24 Electron micrograph. Part of a glomerular lobule showing a large mononuclear cell (Mon) and polymorphonuclear leukocytes (Pmn). The capillary basement membrane, which is stained black, presents a small defect ("break") (Br) and carries a flame-shaped hump (D). Cytoplasm of the podocyte (P) and the foot processes are edematous.
PASM stain. x 13,000.

Fig. 4-25 Electron micrograph. Part of a glomerular lobule in a later stage of endocapillary proliferative glomerulonephritis. Polymorphonuclear leukocytes and humps have disappeard and the capillaries are partly reopened. The expanded mesangium contains many mononuclear cells and considerable amount of quite dense mesangial matrix (MM). x 3,000.

En: endothelial cell, MC: mesangial cell.

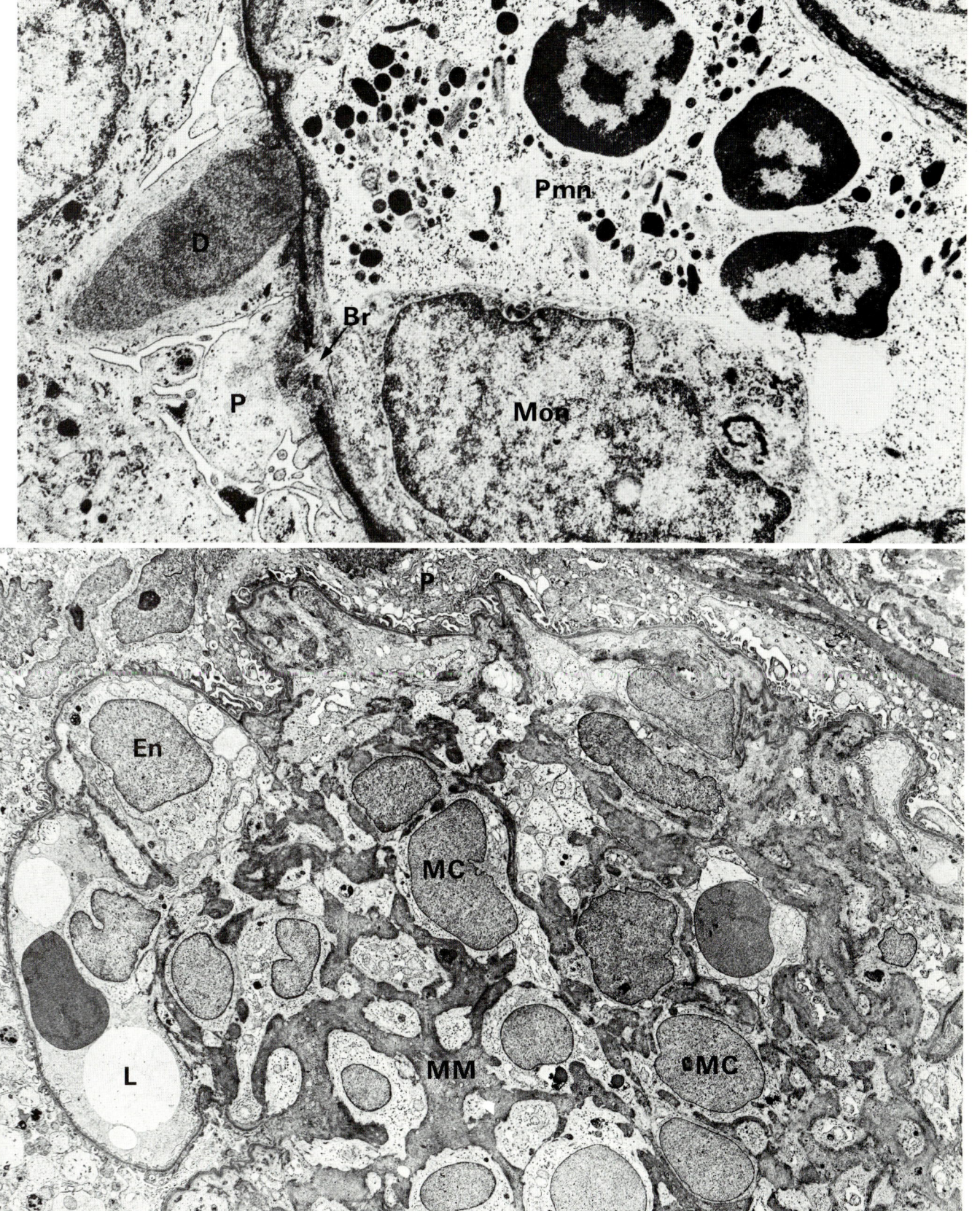

ENDOCAPILLARY PROLIFERATIVE GLOMERULONEPHRITIS

Fig. 4-26 Electron micrograph. Same case as Fig. 4-15. Focal reappearance of subepithelial and intramembranous deposits (D) and formation of spikes (S) in a manner resembling membranous glomerulonephritis.   x 16,000.

BM: basement membrane, P: podocyte.

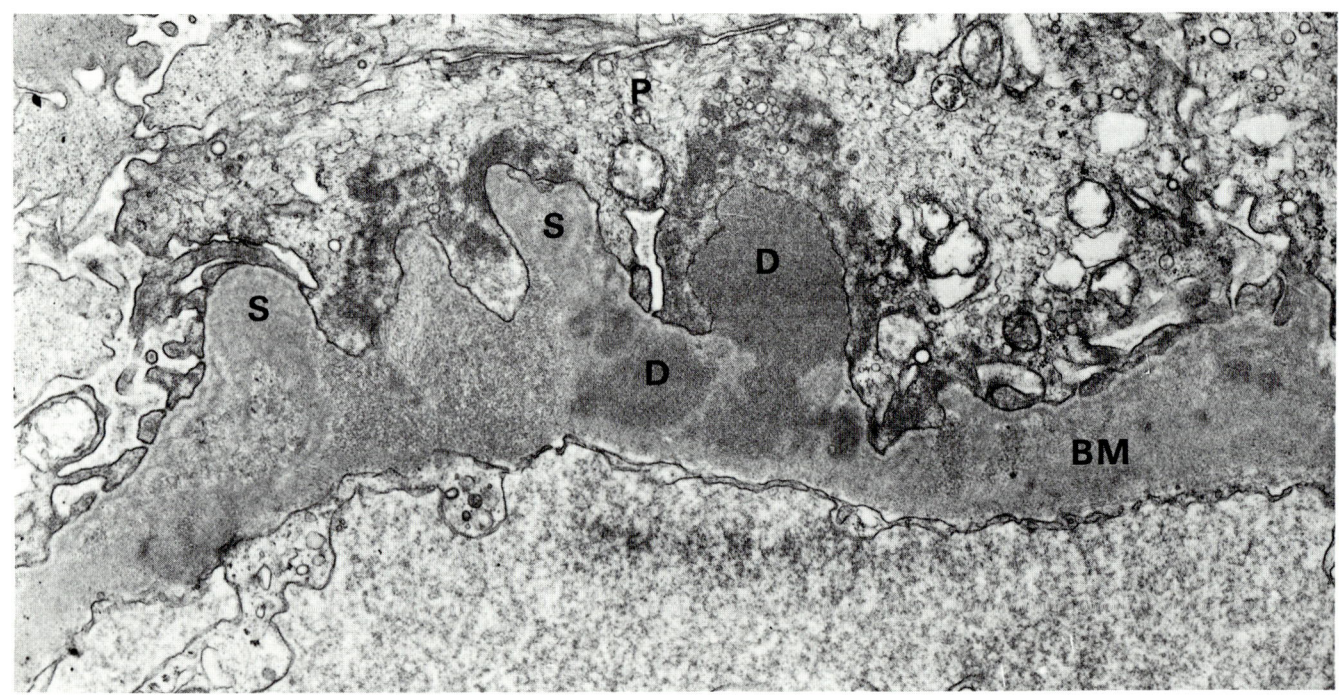

CHAPTER 5

Diffuse Mesangiocapillary Glomerulonephritis Type 1
(Figs. 5-1 to 5-9 and Figs. 5-25 to 5-33)
Diffuse Mesangiocapillary Glomerulonephritis Type 3
(Figs. 5-10 to 5-17 and Figs. 5-34 to 5-36)
Dense Deposit Glomerulonephritis (Type 2)
(Figs. 5-18 to 5-24 and Figs. 5-37 to 5-40)

Diffuse Mesangiocapillary Glomerulonephritis
(Membranoproliferative Glomerulonephritis, Types 1 and 3)

Definition: All or nearly all glomeruli show a combination of capillary wall thickening with a variable amount of mesangial cell proliferation and increased matrix. This may lead to accentuation of the normal lobular structure of the glomerulus (lobular glomerulonephritis). The capillary wall thickening is due to the presence of deposits and to mesangial interposition and frequently takes the form of duplicated or "split" basement membrane, ("double contour") best seen with periodic acid silver methenamine technique. The deposits are sometimes genuinely subendothelial but more often they lie in the interposed subendothelial mesangium; they are also present in the mesangial areas. Occasionally they may be identified by light microscopy. The lamina densa is usually normal as seen in PASM stain but occasionally it may be disrupted by deposits with loss of argyrophilia (Type III). Although the lesions of mesangiocapillary glomerulonephritis are usually diffuse, in a small percentage of cases they are focally distributed.

Examples of additional features from Table II: diffuse mesangiocapillary glomerulonephritis with subepithelial deposits; diffuse mesangiocapillary glomerulonephritis with focal crescents in 25% of glomeruli (see Section I).

Clinical Manifestations: Mesangiocapillary glomerulonephritis is a chronic progressive disease. It occurs at any age but is most common in older children and young adults and is slightly more common in females. It usually begins insidiously with proteinuria and nephrotic syndrome, but in about 1/4–1/3 of patients, particularly in the younger age groups, the initial manifestation is acute nephritic syndrome or sometimes gross hematuria. Another 30% of patients have only isolated proteinuria and/or microscopic hematuria at first examination. Nephrotic syndrome is seen at the onset in about half the patients, but eventually develops in the majority. Hematuria, gross or microscopic, is found in nearly all patients, and both hypertension and renal insufficiency are frequent. A very important finding is depression of the complement in the serum, particularly of C3 but also of the early components, that is C1q, C4 and C2. This depression is not always present at the onset of disease but eventually develops in the majority of patients. In addition the serum contains a globulin called "C3 nephritic factor" (C3 NeF) which is an indirect activator of C3, and is possibly responsible for its excessive utilization.

The clinical course is characterized by periods of improvement and exacerbation, particularly of the nephrotic syndrome and of serum complement levels. Chronic renal failure develops in the majority of patients in 5–10 years, and few survive more than 15 years. A sizable minority develops rapidly progressive renal failure signaled by the appearance of glomerular crescents. Recovery, whether spontaneous or therapeutically induced, is infrequent.

Light Microscopy: The glomeruli are enlarged, often strikingly so. The mesangial areas are expanded by increased numbers of cells and amount of mesangial matrix, sometimes forming distinct nodules in the centers of glomerular lobules ("lobular" form). The cells are mostly mesangial, but polymorphonuclear leukocytes are often present and may be numerous. The proportion of cells to matrix varies with the duration of the disease. In advanced cases lobular centers may become completely sclerosed simulating the Kimmelstiel-Wilson nodules of diabetes.

A very characteristic feature is thickening of the capillary wall. With special stains, such as PASM, this thickening has the appearance of "double contour", that is of two dark lines separated by a pale zone. This change is not necessarily present in all capillaries and often involves only segments of the wall. Sometimes deposits can be demonstrated in the thickened segment by means of trichrome stain or C-SM (Chromotrope – silver methenamine).

Small crescents are not uncommon, but in about 10–20% of cases they are large and numerous. Various types of crescents, from cellular to fibrous, may be present, sometimes all of one type or age and in other cases of several types, suggesting repeated attacks.

Electron Microscopy: The expanded mesangium contains cells and matrix and often also deposits of electron dense material. The foot processes of the epithelial cells are often effaced and the cell bodies show changes associated with nephrotic syndrome (see under Minor Glomerular Abnormalities). The lamina densa of the capillary basement membrane is usually thin and uniform. The subendothelial space is widened, often markedly so, and is filled with mesangial cells and matrix continuous with those in the centrilobular mesangial area and sometimes extending along the entire capillary perimeter (mesangial interposition). Electron dense deposits lie in the subendothelial mesangium, sometimes small and scattered and occasionally quite massive. Large deposits tend to infiltrate the lamina densa. On the endothelial side, the interposed mesangium is delimited by a thin layer of basement membrane-like material, either condensed mesangial matrix or a new basement membrane formed by the endothelial cells. In addition to the "subendothelial" deposits (more accurately deposits in the subendothelial mesangium), in some 15–20% of cases one can find subepithelial deposits, either scattered and fairly scanty, resembling the "humps" of diffuse endocapillary glomerulonephritis, or quite numerous and uniform similar to those in membranous glomerulonephritis.

In Type III of mesangiocapillary glomerulonephritis the deposits are mainly located in the markedly disrupted lamina densa. Whether Type III is a distinct entity or merely a variant of Type I has not been definitely established.

Immunofluorescence Microscopy: The deposits vary in amount, distribution and appearance. They may be granular, "lumpy", short linear or a combination of all three, and are located along the capillary wall, and in the mesangium. The third component of complement (C3) is almost invariably present particularly as prominent granular mesangial deposits, and is usually accompanied by properdin and less frequently by the early components – C1q, C4 and C2. Immunoglobulins are found less consistently, mainly IgG and IgM, occasionally IgA. Fibrin is rarely seen, except in the crescents.

Dense Deposit Glomerulonephritis
(Dense Deposit Disease) (Membranoproliferative Glomerulonephritis Type 2 with Intramembranous Deposits)

Definition: All or nearly all glomeruli are characterized by a combination of capillary wall thickening with a variable amount of mesangial cell proliferation and increased matrix. This may lead to an accentuation of the normal lobular form of the glomeruli. The capillary wall thickening is due principally to the presence of deposits within the lamina densa; mesangial interposition with double outline is occasionally also present.

Although this lesion is usually diffuse, in a small

percentage of cases the changes may be focally distributed.

Example of additional features from Table II: dense deposit glomerulonephritis with diffuse cellular crescents (see Section I).

Clinical Manifestations: The disease is seen mainly in young people, children and young adults. Like mesangiocapillary glomerulonephritis, dense deposit glomerulonephritis is a chronic progressive process, manifested most frequently by proteinuria and nephrotic syndrome, combined with hematuria and often also with hypertension and renal insufficiency. In some cases macroscopic hematuria is the presenting symptom. Other patients have only asymptomatic proteinuria and/or microscopic hematuria and are discovered on routine urinalysis. Rapidly progressive renal failure is more frequent than in mesangiocapillary glomerulonephritis and again, is usually associated with the development of crescents in the glomeruli. For this reason prognosis of dense deposit glomerulonephritis is generally poorer than in mesangiocapillary glomerulonephritis.

Depression of serum complement is a persistent feature of dense deposit glomerulonephritis. It is due almost exclusively to the lowering of C3 levels, while early components remain normal. The complement activating gamma globulin (C3 NeF) is almost invariably present in the serum. An unusual association of complement depression and dense deposit glomerulonephritis with a syndrome of partial lipodystrophy has been described. The latter may also be accompanied by complement depression but without glomerulonephritis.

Light Microscopy: The glomeruli show two essential changes: mesangial cellularity and sclerosis, and abnormalities of the capillary walls. Cellular proliferation is generally mild or moderate and sometimes minimal; mesangial sclerosis also varies but becomes more pronounced with progression of the disease. The capillary basement membranes appear thickened and refractile; they stain strongly with eosin, with PAS and with the green or blue component of the trichrome stain, but show little affinity for a silver in PASM. Tubular basement membranes may also be thickened. The fluorescent dye thioflavin T imparts a yellowish green coloration to the basement membranes when viewed with the fluorescence microscope. This change is usually diffuse, but sometimes only focal and segmental. Similar staining may be observed in the Bowman's capsule, tubular basement membrane and occasionally in the mesangium. In addition, mesangial interposition may be present in the capillary walls, but is seldom striking.

Crescents — cellular, fibrocellular or fibrous — are seen in about one-third of cases, and may be large and numerous.

Electron Microscopy: The most striking change is the presence of very electron dense deposits in the lamina densa of the capillary basement membrane. Lamina densa may remain normal in thickness, but more often it is widened by the deposits which form long continuous ribbons or discontinuous shorter stretches. In less advanced cases the deposits occupy only short segments irregularly distributed in the glomerulus. In addition, deposits of lesser density may be seen under the endothelium or, in the form of "humps" under the epithelium. The dense deposits also occur in the mesangium, but are usually few in number. Tubular, or more accurately peritubular deposits are not infrequent. The Bowman's capsule may be involved in an interrupted fashion, and sometimes a few deposits are seen in the walls of the arterioles at the glomerular hilus.

It is of interest that dense deposits tend to recur in the transplanted kidney, first appearing in the capillaries near the hilus and spreading towards the periphery. These deposits, at least in the early stages, do not provoke a proliferative reaction nor cause urinary abnormalities.

Immunofluorescence Microscopy: The most constant finding is extensive deposition of C3 in the mesangium. In the capillary wall these deposits form interrupted double tracked linear stretches and granules. Lesser deposits are seen in the Bowman's capsule. Immunoglobulins are usually absent, or are present only in a few glomerular segments.

PRIMARY GLOMERULAR DISEASES

MESANGIOCAPILLARY GLOMERULONEPHRITIS

Membranoproliferative Glomerulonephritis, Type 1

Fig. 5-1   Typical mesangiocapillary glomerulonephritis showing increase in number of cells and intercellular substances. Some lobulation is evident.
H&E stain.   x 260.

Fig. 5-2   Same case as Fig. 5-1. Large amount of mesangial matrix is evident (stained red).
PAS stain.   x 260.

Fig. 5-3   Mesangiocapillary glomerulonephritis showing mesangial enlargement and thickening of capillary walls. In some places these walls have double outlines.
PAS stain.   x 260.

Fig. 5-4   High magnification of a case similar to that in Fig. 5-3 showing distinct double outlines.
PAS stain.   x 1,000.

Fig. 5-5   Lobular form of mesangiocapillary glomerulonephritis. Note also focal tubular atrophy with interstitial fibrosis and inflammatory infiltration.
PAS stain.   x 100.

Fig. 5-6   Sclerosing stage of lobular mesangiocapillary glomerulonephritis. There is some resemblance to diabetic glomerulosclerosis but the nodules involve the whole glomerulus and are inhomogeneous in structure.
PAS stain.   x 260.

MESANGIOCAPILLARY GLOMERULONEPHRITIS

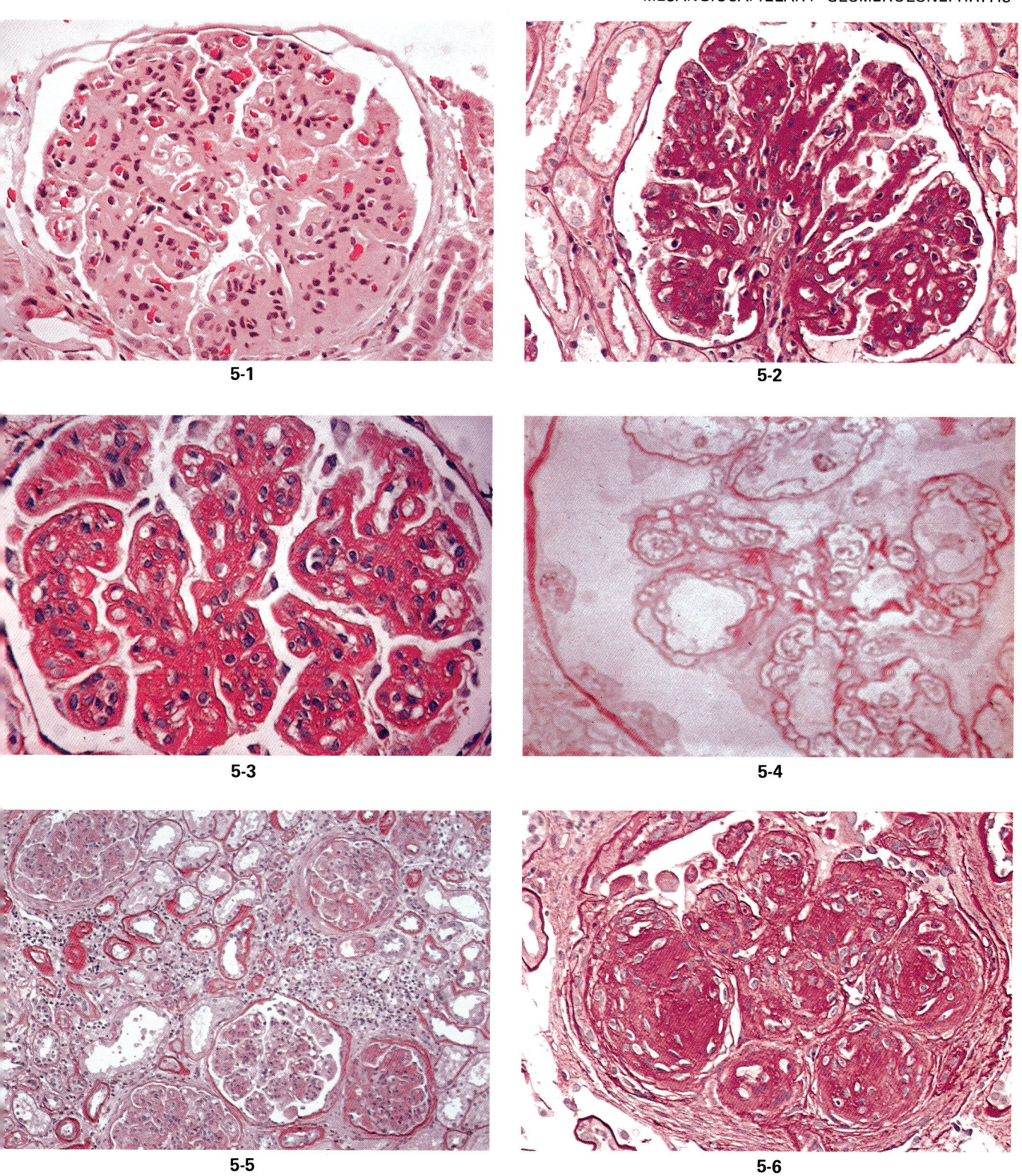

5-1

5-2

5-3

5-4

5-5

5-6

MESANGIOCAPILLARY GLOMERULONEPHRITIS

Membranoproliferative Glomerulonephritis, Type 1

Fig. 5-7 Immunofluorescence microscopy. Extensive deposits of complement (C3) in the mesangium and along the capillary walls. x 260.

Fig. 5-8 Immunofluorescence microscopy. Same case as Fig. 5-7. Rather scanty deposits of IgG mainly along the capillary walls. x 260.

Fig. 5-9 Immunofluorescence microscopy. Another case of mesangiocapillary glomerulonephritis showing nodular deposits of C3 along the capillary walls. x 260.

Membranoproliferative Glomerulonephritis, Type 3

Fig. 5-10 Glomerulus showing moderate mesangial widening and thickening of capillary walls. There is relatively little cellularity.
H&E stain. x 260.

Fig. 5-11 Same case as Fig. 5-10. Mesangial widening and capillary wall thickening are evident.
PAS stain. x 260.

Fig. 5-12 Same case as Fig. 5-10 under high magnification. Part of the glomerular tuft showing markedly thickened capillary walls. This thickening is mainly caused by deposits in and on the outside of the basement membrane. Deposits stain red; basement membrane and mesangial matrix stain blue.
Trichrome stain. x 1,000.

MESANGIOCAPILLARY GLOMERULONEPHRITIS

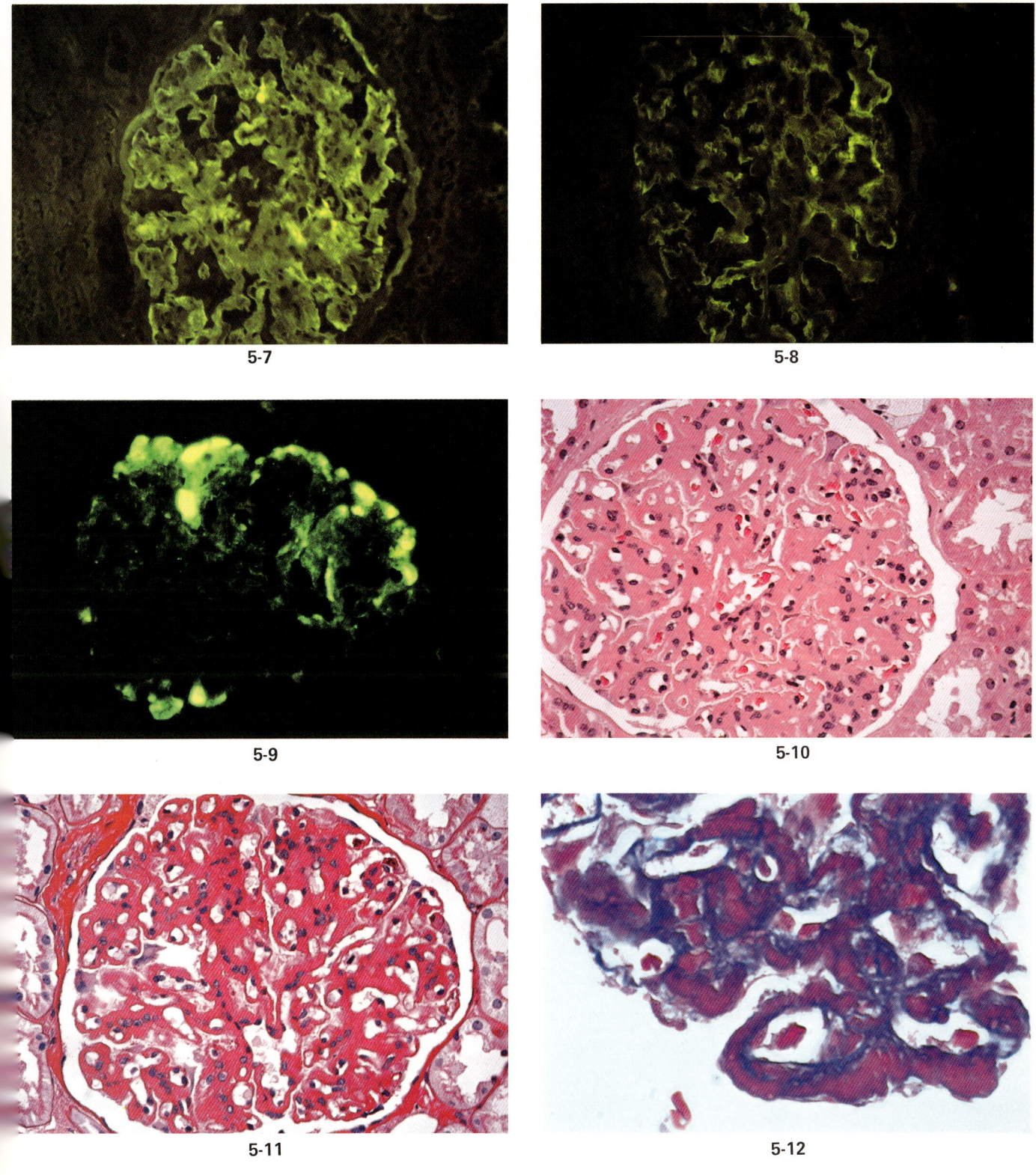

PRIMARY GLOMERULAR DISEASES

MESANGIOCAPILLARY GLOMERULONEPHRITIS

Membranoproliferative Glomerulonephritis, Type 3

Fig. 5-13 Same case as Fig. 5-10 under high magnification. Thick deposits in the glomerular capillary walls disrupting the basement membranes. Deposits are stained pink; basement membranes are black.
PASM counterstained with H&E. × 1,000.

Fig. 5-14 Another example of mesangiocapillary glomerulonephritis type 3 showing more cellular proliferation as well as mesangial widening.
H&E stain. × 260.

Fig. 5-15 Same case as Fig. 5-14 showing increase in mesangial matrix and irregular staining of capillary basement membranes.
PASM stain.

Fig. 5-16 and 5-17 Immunofluorescence microscopy in a case of mesangiocapillary glomerulonephritis type 3.
Fig. 5-16 — Deposits of alpha 2D fraction of complement mainly along the capillary walls.
Fig. 5-17 — Deposits of properdin in the mesangium and along capillary walls.

Dense Deposit Glomerulonephritis

Fig. 5-18 Dense deposit disease. Section of renal cortex showing tubular atrophy, one completely sclerosed glomerulus and one fairly well preserved glomerulus.
PAS stain. × 100.

MESANGIOCAPILLARY GLOMERULONEPHRITIS

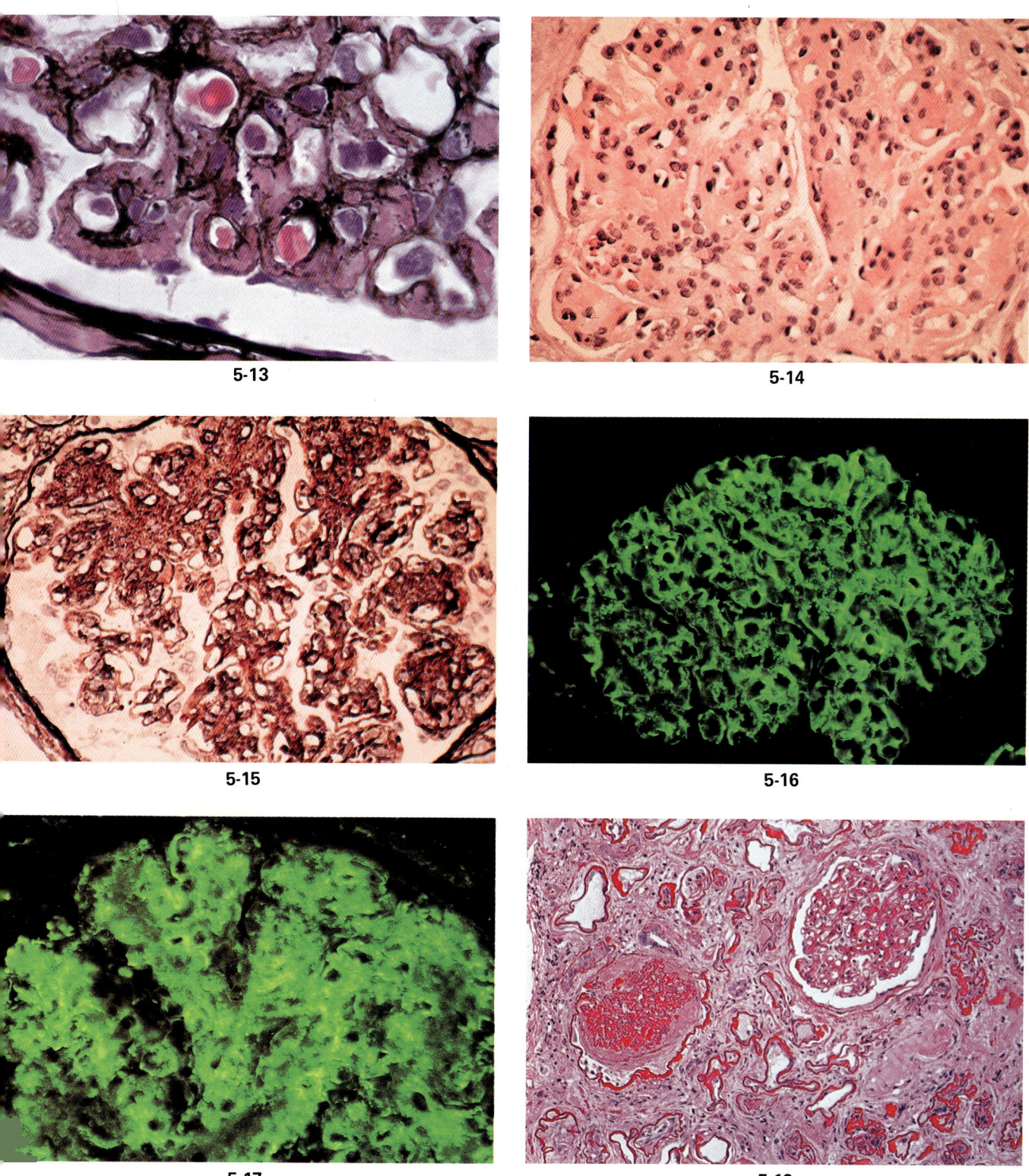

PRIMARY GLOMERULAR DISEASES

Dense Deposit Glomerulonephritis

Fig. 5-19   Another case of dense deposit disease showing mild cellular proliferation and conspicuous thickening of capillary walls.   × 260.
PAS stain.

Fig. 5-20   Same case as Fig. 5-19 showing a large crescent partly compressing the tuft.
PAS stain.   × 260.

Fig. 5-21   Same case as Fig. 5-19. Prominent staining of capillary walls and segmental staining of Bowman's capsule.
Thioflavin T stain.   × 260.

Fig. 5-22   Another case of dense deposit disease showing strong staining of the mesangial matrix and weak staining of capillary basement membranes.
PASM stain.   × 510.

Fig. 5-23   Immunofluorescence microscopy. Same case as Fig. 5-19. Deposits of complement (C3) along the capillary basement membranes.   × 260.

Fig. 5-24   Immunofluorescence microscopy. Another case of dense deposit disease showing intense deposits of complement (C3) in the mesangium.   × 1,000.

DENSE DEPOSIT GLOMERULONEPHRITIS

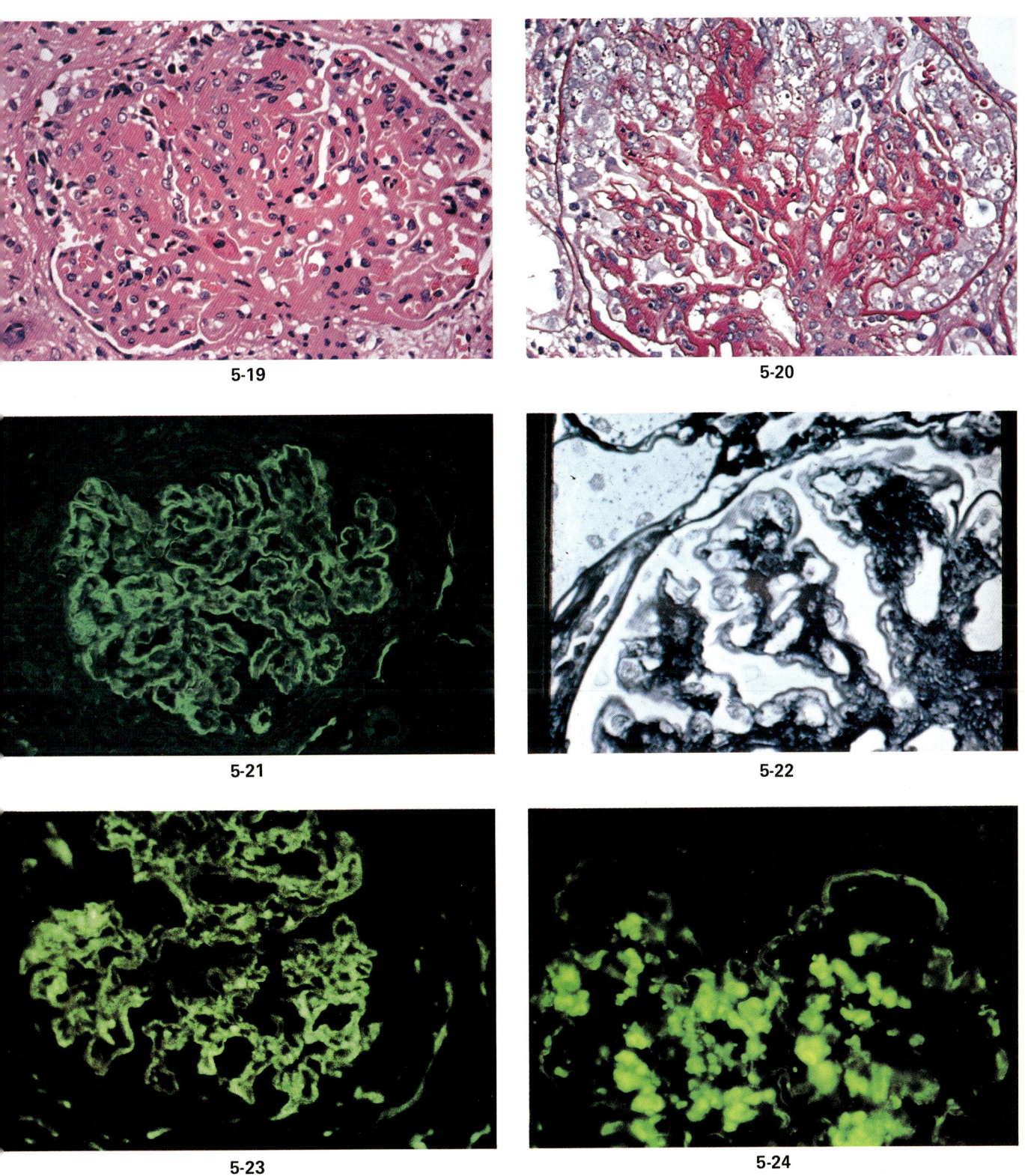

5-19

5-20

5-21

5-22

5-23

5-24

PRIMARY GLOMERULAR DISEASES

MESANGIOCAPILLARY GLOMERULONEPHRITIS

Membranoproliferative Glomerulonephritis, Type 1

Fig. 5-25 Electron micrograph. Part of a glomerulus showing double outlines of capillary walls with mesangial interposition (MI).
PASM stain.   x 4,600.

Fig. 5-26 Electron micrograph. Same case as Fig. 5-9. Striking mesangial interposition. Large mononuclear cells (Mon) and a single red blood cell (RBC) are seen in the capillary lumen (L).   x 6,400.

U: urinary space, MC: mesangial cell, MM: mesangial matrix, BM: basement membrane.

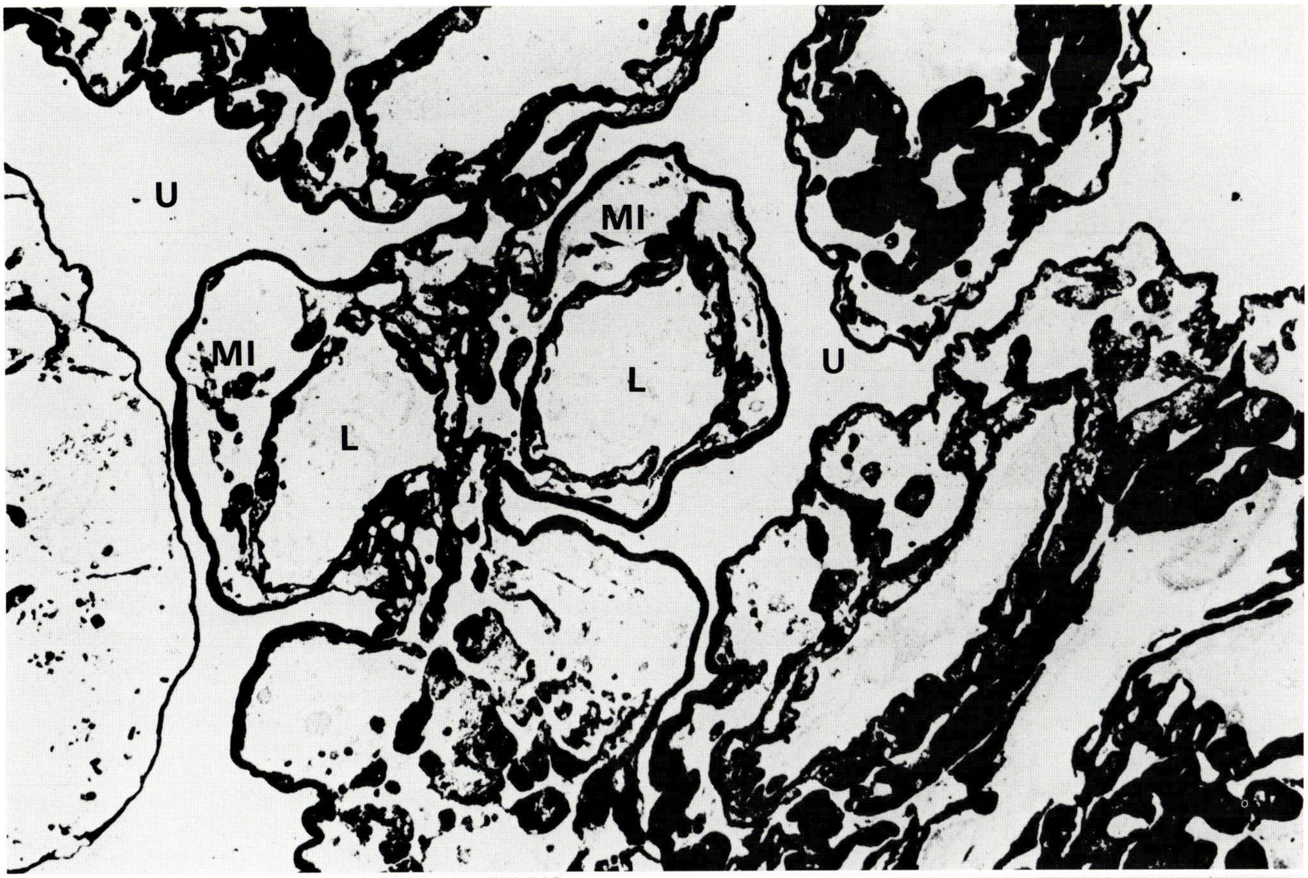

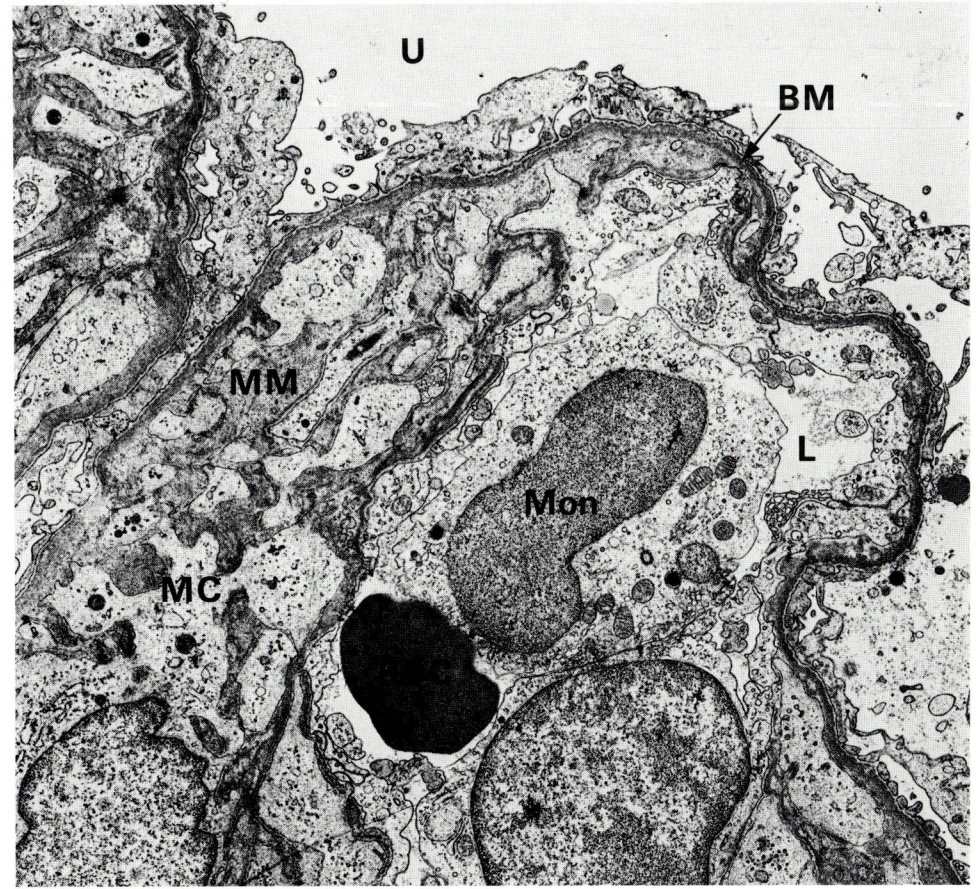

PRIMARY GLOMERULAR DISEASES

MESANGIOCAPILLARY GLOMERULONEPHRITIS

Membranoproliferative Glomerulonephritis, Type 1

Fig. 5-27 Electron micrograph. Same case as Fig. 5-5. Double outline of capillary walls. Original basement membrane (BM) on the outside and a new basement membrane (mesangial matrix ?) (MM) on the inside adjoining the endothelium. The space between the two layers contains cytoplasm of mesangial cells (MC). x 9,600.

Fig. 5-28 Electron micrograph. So-called "subendothelial" electron dense deposits (D). These deposits are actually located in the interposed mesangium.
x 12,000.

P: podocyte, L: capillary lumen.

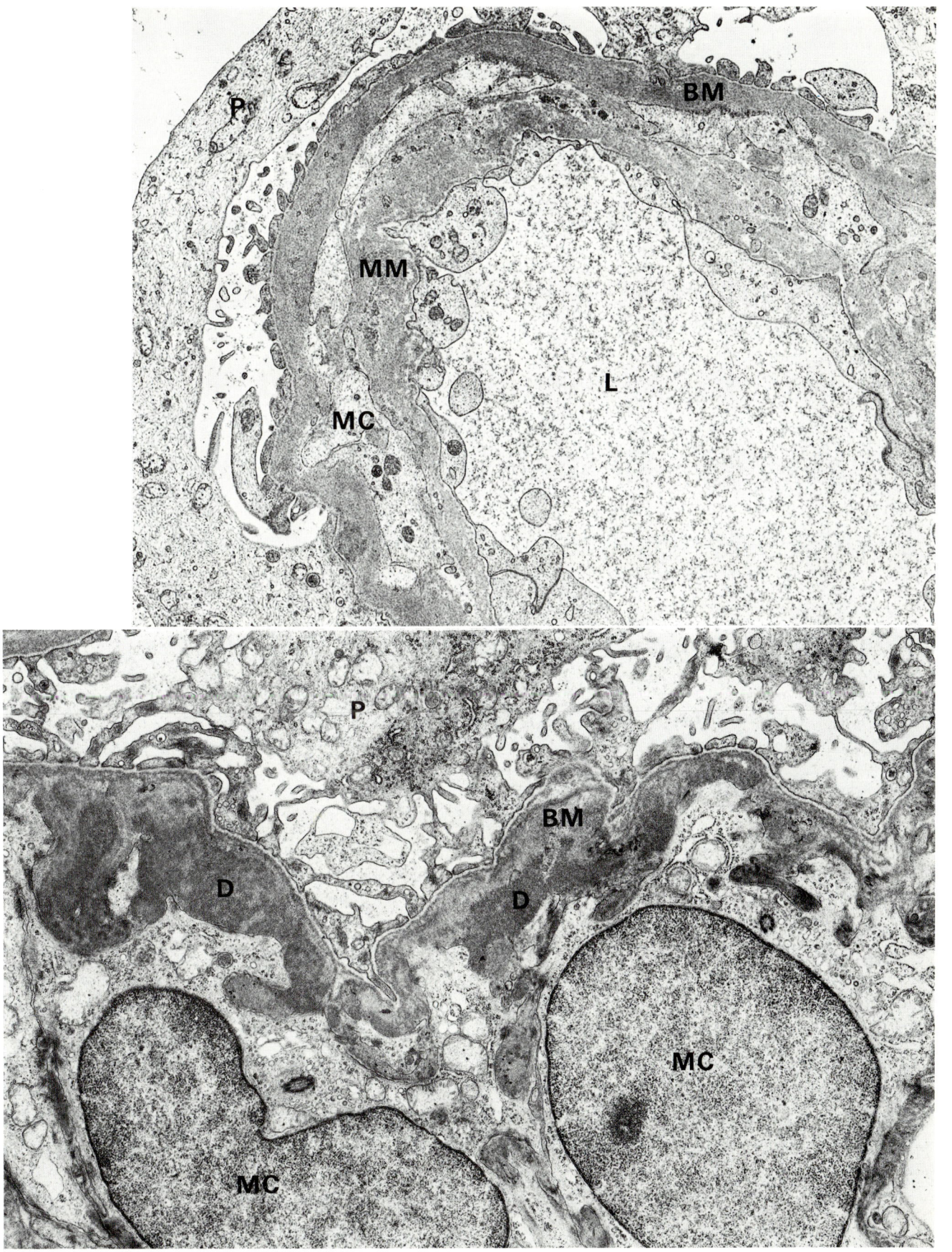

MESANGIOCAPILLARY GLOMERULONEPHRITIS

Membranoproliferative Glomerulonephritis, Type 1

Fig. 5-29 Electron micrograph. Massive subendothelial as well as intramembranous and subepithelial deposits (D). × 11,000.

Fig. 5-30 Electron micrograph. Same case as Fig. 5-29. Markedly expanded mesangium showing cells (MC) and mesangial matrix (MM). Electron dense deposits (D) are present in the matrix and in the interposed mesangium along the capillary walls. × 9,500.

P: podocyte, BM: basement membrane.

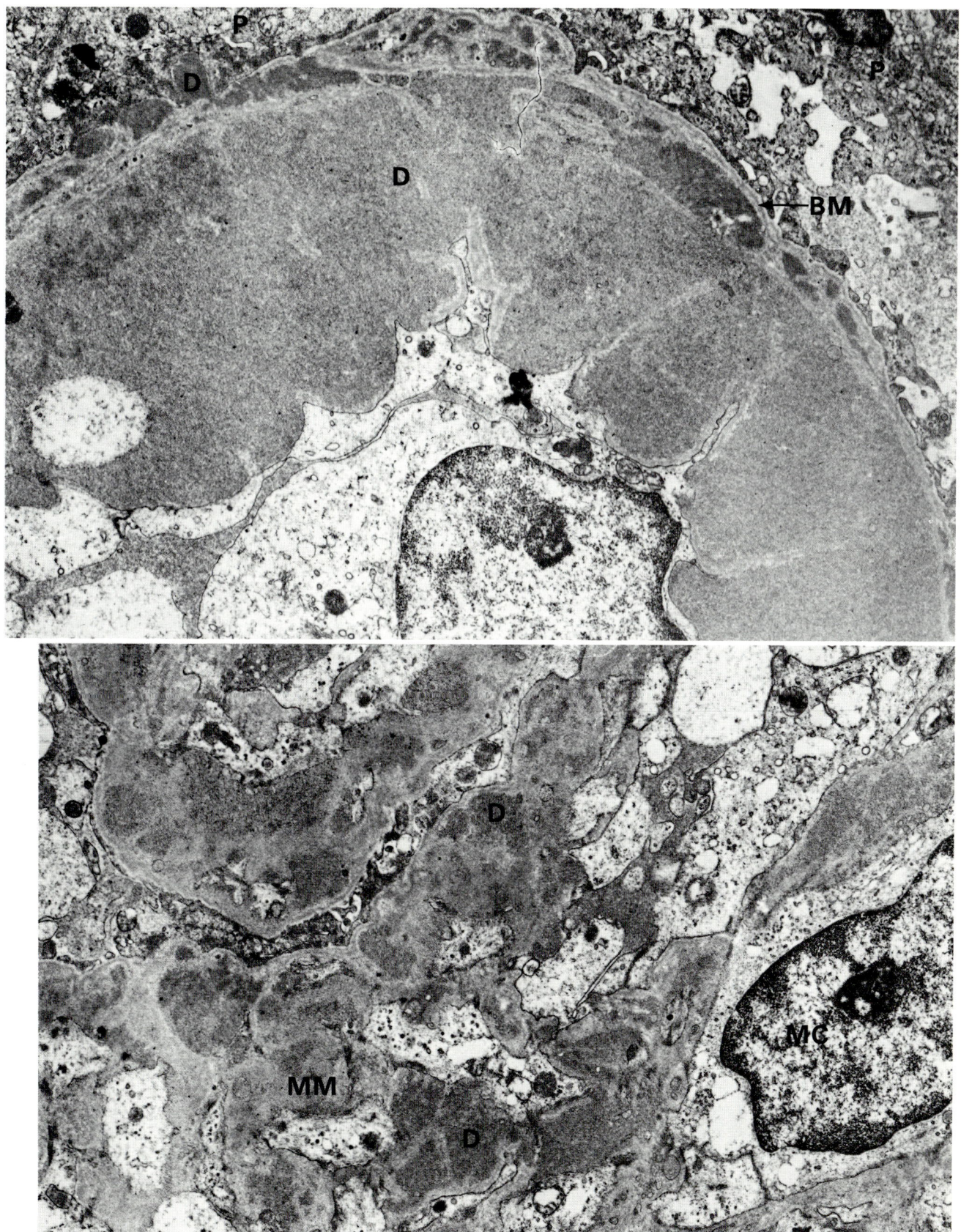

PRIMARY GLOMERULAR DISEASES

MESANGIOCAPILLARY GLOMERULONEPHRITIS

Membranoproliferative Glomerulonephritis, Type 1

Fig. 5-31   Electron micrograph. Part of a glomerular lobule showing mesangial proliferation and numerous subepithelial deposits (D) accompanied by spikes. The mesangial cells (MC) contain scattered lipid droplets.   x 7,400

Fig. 5-32   Electron micrograph. Part of a glomerular lobule showing mesangial cells and large amount of matrix (MM). Hump-like scattered subepithelial deposits are seen along the capillary walls.   x 3,200.

U: urinary space, BM: basement membrane, L: capillary lumen, P: podocyte.

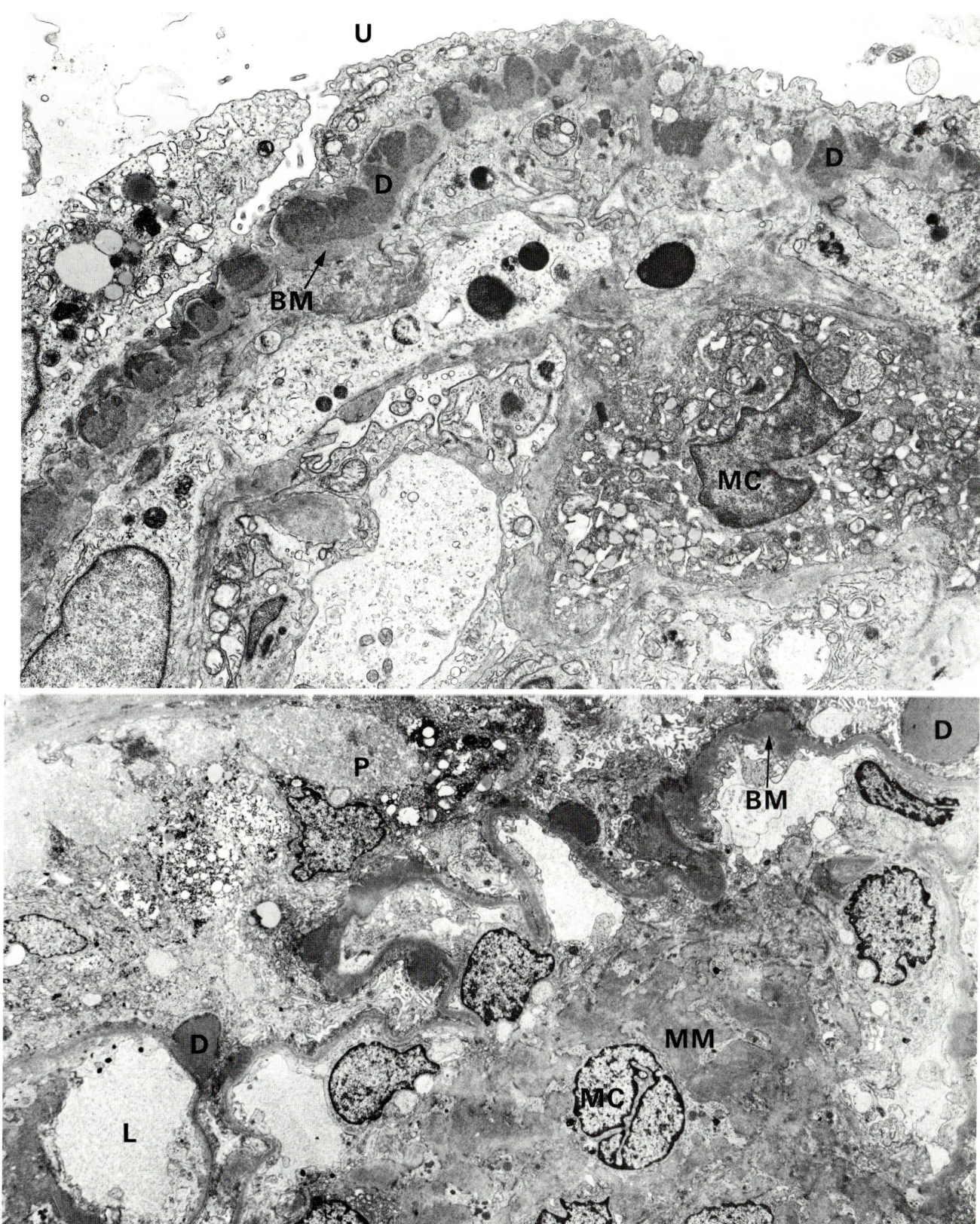

MESANGIOCAPILLARY GLOMERULONEPHRITIS

Membranoproliferative Glomerulonephritis, Type 1

Fig. 5-33 Electron micrograph. Advanced lobular glomerulonephritis showing remnants of cells and fused masses of mesangial matrix (MM). Note thin basement membrane (BM)　　　　　　　　　　　　　　　　　　　　　　× 6,700.

Membranoproliferative Glomerulonephritis, Type 3

Fig. 5-34 Electron micrograph. Same case as Fig. 5-10. Electron dense deposits (D) in the capillary basement membrane (BM) and in the mesangial matrix.
　　　　　　　　　　　　　　　　　　　　　　× 7,500.

L: capillary lumen,　FP: foot process,　MC: mesangial cell,
U: urinary space.

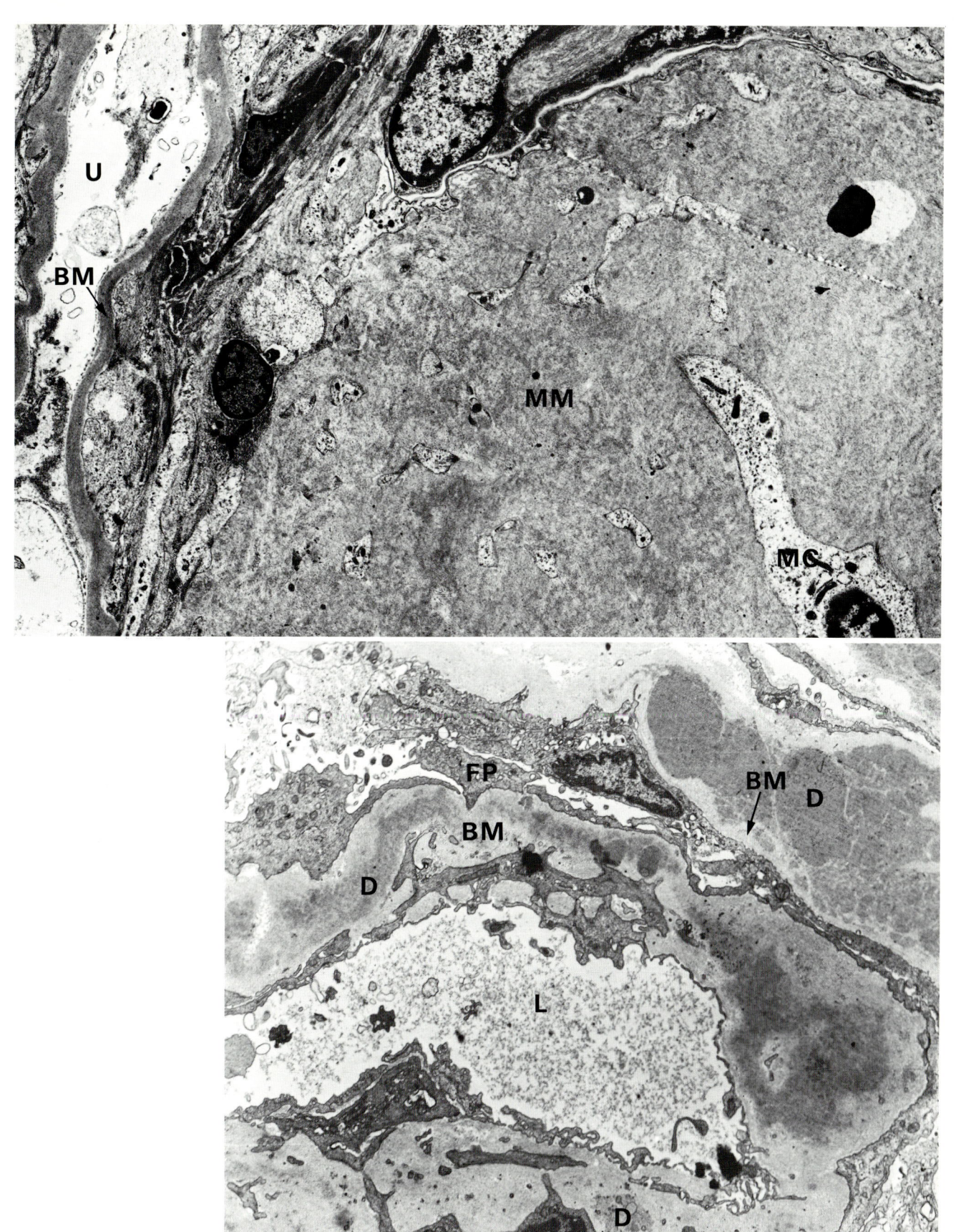

PRIMARY GLOMERULAR DISEASES

MESANGIOCAPILLARY GLOMERULONEPHRITIS

Membranoproliferative Glomerulonephritis, Type 3

Fig. 5-35 Electon micrograph. Same case as Fig. 5-14. Electron dense deposits within a markedly thickened capillary basement membrane (BM).   x 16,000.

Fig. 5-36 Electron micrograph. Marked disruption of basement membrane by gray staining deposits (D). Remnants of lamina densa are represented by thin strands which stain black. Mesangial matrix is stained mostly in a normal fashion (black).
PASM stain.   x 15,000.

U: urinary space, En: endothelial cell, MC: mesangial cell, FP: foot process.

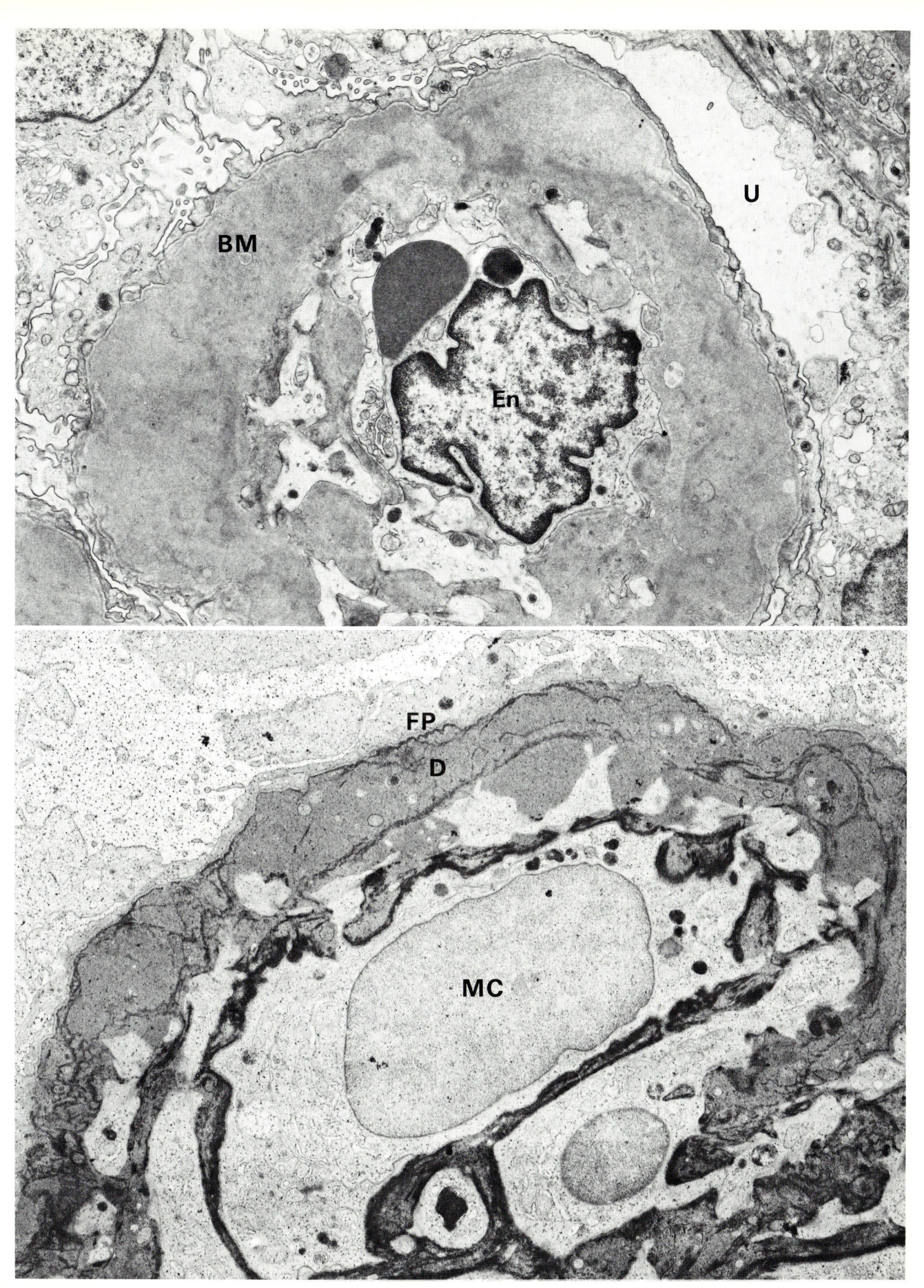

PRIMARY GLOMERULAR DISEASES

Dense Deposit Glomerulonephritis

Fig. 5-37   Electron micrograph. Very dark deposits (D) following the outlines of the capillary basement membrane (BM).   x 7,000.

Fig. 5-38   Electron micrograph. Discontinuous dense deposits (D) lying within and expanding the capillary basement membrane.   x 13,000.

P: podocyte, BMM: basement membrane material, MM: mesangial matrix, FP: foot process, L: capillary lumen.

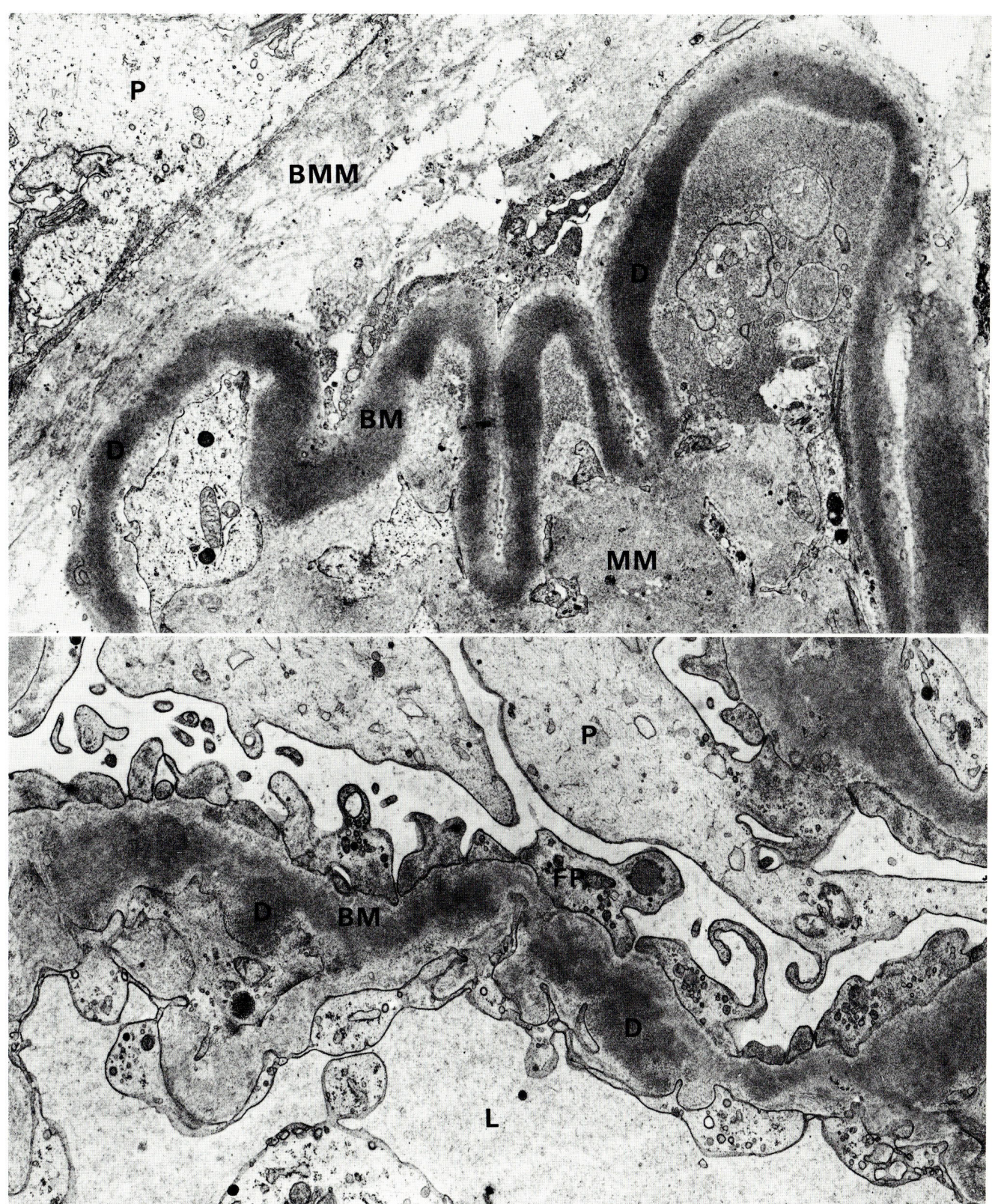

PRIMARY GLOMERULAR DISEASES

Dense Deposit Glomerulonephritis

Fig. 5-39   Electron micrograph. Irregularly thickened capillary basement membrane stains dark gray. The mesangial matrix and the inner layer of Bowman's capsule stain black. Paraformaldehyde fixation, methacrylate embedding, PASM stain.   x 14,000.

Fig. 5-40   Electron micrograph. Irregular layer of dense deposit (D) on the outside of the tubular basement membrane (TBM).   x 11,000.

U: urinary space, L: capillary lumen, TC: tubular cell.

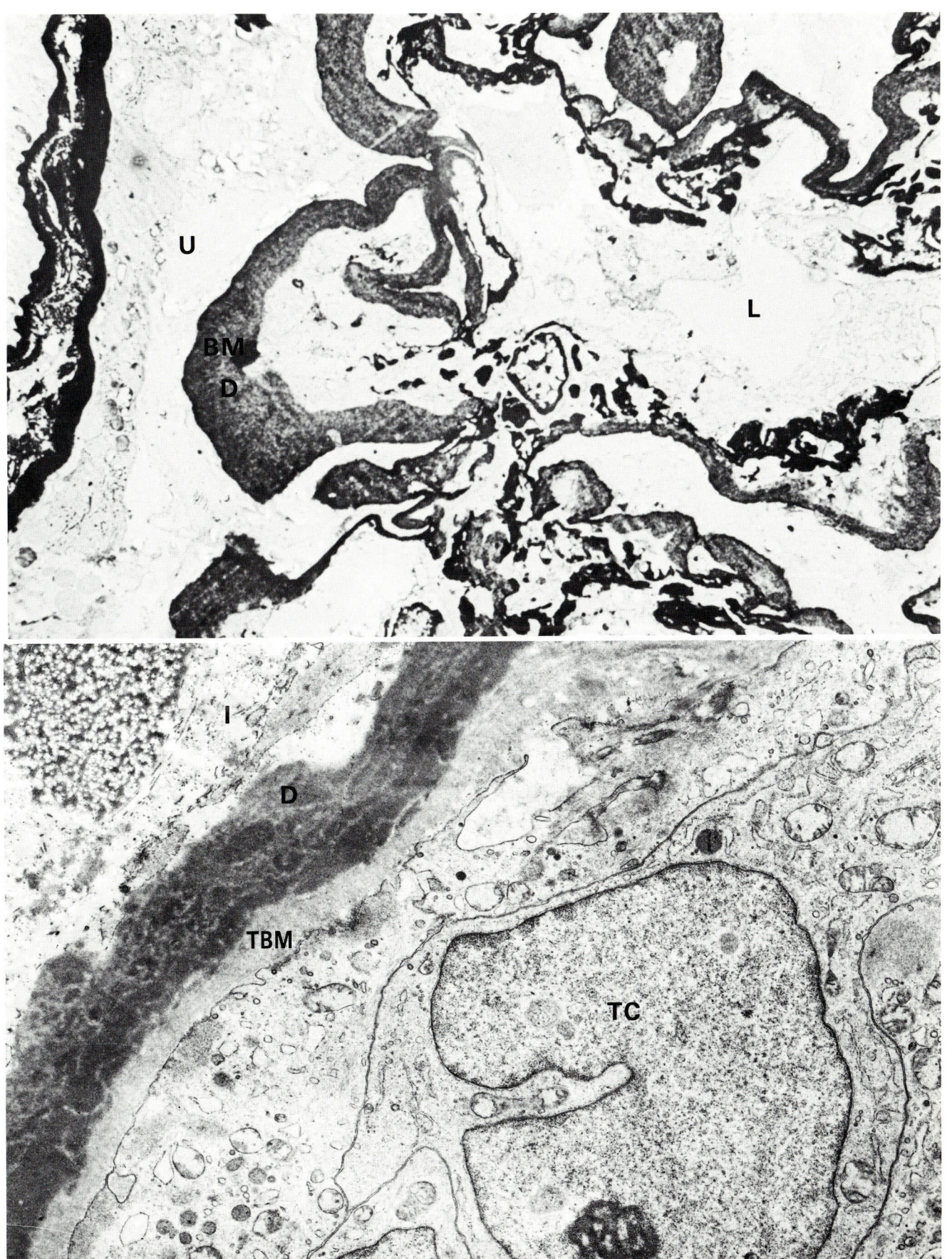

CHAPTER 6

Diffuse Crescentic Glomerulonephritis
(Figs. 6-1 to 6-12 and Figs. 6-19 to 6-21)
Diffuse Sclerosing Glomerulonephritis
(Figs. 6-13 to 6-18 and Figs 6-22)

Diffuse Crescentic Glomerulonephritis
(Extracapillary Glomerulonephritis)

Definition: This is characterized by the presence of crescents in the majority of glomeruli. The crescents may be cellular, fibrocellular or fibrous. The category is reserved for cases in which either no abnormality can be discerned in underlying (or uninvolved) glomeruli or crescentic disease is so extensive that identification of the primary glomerular lesion is impossible. Where specific morphologic changes are recognizable, the lesion should be included under the appropriate category.

Clinical Manifestations: The disease is rare in children. It is mostly seen in young and middle aged adults, but the old age is not exempt. Men are affected more often than women.

The onset may be acute, with symptoms of the acute nephritic syndrome, but more often it is insidious. (If accompanied by pulmonary hemorrhages, see Goodpasture's syndrome.) An upper respiratory illness often precedes the onset, but there is no evidence of specific infection, such as due to Streptococcus. The nephritic syndrome is characterized by tendency to severe oliguria, but rather mild hypertension. With insidious onset, general weakness and anemia may be the presenting symptoms, accompanied by nausea and vomiting and in some cases, by edema. Azotemia and hematuria are almost invariably present; proteinuria is moderate, rarely massive. Complement levels in the serum are usually within normal range.

The disease runs a relentlessly progressive course. Before the days of dialysis patients died within a few weeks or a few months. Those who improved either had a lesser degree of involvement (focal crescentic glomerulonephritis) or belonged to other categories of glomerular disease, mainly those with endocapillary proliferation. Some of the patients with focal crescentic glomerulonephritis develop a second attack within a few months and may progress to a diffuse disease. A proportion of patients with apparently idiopathic crescentic glomerulonephritis have systemic features suggesting vasculitis.

Light Microscopy: Those patients who are biopsied (or who die of pulmonary hemorrhages) during the early stages of the disease, may show only limited glomerular involvement. This consists of segmental areas of thrombosis and necrosis, with spilling of fibrin into Bowman's space and the beginning of crescent formation. The uninvolved glomeruli show practically no changes. Within a short time crescents appear in nearly all glomeruli, grow in size (occluding crescents) and surround and compress the capillary tufts. The original necrotic segments are converted into collapsed compacted areas of the tuft or are incorporated into the crescents as deposits of fibrin and debris.

The crescents at first consist almost exclusively of cells (cellular crescents). The cells are mainly derived from the proliferating lining of the Bowman's capsule (parietal epithelium) with some participation of the podocytes (visceral epithelium), macrophages or monocytes and polymorphonuclears. Basement membrane-like strands (stainable with PAS) and collagen fibers rapidly appear among the cells and increase in bulk thus creating fibrocellular crescents. Eventually the cells disappear completely or almost completely, and the crescents become purely fibrous. Apparently in the early stages some crescents can resolve. In less involved glomeruli segmental damage results in localized adhesions via fibrous transformation of small crescents or via direct organization of fibrinous exudate. The capillary tufts show few changes except rapid or gradual collapse proportional to the size of the crescents. There is little or no endocapillary proliferation and focal increases of mesangial matrix probably represent condensation of the original material rather than formation of new matrix. Often mild or moderate periglomerular inflammation or more diffuse interstitial inflammation is noted. Tubular degeneration may be present.

Electron Microscopy: Fibrin may be seen in the capillary lumina or in the Bowman's space. The composition of the crescent corresponds to what is seen by light microscopy. Two types of cells may be noted, often connected by desmosomes: light, which contain only a few organelles, and dark, rich in rough-surfaced endoplasmic reticulum. Some of the cells are probably monocytes or macrophages. Some of the strands of intercellular material have the appearance of basement membranes and some show the periodicity of collagen. The capillary walls often show "breaks", particularly in the areas of crescents, but also elsewhere. In some cases small dense deposits are present under the capillary endothelium. In other cases, continuous "translucent deposits" may occupy the lamina rara interna. Frequently no deposits can be recognized.

Immunofluorescence Microscopy: Fibrin is usually present in the Bowman's space, in the crescents and occasionally in the capillary tuft. The pattern of immunoglobulin deposition is quite variable. In some cases linear deposits of IgG with or without C3 are found along the capillary walls. (This pattern is more common in Goodpasture's syndrome – see there). Other cases show granular deposits of IgG, IgM or IgA and C3. Some of these may represent endocapillary glomerulonephritis (see there). In about 50% of cases the immune deposits are very scanty or absent.

Diffuse Sclerosing Glomerulonephritis

Definition: This lesion is characterized by widespread sclerosis of glomeruli with evidence that the basic process is of glomerular origin, although the type of glomerular disease can no longer be identified precisely. Diffuse sclerosing glomerulonephritis is not a specific entity, but an end result of a variety of glomerular diseases, from unresolved post-infectious glomerulonephritis to focal segmental glomerulosclerosis and to hereditary nephritides. If the nature of the original disease can be identified by additional studies (electron microscopy, immunofluorescence microscopy), it should be transferred to the appropriate diagnostic category and additional qualifying features specified from Table II (see Section I).

Clinical Manifestations: The main clinical manifestation is chronic renal failure ending in uremia. In a minority of patients a history of "acute glomerulonephritis" can be obtained. This progresses to chronic renal failure either directly or after an apparent improvement and a "latent period" of varying length (2–30 years). In the majority, the onset is insidious, with proteinuria, sometimes in the nephrotic range, variable hematuria, hypertension and reduced glomerular filtration rate. A renal biopsy at this stage may reveal a specific glomerular lesion; however in many cases, only mesangial proliferative glomerulonephritis is seen which cannot be further defined. The disease progresses slowly over a period of many years. In a proportion of patients, acute exacerbations occur with aggravation of hematuria and proteinuria. Such attacks usually follow a non-specific respiratory infection. Once the renal insufficiency reaches the clinical state of uremia, progression to terminal renal failure is rapid, with an average of one year (6–24 months).

Gross Features and Light Microscopy: The kidney is generally small and on the average half its normal weight. The surface is finely granular, but may also show larger scars presumably of vascular origin. On section the cortex is markedly thinned.

Under the microscope, the glomeruli often appear crowded because of the concomitant tubular atrophy, but actually their total number is reduced. Sometimes all glomeruli have been converted into small sclerotic nodules, but more often a few remain partly or nearly completely preserved. The sclerotic tufts may be surrounded by a thick layer of fibrous tissue apparently originating from the Bowman's capsule. Occasionally true epithelial or fibroepithelial crescents are seen, probably evidence of acute exacerbation. In the partly preserved glomeruli one may observe segmental areas of sclerosis with adhesions to the capsule. Sometimes narrow spaces lined by cuboidal epithelium ("pseudotubules") lie between the sclerosed tuft and Bowman's capsule. Some of the partly collapsed capillary lumina are filled with hyaline material (exudative or hyaline lesions). Nests of dilated hypertrophic tubules may be scattered in the generally atrophic cortex. There is considerable interstitial fibrosis together with variable collections of mononuclear inflammatory cells. Arteries and arterioles show moderate to severe sclerosis.

Electron Microscopy: Electron microscopy generally contributes little, mainly recapitulating the changes seen on light microscopy. However, it may be helpful in identifying specific lesions, e.g. those of membranous glomerulonephritis.

Immunofluorescence Microscopy: Deposits of immunoglobulins and of complement components are frequently present. Again they may be helpful in establishing a specific diagnosis such as Berger's disease, but findings must be interpreted with caution. In the majority of cases granular and lumpy deposits are seen in a segmental and focal distribution. Most often they contain IgM and C3, occasionally also IgG or IgA and early complement components. This pattern is more suggestive of a non-specific trapping rather than immune complex deposition.

Unclassified Glomerulonephritis

Definition: This category is reserved for cases of glomerulonephritis which cannot be fitted into any of the above groups.

PRIMARY GLOMERULAR DISEASES

CRESCENTIC GLOMERULONEPHRITIS

Fig. 6-1 Early stage of crescentic glomerulonephritis. Pink deposits of fibrin between capillary loops.
H&E stain. x 260.

Fig. 6-2 Similar case to Fig. 6-1. Fibrin deposits between the loops of the capillary tuft.
PTAH stain. x 260.

Fig. 6-3 Crescentic glomerulonephritis. Cellular crescent partly covering glomerular tuft. Pink fibrin deposits are noted toward 8 o'clock.
Trichrome stain. x 260.

Fig. 6-4 Same case as Fig. 6-2. More advanced stage. Large crescent compressing capillary tuft.
PAS stain. x 260.

Fig. 6-5 Same case as Fig. 6-4. Cellular crescent and fibrin strands.
PTAH stain. x 260.

Fig. 6-6 Immunofluorescence microscopy. Another case of crescentic glomerulonephritis showing deposits of fibrin along the capillary walls. x 260.

CRESCENTIC GLOMERULONEPHRITIS

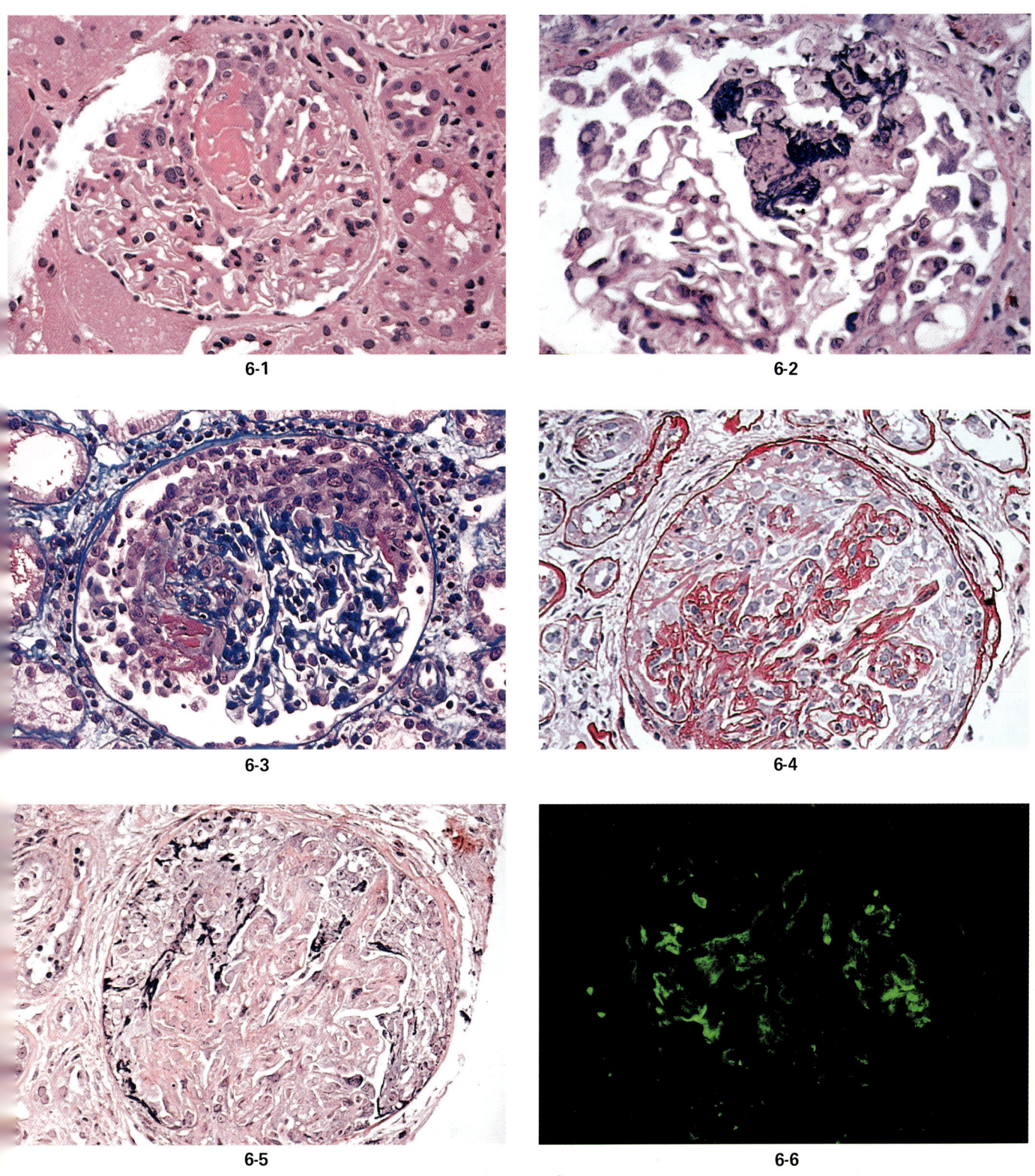

6-1

6-2

6-3

6-4

6-5

6-6

PRIMARY GLOMERULAR DISEASES

CRESCENTIC GLOMERULONEPHRITIS

Fig. 6-7   Same case as Fig. 6-6 showing scattered deposits of IgG.   x 260.

Fig. 6-8   Advanced stage of crescentic glomerulonephritis showing sclerosed glomeruli surrounded by inflammatory cells.
H&E stain.   x 100.

Fig. 6-9   Same case as Fig. 6-8. Sclerosed glomerulus showing a large fibrous crescent and collapsed remnants of capillary tuft.
PAS stain.   x 410.

Fig. 6-10   Small fibrous crescent enveloping a segment of capillary tuft.
PAS stain.   x 260.

Fig. 6-11   Secondary crescentic glomerulonephritis. Proliferative endocapillary glomerulonephritis with a small crescent along the left border of the tuft.
PAS stain.   x 260.

Fig. 6-12   Secondary crescentic glomerulonephritis. Glomerulus showing proliferation and sclerosis in the capillary tuft and a thin fibrocellular crescent along the periphery.
PAS stain.   x 260.

CRESCENTIC GLOMERULONEPHRITIS

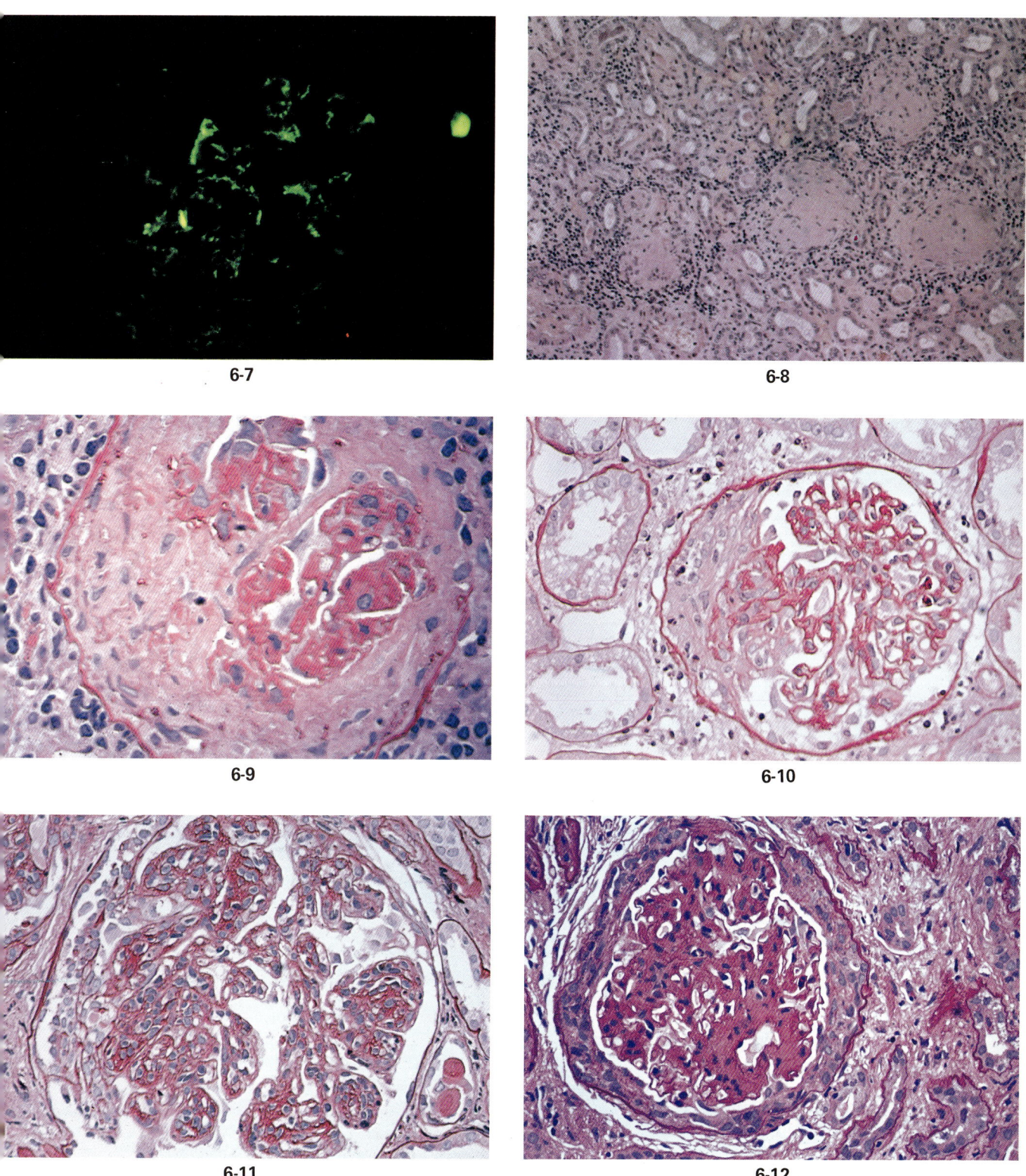

PRIMARY GLOMERULAR DISEASES

SCLEROSING GLOMERULONEPHRITIS

Fig. 6-13 Advanced sclerosing glomerulonephritis. Section of renal cortex showing two completely or almost completely sclerosed glomeruli and a third glomerulus with partial sclerosis. Note atrophy as well as dilatation of tubules.
PAS stain. × 100.

Fig. 6-14 Sclerosing glomerulonephritis. Glomerulus showing moderate cellularity and large amount of intercellular matrix. Note adhesions to the Bowman's capsule and proliferation of cells in the remaining urinary space.
H&E stain. × 260.

Fig. 6-15 Same case as Fig. 6-14. Partly sclerotic glomerular tuft overlaid by a fibrocellular crescent.
PAS stain. × 260.

Fig. 6-16 Sclerosing glomerulonephritis showing mesangial proliferation, increase in matrix and adhesion to the Bowman's capsule with formation of pseudotubles.
PAS stain. × 410.

Fig. 6-17 Immunofluorescence microscopy. Same case as Fig. 6-16 showing irregular distribution of IgG. × 260.

Fig. 6-18 Same case as Figs. 6-14 and 6-15 showing completely sclerosed glomerulus surrounded by an infiltrate of inflammatory cells, mainly lymphocytes.
H&E stain. × 260.

SCLEROSING GLOMERULONEPHRITIS

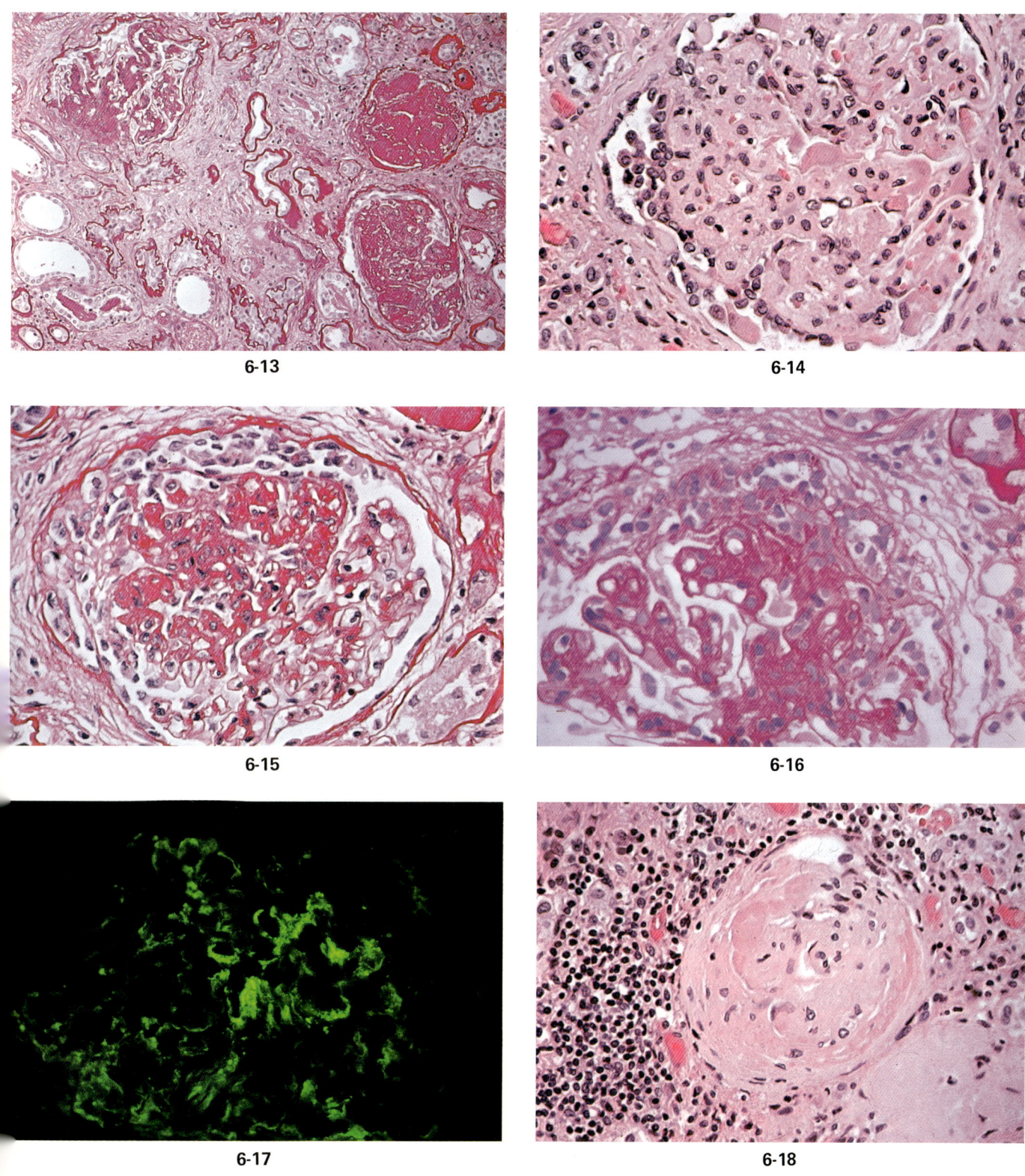

6-13

6-14

6-15

6-16

6-17

6-18

PRIMARY GLOMERULAR DISEASES

CRESCENTIC GLOMERULONEPHRITIS

Fig. 6-19   Electron micrograph showing disruption (between arrows) of the capillary basement membrane (BM) and spilling of fibrin (F) into the urinary space (U).   x 6,400.

Fig. 6-20   Electron micrograph. Crescentic glomerulonephritis. Cellular crescent overlying a partly collapsed capillary. The crescent consists of parallel arrays of flattened cells extending from the Bowman's capsule (BC) on the left to the capillary tuft on the right. Note electron dense deposits (D) in the tuft in the mesangial or subendothelial location.   x 7,000.

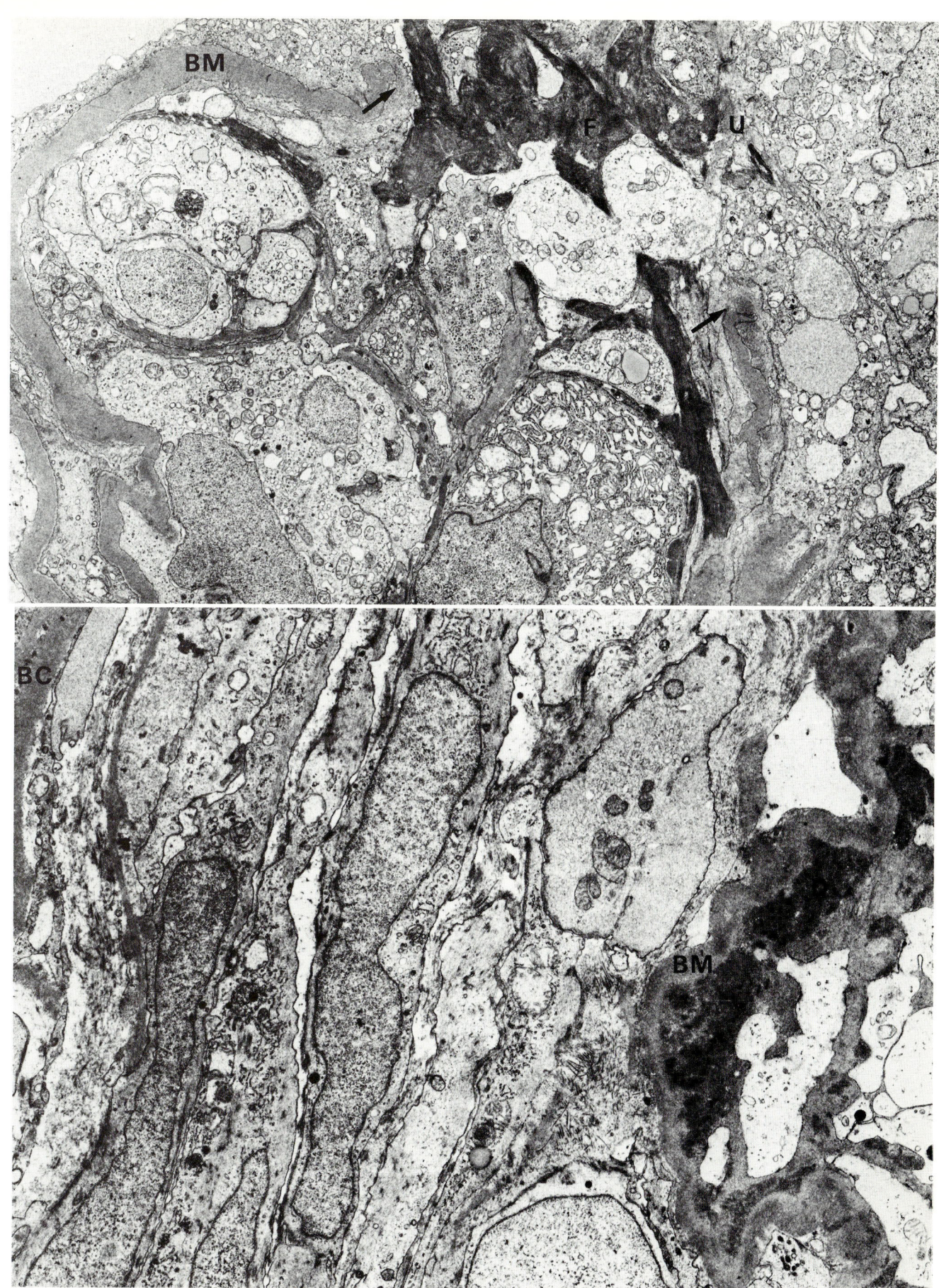

PRIMARY GLOMERULAR DISEASES

CRESCENTIC GLOMERULONEPHRITIS

Fig. 6-21 Electron micrograph. Fibrocellular crescent consisting of cells and numerous collagen (Col) fibrils. Part of a collapsed glomerular capillary (Cap) at the bottom of the picture. x 6,400.

SCLEROSING GLOMERULONEPHRITIS

Fig. 6-22 Electron micrograph. Part of a glomerular tuft extensively replaced by mesangial matrix (MM). Note a few cells between the strands of matrix, scattered dense deposits, effacement of the foot processes over the surface of the tuft and prominent parietal cells of the Bowman's capsule (BC), containing vacuoles and lipid droplets. x 6,400.

Cr cell: cell of Crescent, MC: mesangial cell.

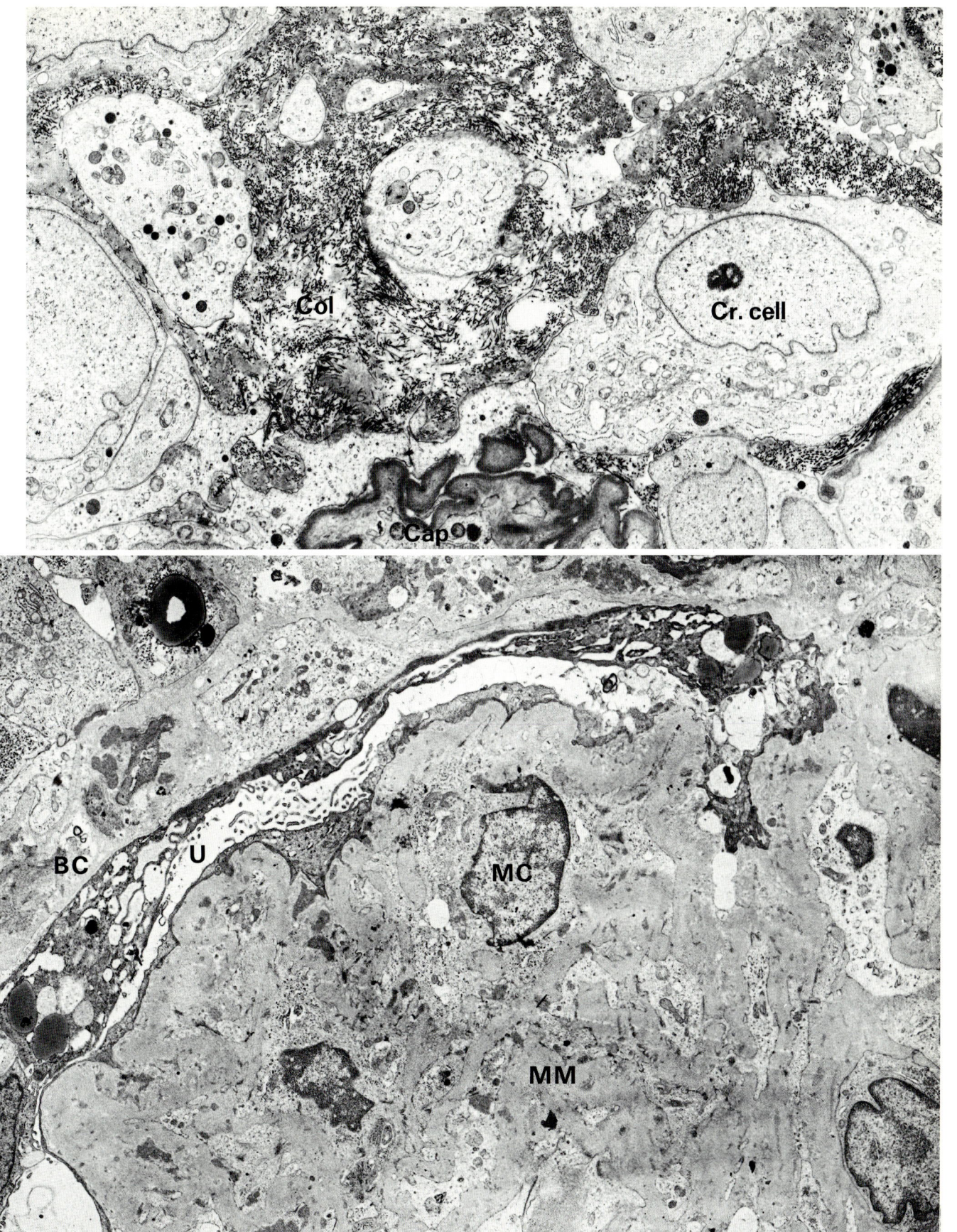

Glomerulonephritis of Systemic Diseases

CHAPTER 7

Lupus Nephritis
(Figs. 7-1 to 7-37)

Lupus Nephritis

Definition: This term is applied to renal involvement accompanying systemic lupus erythematosus (SLE). The involvement may be very mild with no or only very slight clinical manifestations, or on the contrary it may be very severe, leading to irreversible renal failure. The various forms of lupus nephritis are presented in Table VI.

Clinical Manifestations: Systemic lupus erythematosus (SLE) affects primarily the young members of the population particularly young women in their 20's, but can occur at almost any age. The female to male ratio is of the order of 5–10:1. It is more common, at least in the United States, in the black race.

The clinical manifestations are an expression of multisystem involvement and include skin rashes, particularly over the areas exposed to sunlight; arthralgias and arthritis; inflammation of serosal surfaces, such as pleura and pericardium; anemia and thrombocytopenia. Involvement of the central nervous system and of the kidneys accounts for most of the cases with an unfavorable outcome. Fever is not uncommon but severe acute lupus with high fever and constitutional toxicity nowadays seldom leads to death, because it is readily controlled by therapy. On the other hand, patients with mild manifestations, such as arthralgias, pleurisy and evanescent skin rashes may go on for years and never come to the attention of a physician. It had been suggested in fact that this is the most frequent course of SLE. However a sudden exacerbation of symptoms may occur after many years of nearly asymptomatic disease.

Renal involvement is very common in lupus and can be demonstrated in renal biopsies in almost 100% of patients by means of electron microscopy and immunofluorescence microscopy. However not all patients have clinical manifestations. The most frequent abnormality is proteinuria varying from trace amounts to those in the nephrotic range. The degree of proteinuria generally correlates with the severity and the histologic type of the glomerular lesion, the nephrotic syndrome being most common in membranous and in diffuse proliferative forms, but occurring on occasion with milder disease, that is focal and mesangial lupus nephritis. Hematuria is uncommon in milder cases, but is frequent in severe disease where red and white cells together with hyaline, granular and broad casts may be present simultaneously (so-called "telescoped" urinary sediment). A few patients will present themselves with acute nephritic syndrome. Reduced glomerular filtration rate is characteristic of severe disease and may progress rapidly to complete renal failure. Hypertension is usually a later development, but in some patients may be the dominant feature even in the absence of severe renal involvement. In general, individual patients tend to maintain a constant pattern of clinical manifestations, but are liable to exacerbation of symptoms. Spontaneous regression is uncommon.

Table VI WHO MORPHOLOGIC CLASSIFICATION OF LUPUS NEPHRITIS (MODIFIED).

I. Normal Glomeruli
   a) Nil (by all techniques)
   b) Normal by light microscopy, but deposits by electron or immunofluorescence microscopy

II. Pure Mesangial Alterations (Mesangiopathy)
   a) Mesangial widening and/or mild hypercellularity (+)
   b) Moderate hypercellularity (++)

III. Focal Segmental Glomerulonephritis (associated with mild or moderate mesangial alterations)
   a) "Active" necrotizing lesions
   b) "Active" and sclerosing lesions
   c) Sclerosing lesions

IV. Diffuse Glomerulonephritis (severe mesangial, endocapillary or mesangio-capillary proliferation and/or extensive subendothelial deposits)
   a) Without segmental lesions
   b) With "active" necrotizing lesions
   c) With "active" and sclerosing lesions
   d) With sclerosing lesions

V. Diffuse membranous Glomerulonephritis
   a) Pure membranous glomerulonephritis
   b) Associated with lesions of Category II (a or b)
   c) Associated with lesions of Category III (a–c) *
   d) Associated with lesions of Category IV (a–d) *

VI. Advanced Sclerosing Glomerulonephritis

* Alternately cases in these two subcategories may be classified under category *IV*. *Diffuse Glomerulonephritis.*

Table VI-A ACTIVE LESIONS

1. Disruption of capillary walls
2. Polymorphs and karyorrhexis
3. Hematoxyphil bodies
4. Crescents, cellular or fibrocellular
5. "Wire-loops" (*by light microscopy*)
6. Hyaline thrombi
7. Fibrin thrombi
8. Segmental fibrin deposition

Table VI-B SCLEROSING LESIONS.

1. Segmental
2. Mesangial
3. Global

Serological abnormalities that accompany SLE are numerous and may be seen in all forms of renal involvement. With a few exceptions they do not correlate well with the specific type of glomerular disease. Rather, they are a measure of the activity of the lupus process throughout the body. These abnormalities include false positive tests for syphilis, depression of complement levels, particularly of C3 and C4, and the presence of antinuclear antibodies, antibodies to DNA, RNA, nucleoproteins, of rheumatoid factor and of other autoantibodies (against erythrocytes, lymphocytes and platelets). Some patients present with a clinical picture reminiscent of hemolytic uremic syndrome or thrombotic thrombocytopenic purpura, concomitant with other manifestations, or as an isolated early phenomenon. Among serological changes that are believed to correlate fairly well with the severity of renal disease is the presence of antibodies to double-stranded DNA, of immune complexes and of marked depression of C3. The immune complexes, especially DNA-anti-DNA probably play a crucial role in the pathogenesis of lupus.

Light Microscopy: The patterns of glomerular involvement are enumerated in Table IV and in greater detail, in Table VI. Practically any form of glomerulonephritis from the mildest to the most severe can be seen in SLE but the separation between categories is not always sharp and various transitional and combination forms are not unusual.

Minor glomerular abnormalities are relatively uncommon, perhaps because such patients have few clinical manifestations and are seldom biopsied. When examined by electron and immunofluorescence microscopy definite abnormalities are seen in almost all instances (see later).

Mesangial lupus nephritis is characterized by widening of the mesangial stalk due to an increase in the number of cells and the amount of mesangial matrix. At its mildest it merges imperceptibly with the Minor category; at the other end, it forms a transition to severe diffuse disease. Mesangial lupus nephritis is not very common among the hospitalized patients, but much more common among ambulatory patients with mild clinical disease. The histological changes apparently remain stable in the majority of patients. They may regress, perhaps spontaneously, but more often under the influence of steroid and immunosuppressive therapy. On the other hand in a fair proportion of cases, perhaps 20%, they progress to diffuse lupus nephritis. This statement, though, applies only to renal biopsies performed before institution of therapy. There is evidence to suggest that in treated patients, mild or moderate diffuse disease can be reduced in intensity to that of mesangial proliferation, only to rebound despite continuing treatment.

Focal lupus nephritis is characterized by focal and segmental lesions of proliferation, inflammation, necrosis and sclerosis. Inflammation is accompanied by exudation of polymorphonuclear leukocytes which tend to undergo fragmentation. Necrosis, when present, is of fibrinoid type and may be due to thrombosis. Sclerosis results in formation of acellular scars which are often adherent to Bowman's capsule. It is uncertain whether focal lupus nephritis as defined, is produced by the same immunological mechanism as Mesangial and Diffuse forms, because in some instances immune deposits are absent from the focal lesion though present elsewhere in the glomerulus (see later).

Isolated lesions of focal lupus nephritis have apparently little effect on the renal function and are compatible with long survival. When numerous they may reduce the reserve capacity of the kidney and indicate poorer prognosis. However, most of the time focal lesions are superimposed upon another form, usually mesangial lupus nephritis, and represent a stage in progression to diffuse lupus nephritis.

Diffuse lupus nephritis involves all or nearly all glomeruli and occurs in several histological forms.

a) Endocapillary proliferative process, similar to that seen in post-infectious glomerulonephritis, including prominent exudation of polymorphonuclears, but few if any changes specific for lupus, at least on light microscopy. This process develops acutely and is clinically difficult to distinguish from post-infectious glomerulonephritis, except with the help of laboratory studies and electron microscopic and immunofluorescence examination of glomeruli. It apparently resolves to a considerable degree with steroid therapy.

b) Proliferative, necrotizing and sclerosing glomerulonephritis. This is the most common variety of diffuse lupus glomerulonephritis. It is characterized by mononuclear, mainly mesangial cell proliferation combined with variable degrees of necrosis and sclerosis. Typically the process is non-homogeneous varying from glomerulus to glomerulus and from lobule to lobule within the glomerulus Polymorphonuclear leukocytes are present mainly within the scattered areas of necrosis. The less involved glomerular areas often show striking eosinophilic thickening of the capillary walls caused by subendothelial immune deposits ("wire loops"). The "wire loops" are not infrequently accompanied by intraluminal thrombi consisting of similar material. A very characteristic but an infrequent finding are "hematoxylin bodies" which represent fragmented and altered nuclear material and are the tissue equivalent of LE cell. Hematoxylin bodies vary in size from that of a single nucleus to fairly large clusters; in standard hematoxylin and eosin preparations they take on a coloring somewhere between that of nuclei and cytoplasm, but usually closer to the former. Hematoxylin bodies may lie extracellularly or within the cytoplasm of macrophages and other cells. Rarely, true LE cells may be found in the capillary lumina.

c) Mesangiocapillary lupus glomerulonephritis is an infrequent variety of proliferative and sclerosing glomerulonephritis. It occurs particularly in treated individuals. It is quite similar to the idiopathic disease and may need confirmatory laboratory and histologic evidence for its identification.

d) Crescentic glomerulonephritis is the most severe variety due to superimposition of crescents upon other forms of diffuse lupus glomerulonephritis described above. As mentioned earlier, this may lead to rapid renal failure.

Progression of diffuse lupus nephritis leads to gradual decrease of cellularity and increase of sclerosis with capillary obliteration, capsular adhesions, pseudotubule formation and other changes similar to those of idiopathic sclerosing glomerulonephritis. Treatment with steroids when undertaken early in the disease often results in resolution of cellular proliferation, disappearance of deposits, healing of necrotic areas and perhaps even decrease in the amount of mesangial matrix. However, the more advanced areas of sclerosis remain unaffected and in fact continue to progress, testifying to the ineffectiveness of therapy in the late stages.

Membranous lupus nephritis in its "pure" form is very similar in appearance to that of idiopathic membranous glomerulonephritis. There is the same thickening of capillary walls with subepithelial deposits interspersed by projections of basement membrane ("spikes"), although distribution of these changes may be less uniform. Segmental or diffuse membranous change is often combined with other forms of lupus nephritis — mesangial, focal or diffuse — and may be masked by them, particularly by the diffuse proliferation. The incidence of membranous lupus nephritis is estimated to lie between 5 and 25%, the higher figure probably representing the mixed, and the lower — the "pure" form. Even in the latter, some mesangial deposits are almost invariably present.

It is said that membranous lupus nephritis runs a slowly progressive course similar in its manifestations and outlook to that of the idiopathic membranous glomerulonephritis, and that it responds poorly to therapy. However in some cases there is a more rapid progression to renal failure perhaps assisted by the development of proliferative and sclerotic lesions. On the other hand, it has been reported that proliferative glomerulonephritis can be transformed by therapy into the membranous form. It is not clear whether this represents true transformation or unmasking of membranous lesion after reduction of the proliferative changes.

Interstitial and Vascular Disease: SLE is a "connective tissue" disease. Involvement of the interstitial tissue and of blood vessels is often seen in the kidney, particularly with the more severe varieties of glomerular involvement. Deposits similar to those in the glomeruli can be found around the tubular basement membranes and in the walls of small arteries, and in the connective tissue and small vessels throughout the body. Interstitial inflammation may be severe, but vascular lesions tend to be "bland" even when the deposits are extensive enough to markedly narrow the lumen. True arteritis is seen occasionally.

Electron Microscopy: In addition to the various degrees of cellular proliferation and mesangial sclerosis, electron microscopy clearly demonstrates two important changes: thickening of capillary basement membranes and formation of electron dense deposits. Basement membrane thickening is segmental and focal; it is seldom striking, perhaps doubling and occasionally quadrupling the normal width of the lamina densa. Deposits are found in all locations — under the endothelium, under the epithelium, in the basement membrane and in the mesangium most often in various combinations. Though they may be demonstrated by light microscopy, small deposits are best recognized by electron microscopy.

The deposits are homogeneous or finely granular, but in perhaps 10% they show an organized whorled "fingerprint" pattern, either pure or mixed with the granular material. "Fingerprints" are quite characteristic of SLE, but not entirely specific. Occasionally the deposits contain arrays of straight tubular structures. Another common but not diagnostic feature are "myxovirus-like particles", fine interlacing tubular structures in the cytoplasm of endothelial cells. Hematoxylin bodies in the form of very dark (black) homogeneous structures about the size and shape of a nucleus can be found on rare occasions.

Immunofluorescence Microscopy: Deposits are found in nearly every case in the mesangium and less consistently in the capillary wall. They may be granular, "lumpy", short linear or massive sausage-like. Their amount, shape and distribution varies with the histological type, activity of disease and intensity of treatment. In minor lupus nephritis scanty granular deposits may be present in the mesangium. They are more prominent in mesangial lupus nephritis and may on occasion extend under the endothelium of the capillary wall. In focal lupus nephritis the segmental lesions may or may not contain deposits, but the mesangium almost invariably does. The characteristic lesion of diffuse lupus nephritis, the "wire loop", forms a thick irregular layer under the endothelium and may encircle the entire capillary in a continuous or discontinuous manner. The subepithelial deposits of membranous lupus nephritis are small and granular. On rare occasion true linear deposits are seen along the basement membrane in patients with mild clinical and histological changes.

The composition of the deposits varies but generally they contain several immunoglobulins, most frequently IgG but also IgM and sometimes also IgA, and several components of the complement system (C3, C1q, C4, properdin). The simultaneous presence of several immunoglobulins and complement components, including C1q, is particularly characteristic of lupus nephritis. Fibrinogen or fibrin is found in the necrotic areas and in the crescents. The presence of the antigen, DNA, can often be demonstrated, and recently antigen related to a type C virus has been identified.

Similar granular deposits also occur along the tubular basement membranes and in the walls of blood vessels. Examination of the skin frequently reveals deposits at the dermoepidermal junction and in the walls of small blood vessels, even in the areas without visible eruption.

GLOMERULONEPHRITIS OF SYSTEMIC DISEASES

LUPUS NEPHRITIS

Fig. 7-1 Minimal lupus nephritis. The glomerulus shows only minimal and segmental mesangial widening. The tubules are without significant changes.
PAS Stain. × 260.

Fig. 7-2 Mesangial lupus nephritis. There is more obvious mesangial widening and mild increase in the number of cells.
PAS stain. × 410.

Fig. 7-3 Immunofluorescence microscopy. Mesangial lupus nephritis. IgG deposits in the mesangium and in the nearby arteriole. × 260.

Fig. 7-4 Focal segmental lupus nephritis. About one-third of the glomerulus is occupied by a necrotic lesion containing fragmented polymorphonuclear leukocytes. The remainder of the glomerular tuft shows only minimal changes.
PAS stain. × 410.

Fig. 7-5 Immunofluorescence microscopy. Focal segmental lupus nephritis showing deposits of fibrinogen in the segmental necrotic area. × 310.

Fig. 7-6 Diffuse "acute" lupus nephritis. Two glomeruli showing diffuse cellular proliferation and exudation of polymorphonuclear leukocytes.
H&E stain. × 260.

LUPUS NEPHRITIS

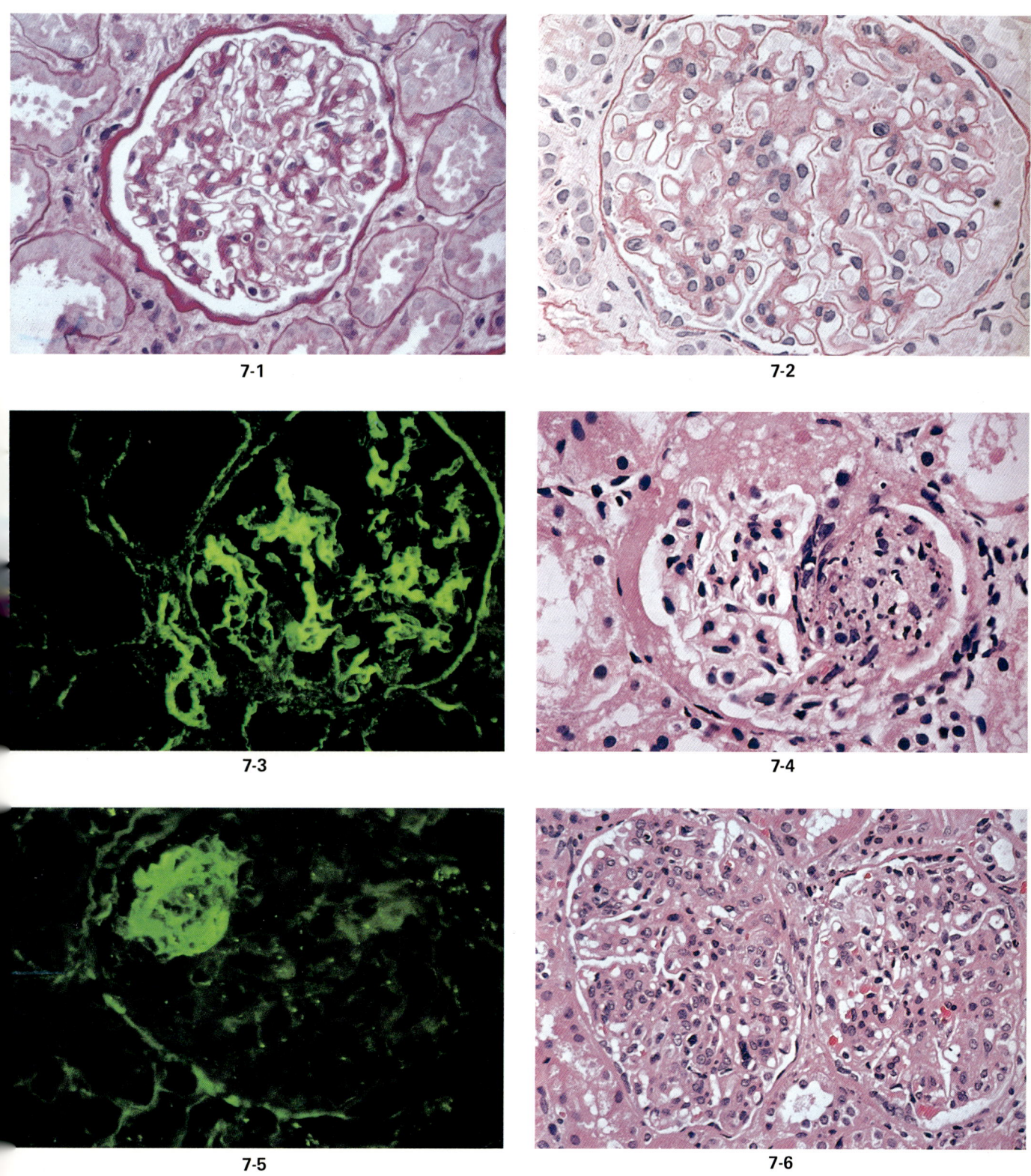

LUPUS NEPHRITIS

Fig. 7-7 Diffuse lupus nephritis, lobular form. The appearance is quite similar to the lobular form of idiopathic mesangiocapillary glomerulonephritis.
H&E stain. × 260.

Fig. 7-8 Diffuse lupus nephritis showing cellular proliferation and sclerosis with adhesions to Bowman's capsule and formation of pseudotubules.
H&E stain. × 260.

Fig. 7-9 Immunofluorescence microscopy. Diffuse lupus nephritis. Mesangial and peripheral deposits of IgM. IgG, IgA and C3 were also present.
× 260.

Fig. 7-10 Diffuse lupus nephritis showing a fibroepithelial crescent.
PAS stain. × 260.

Fig. 7-11 Diffuse lupus nephritis showing cellular proliferation and prominent wire loops (left side of the tuft).
H&E stain. × 260.

Fig. 7-12 Immunofluorescence microscopy. Diffuse lupus nephritis. Massive deposits of IgG along the capillary walls ("wire loops"). × 260.

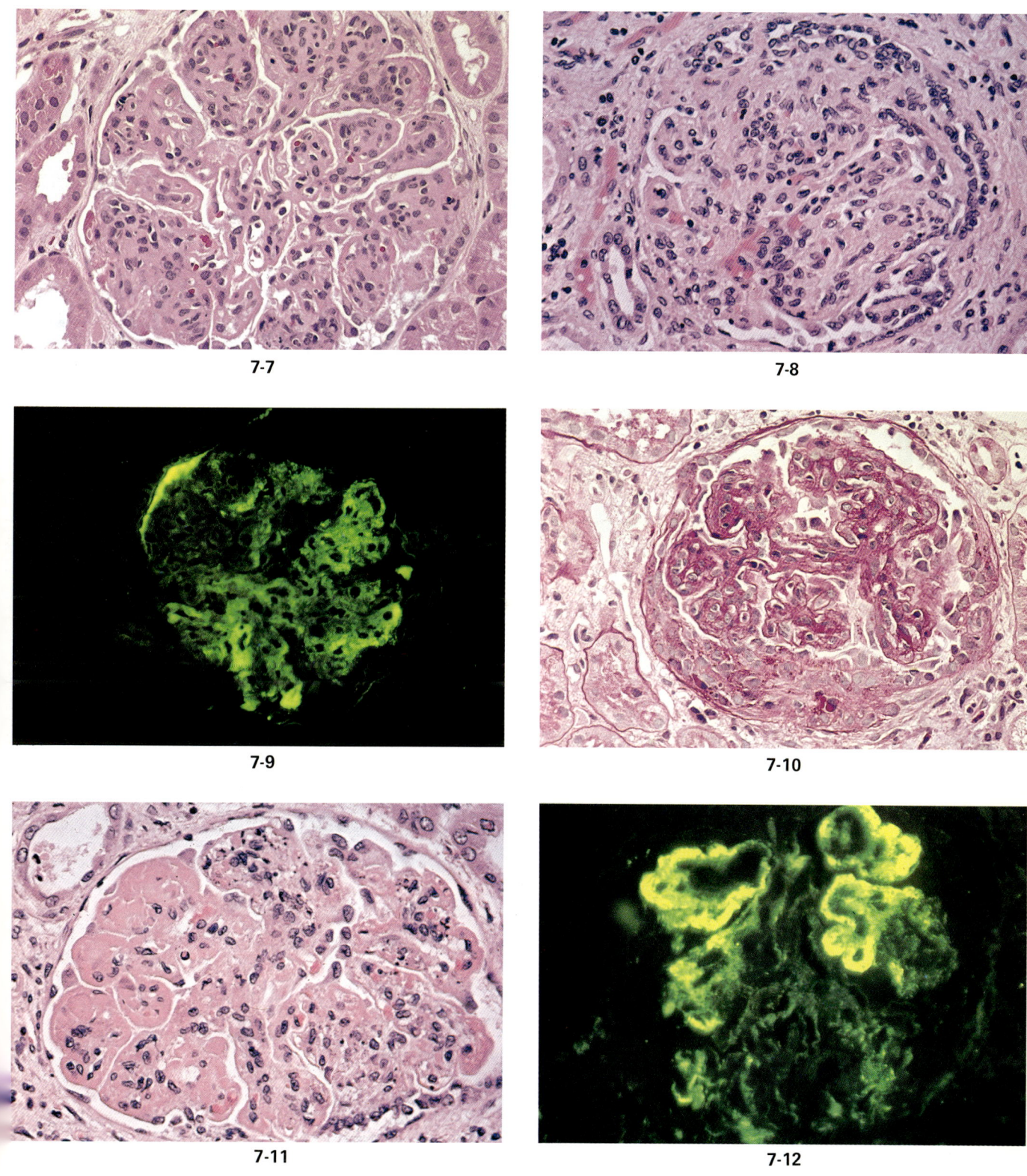

GLOMERULONEPHRITIS OF SYSTEMIC DISEASES

LUPUS NEPHRITIS

Fig. 7-13 Glomerular wire loops under high magnification. Note thick pink deposits on the inside of a thin capillary basement membrane.
PAS stain. × 1,000.

Fig. 7-14 Diffuse lupus nephritis showing cell proliferation and many hyaline thrombi.
H&E stain. × 260.

Fig. 7-15 Membranous lupus nephritis. Capillary walls appear thickened.
PAS stain. × 260.

Fig. 7-16 Membranous lupus nephritis under high magnification. The capillary basement membranes are thickened by a fuzzy subepithelial layer.
PAS stain. × 1,000.

Fig. 7-17 Immunofluorescence microscopy. Membranous lupus nephritis. Finely granular deposits of IgG along the capillary walls. × 260.

Fig. 7-18 Membranous and diffuse lupus nephritis. There is comparatively little cellular proliferation but capillary walls are massively thickened (see Fig. 7-34).
PAS stain. × 260.

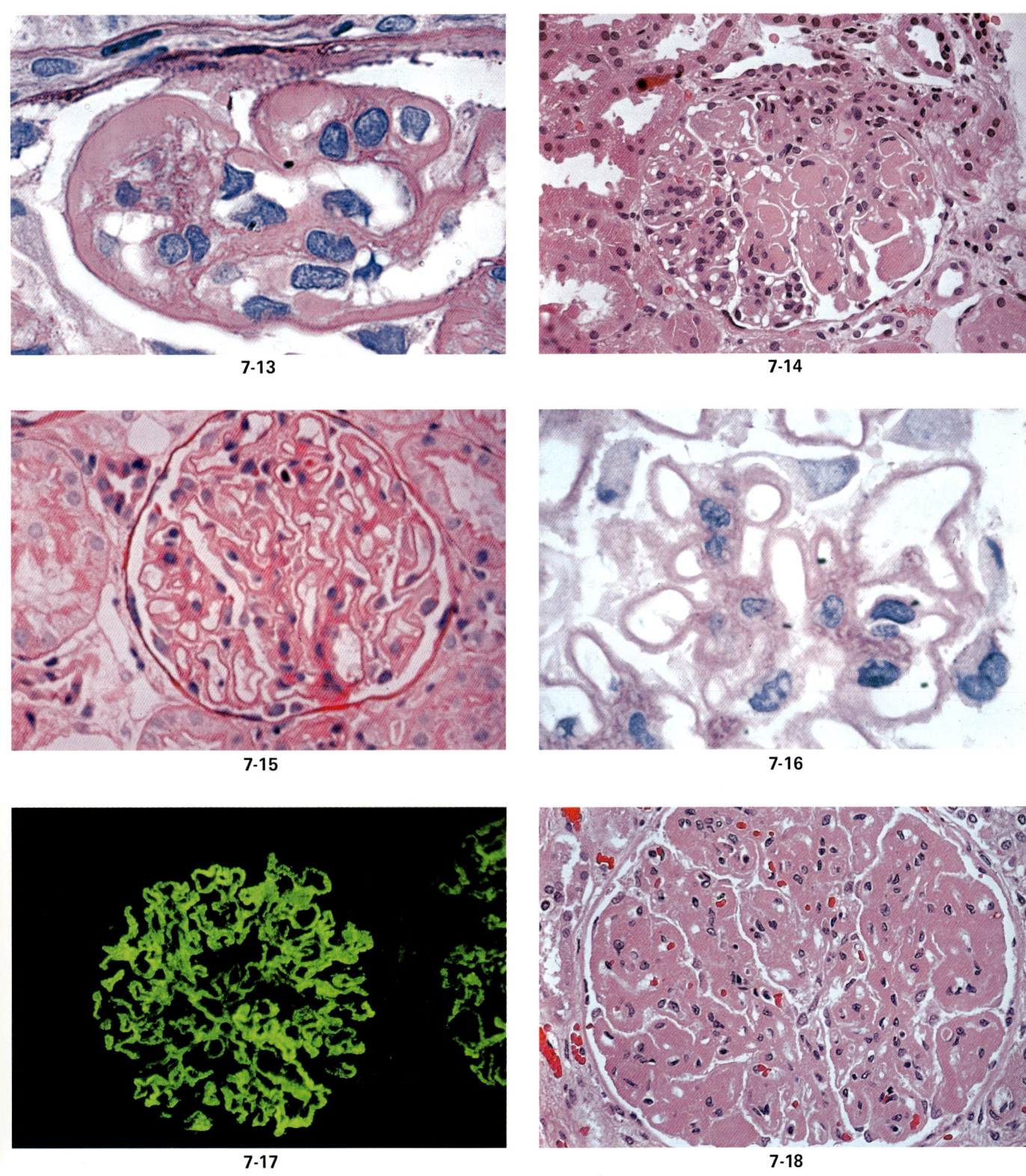

GLOMERULONEPHRITIS OF SYSTEMIC DISEASES

LUPUS NEPHRITIS

Fig. 7-19 Same case as Fig. 7-18 showing mesangial widening with deposition of mesangial matrix and numerous "spikes" along the capillary walls.
PASM stain.   x 410.

Fig. 7-20 Immunofluorescence microscopy. Same case as Fig. 7-18. Prominent deposits of IgG in the capillary walls (left side of the picture) and granular deposits along the tubular basement membrane (right side).   x 260.

Fig. 7-21 Diffuse lupus nephritis showing moderate proliferation and many deposits.
PAS stain.   x 260.

Fig. 7-22 Same case as Fig. 7-21 after six months of steroid therapy. Deposits have mostly disappeared and most capillaries have reopened but mesangial changes are still evident.
PAS stain.   x 260.

Fig. 7-23 Hematoxylin bodies in the wall of a small renal artery.
H&E stain.   x 1,000.

Fig. 7-24 Large hematoxylin body in a glomerulus. Note small dark nucleus in the center of the phagocytic cell, surrounded by many altered purplish-pink ingested nuclei.
H&E stain.   x 1,000.

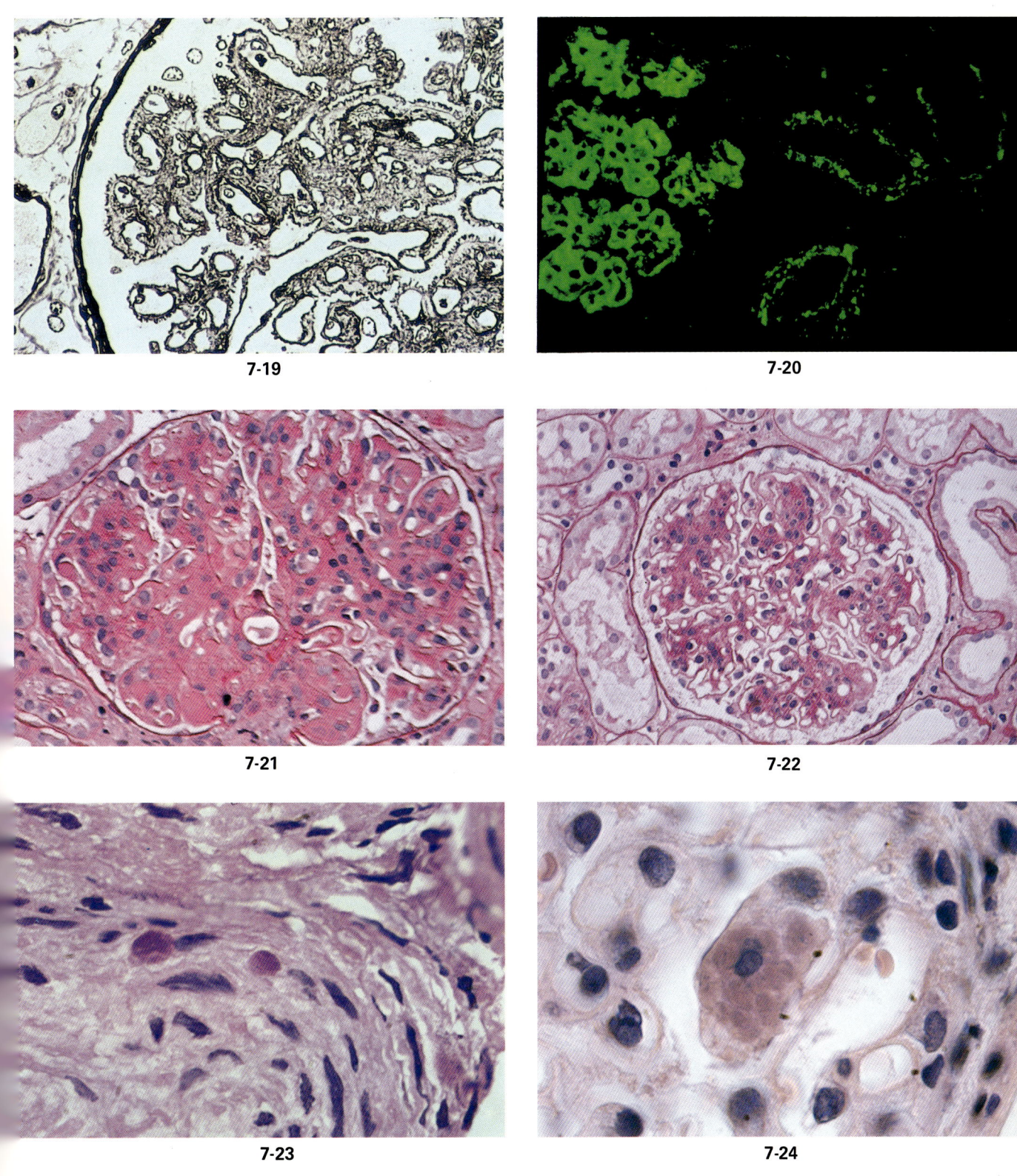

GLOMERULONEPHRITIS OF SYSTEMIC DISEASES

LUPUS NEPHRITIS

Fig. 7-25   Granular deposits of "wire loops" material around intertubular capillaries. PAS stain.   ×1,000.

Fig. 7-26   Massive deposits of wire loop material in a wall of small renal artery. PAS stain.   ×410.

Fig. 7-27   Lupus nephritis. True fibrinoid arteritis. H&E stain.   ×150.

Fig. 7-28   Lupus nephritis showing interstitial inflammation and focal necrosis. H&E stain.   ×260.

Fig. 7-29   Immunofluorescence microscopy. Prominent staining of tubular nuclei for IgG.   ×130.

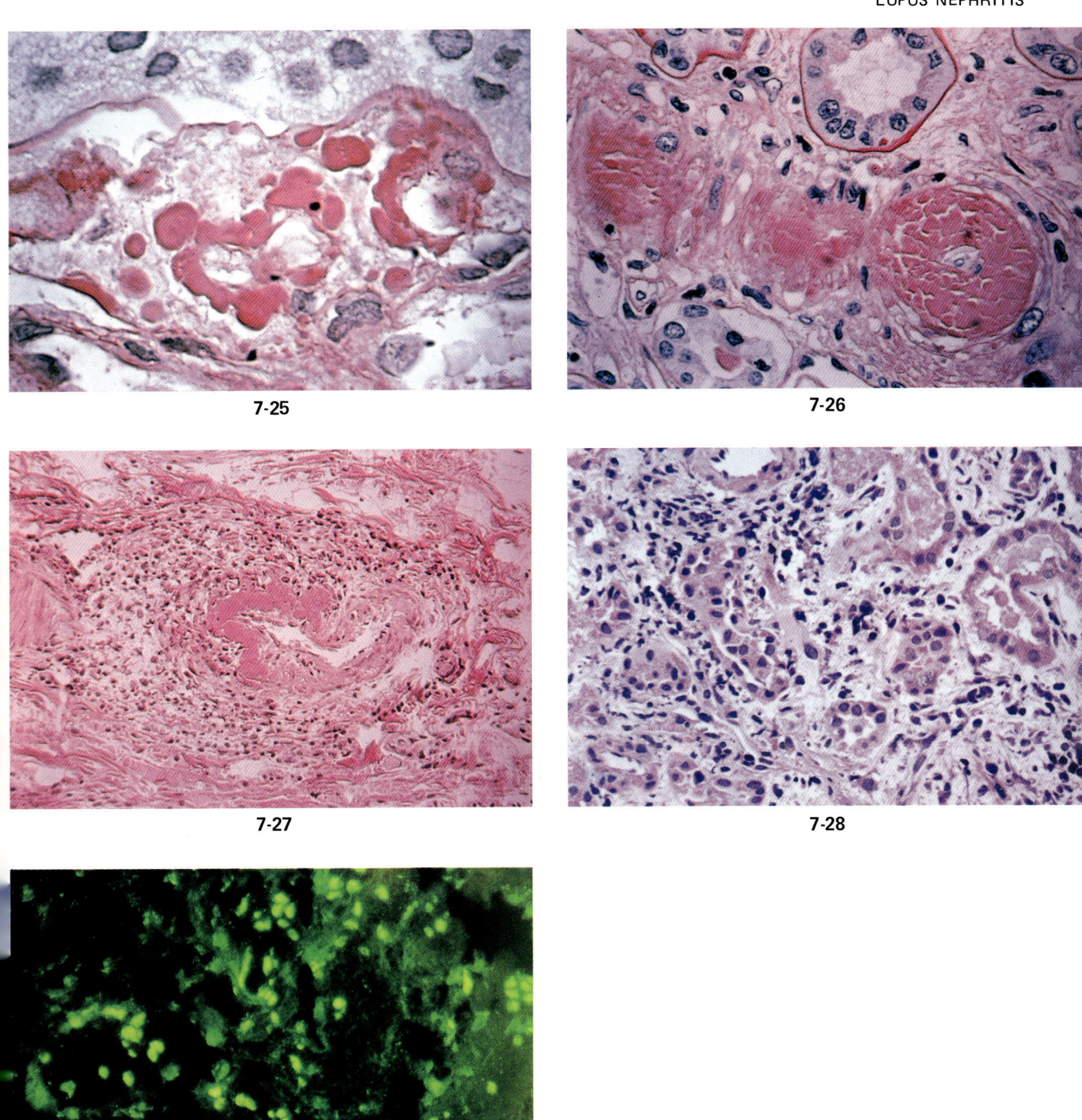

GLOMERULONEPHRITIS OF SYSTEMIC DISEASES

LUPUS NEPHRITIS

Fig. 7-30   Electron micrograph. Mesangial lupus nephritis. Small electron dense deposits (D) in the mesangial area.   × 16,000.

Fig. 7-31   Electron micrograph. Diffuse lupus nephritis. Massive subendothelial electron dense deposits (D) forming a wire loop.   × 14,000.

MM: mesangial matrix, P: podocyte, En: endothelial cell, BM: basement membrane, U: urinary space.

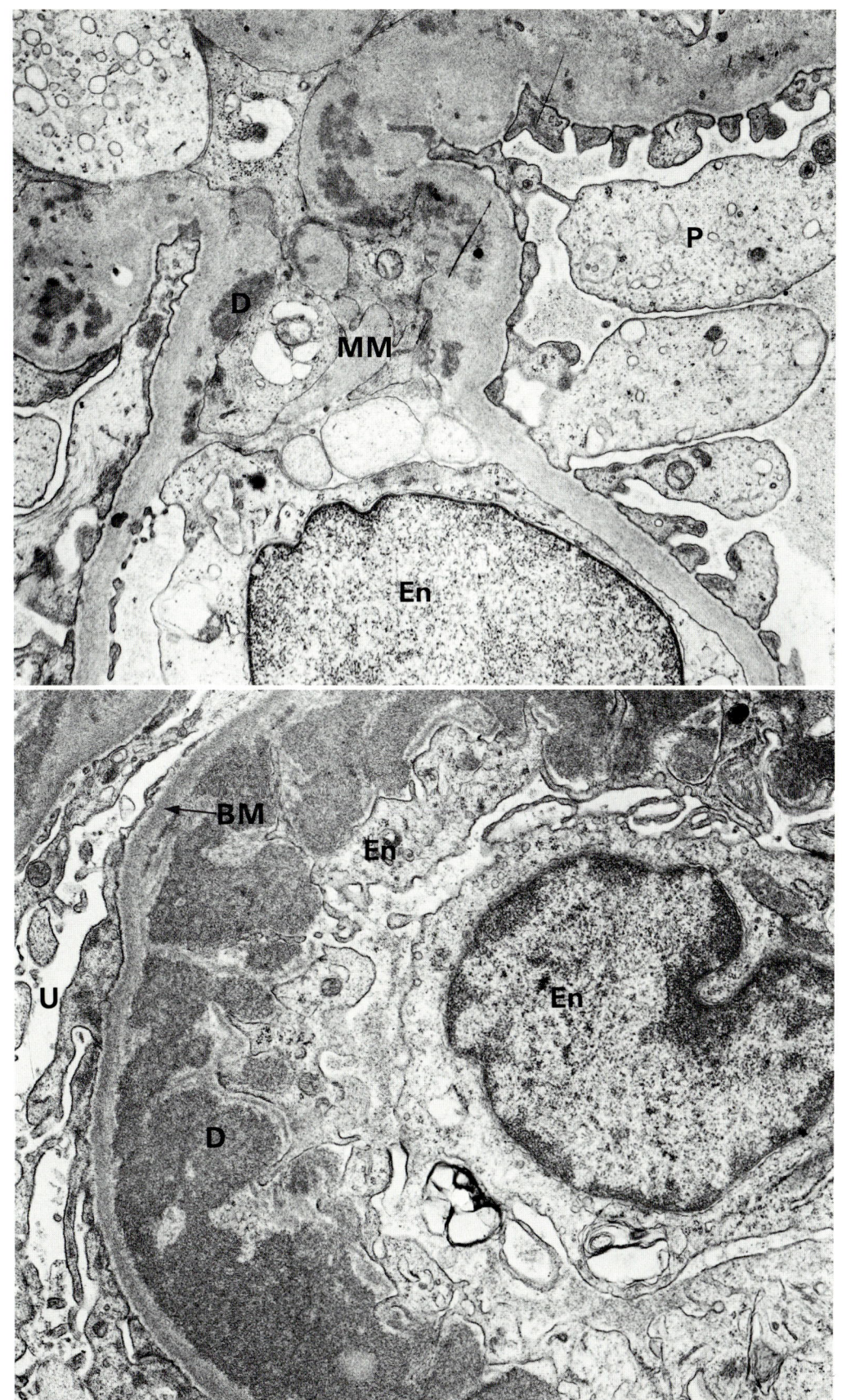

GLOMERULONEPHRITIS OF SYSTEMIC DISEASES

LUPUS NEPHRITIS

Fig. 7-32 Electron micrograph. Membranous lupus nephritis. Small electron dense deposits (D) under the epithelium and in the mesangial matrix (MM).
x 15,000.

Fig. 7-33 Electron micrograph. Membranous lupus nephritis. Subepithelial and intramembranous electron dense deposits (D) and fairly numerous "spikes" (S). x 7,300.

P: podocyte, MC: mesangial cell, BM: basement membrane, L: capillary lumen, U: urinary space.

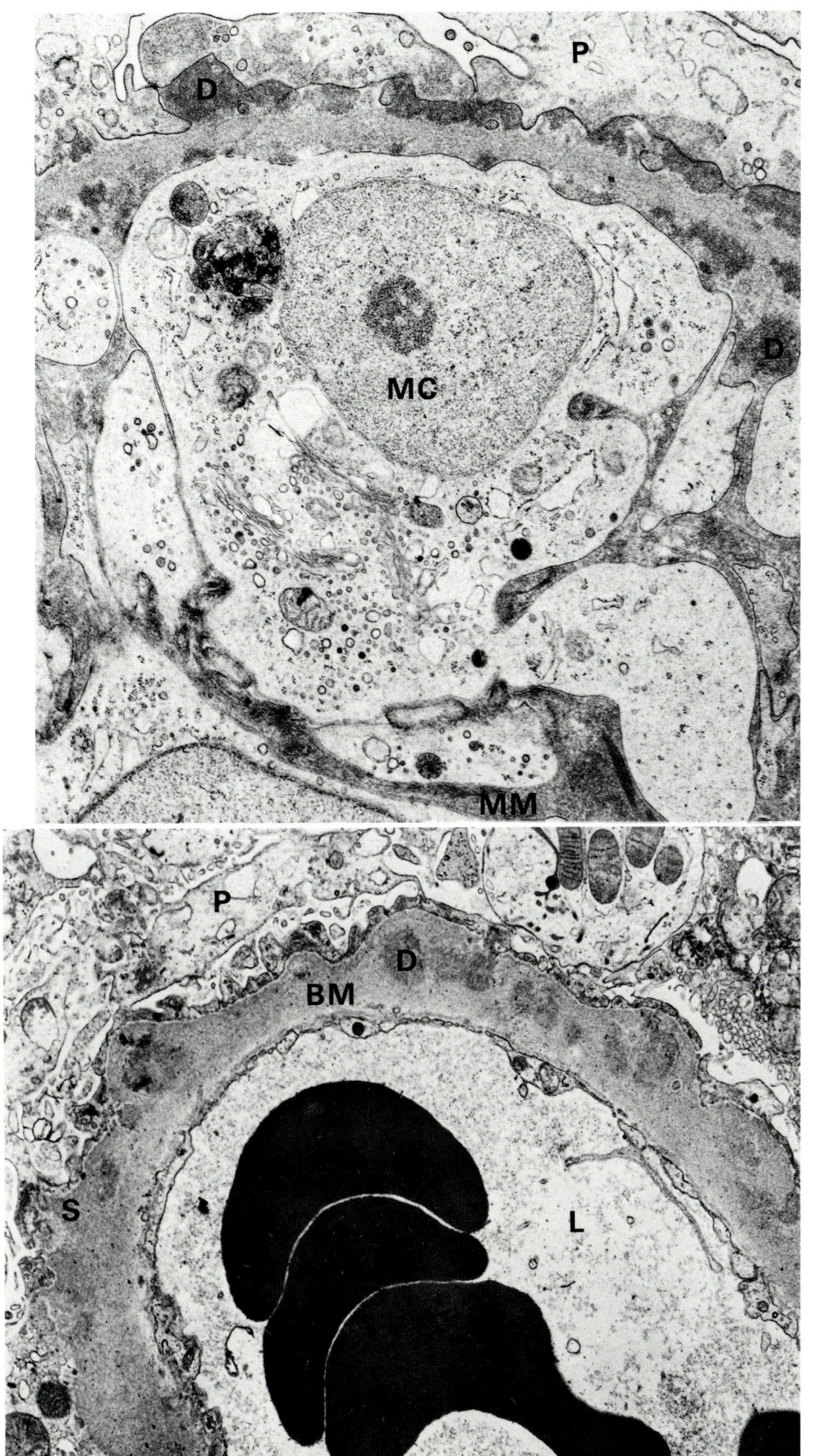

GLOMERULONEPHRITIS OF SYSTEMIC DISEASES

LUPUS NEPHRITIS

Fig. 7-34   Electron micrograph. Membranous and diffuse lupus nephritis. Large subepithelial and subendothelial deposits (D)   x 16,000.

Fig. 7-35   Electron micrograph. Electron dense deposits under the endothelium (EN) of an intertubular capillary and along tubular basement membranes (TBM).
x 6,800.

BM: basement membrane, RBC: red blood cell, U: urinary space.

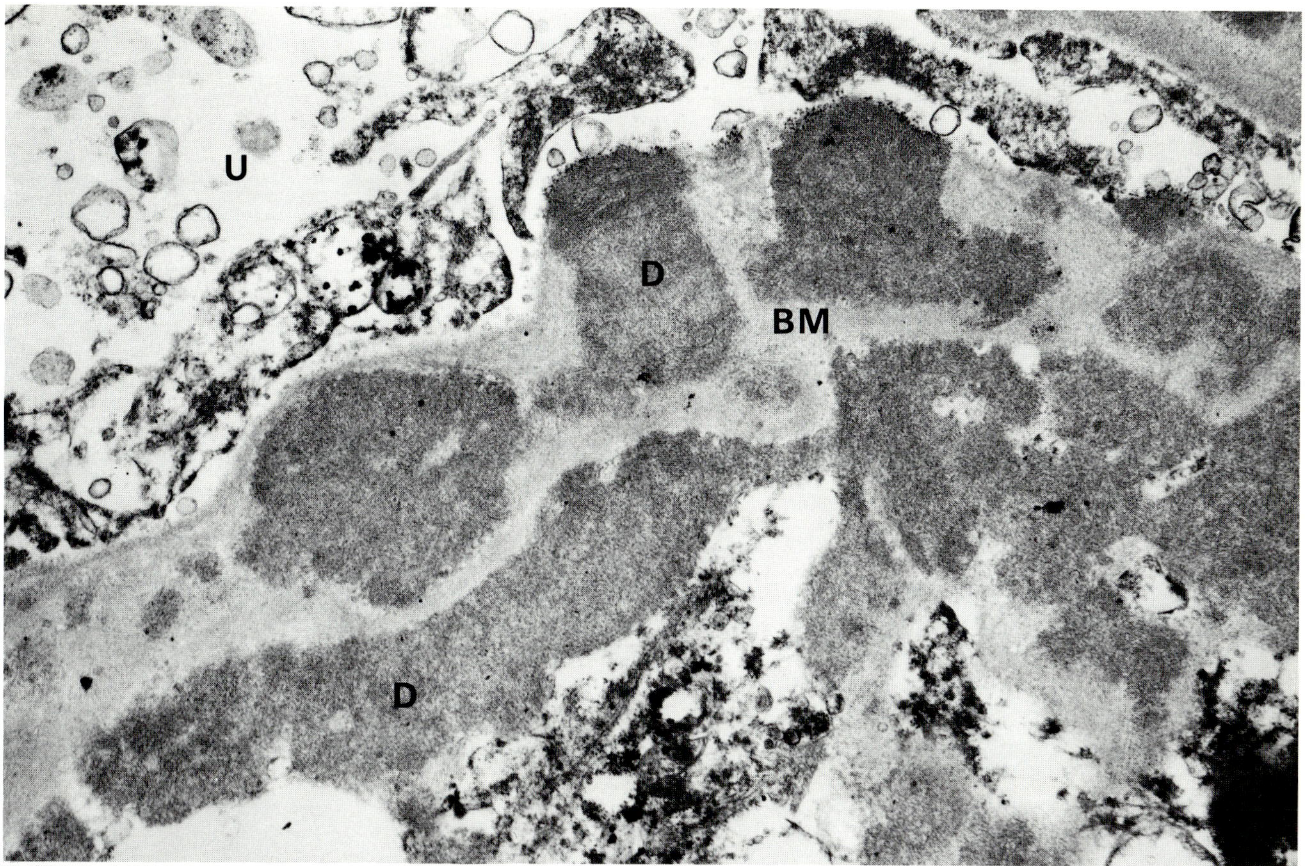

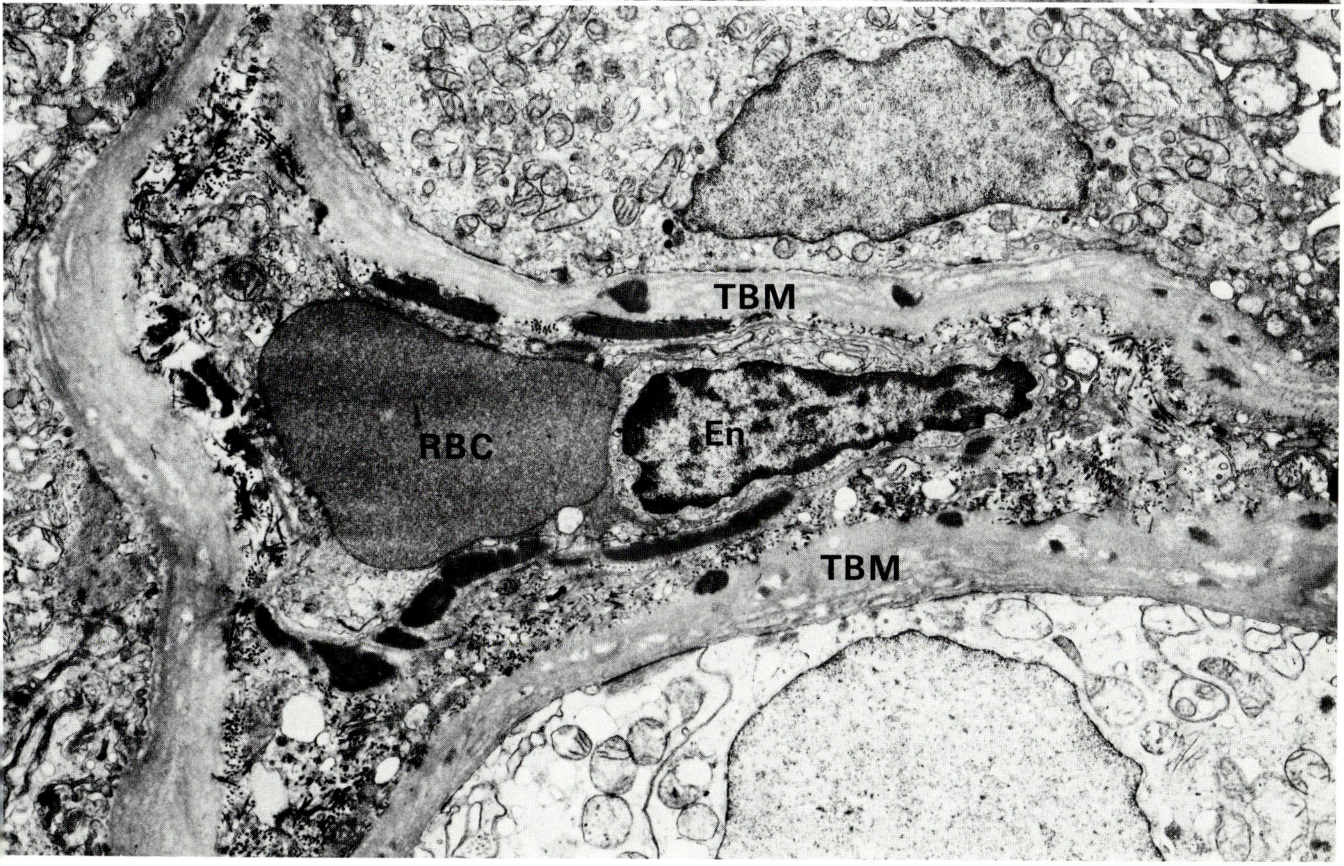

LUPUS NEPHRITIS

Fig. 7-36   Electron micrograph. Electron dense deposits (D) along the tubular basement membrane (TBM)   × 23,000.

Fig. 7-37   Electron micrograph. Lupus nephritis. Organized ("fingerprint") deposits in the glomerulus.   × 62,000.

I: interstitium.

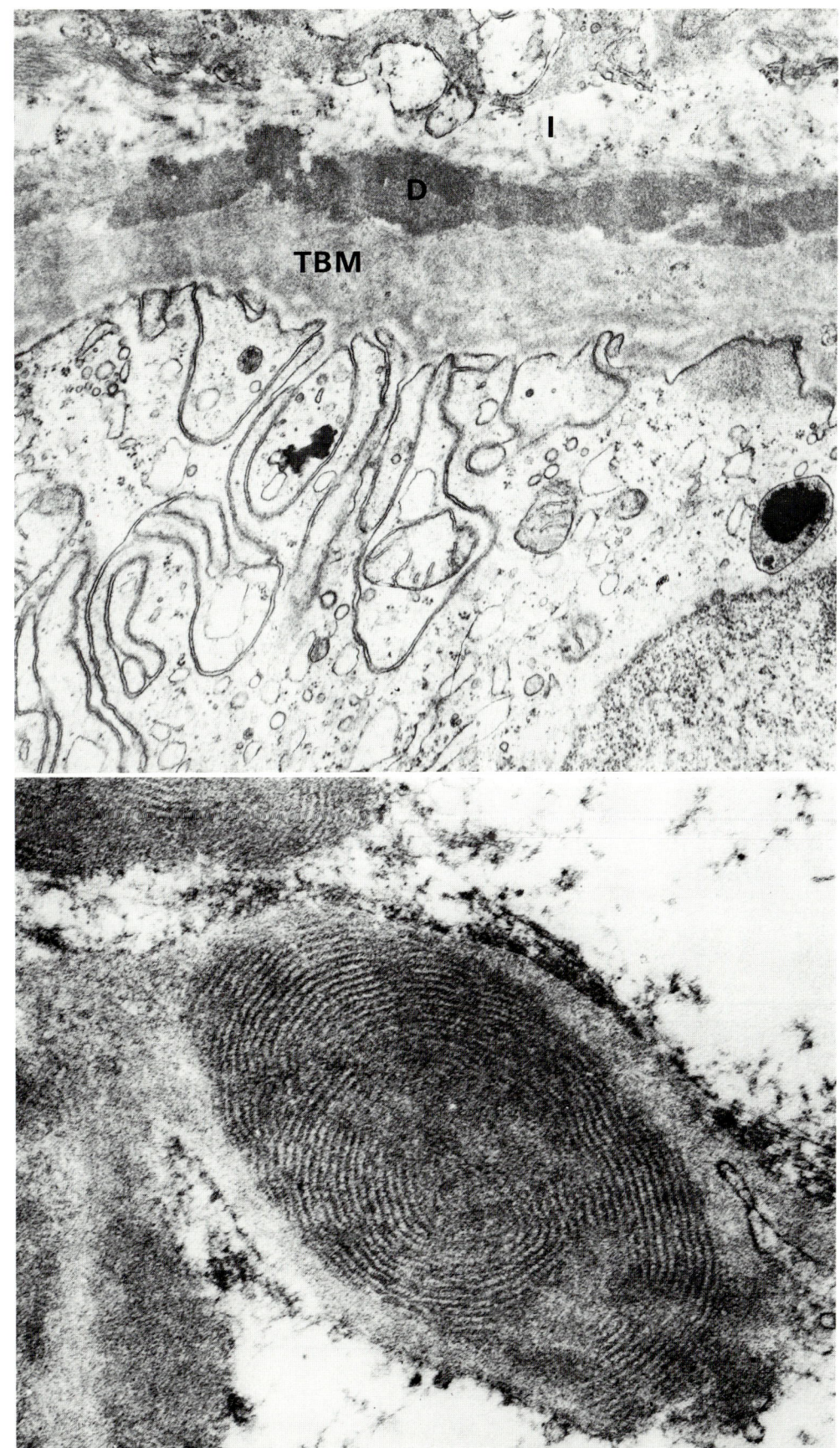

CHAPTER 8

Nephritis of Henoch-Schönlein Purpura
(Figs. 8-1 to 8-6 and Figs. 8-19 to 8-22)
Berger's Disease
(Figs. 8-7 to 8-11 and Figs. 8-23 to 8-24)
Goodpasture's Syndrome
(Figs. 8-12 to 8-18 and Fig. 8-25)

Nephritis of Henoch-Schönlein Purpura
(Anaphylactoid Purpura)

Definition: Glomerular disease accompanying Henoch-Schönlein (anaphylactoid) purpura. It occurs in the minority of patients and is usually mild and self-limited, but on occasion, severe and progressive. The main histological changes consist of various degrees of diffuse mesangial proliferation and of focal and segmental thrombosis, necrosis and crescent formation.

Clinical Manifestations: Henoch-Schönlein purpura is mainly a disease of children, but also occurs in adults. Males are affected considerably more frequently than females. The characteristic skin lesions consist of a purpuric rash especially over the lower extremities and buttocks and occasionally of larger cutaneous hemorrhages. Visceral manifestations are seen in about 1/4 — 1/2 of patients and include hematemesis, melena, hemoptysis and hematuria. Arthritis is not infrequent but usually mild and transient. In most cases all manifestations resolve completely, but may recur at intervals, particularly after an intercurrent upper respiratory infection. In adults a somewhat similar clinical picture may be produced by mixed essential cryoglobulinemia.

It has been estimated that renal disease affects less than one-half of the patients. In addition to gross or microscopic hematuria, proteinuria may be present, sometimes severe enough to cause a nephrotic syndrome. The latter is generally an indication of severe glomerular disease which may leave appreciable residual damage or lead to acute or chronic renal failure. Hypertension is seen occasionally. A few patients develop a rapidly progressive glomerulonephritis. Though antistreptolysin titer is elevated in about 30% of patients, attempts to prove streptococcal etiology have not been successful. Complement levels in the serum are usually normal, but interestingly, IgA immunoglobulin is frequently elevated.

Light Microscopy: Most of the lesions listed in Tables I and II (with the exception of Dense Deposit Disease and Membranous Glomerulonephritis) have been noted in Henoch-Schönlein nephritis. In essence these can be divided into two groups: (1) mesangial proliferation, varying from minor to diffuse endocapillary and on occasion, mesangiocapillary; (2) focal thrombosis, necrosis and crescent formation. The two types of lesions frequently co-exist, but appear to be independent of each other. Mesangial proliferation is generally self-limited, and tends to resolve completely, though its most severe forms, such as diffuse mesangiocapillary and occasionally, diffuse endocapillary may end in mesangial and diffuse glomerular sclerosis. On the contrary, thrombosis and necrosis almost invariably lead to crescentic glomerulonephritis the outcome of which depends upon size and number of crescents. Though some of the crescents resolve, the majority probably heal by fibrosis with segmental or global scarring of the tuft. The more severe glomerular disease is sometimes accompanied by arteritis of small branches. Care should be taken to distinguish idiopathic Henoch-Schönlein purpura from microscopic periarteritis nodosa with crescentic glomerulonephritis and purpuric skin rash. This is best done by immunofluorescence microscopy which demonstrates IgA deposits in Henoch-Schönlein purpura (see below). Early cutaneous lesions of Henoch-Schönlein purpura show capillary thrombosis and subsequent perivascular inflammation with fragmentation of leukocytes (leukocytoclastic vasculitis).

Electron Microscopy: In addition to mesangial proliferation and crescent formation, electron dense deposits are found in the mesangium, to a lesser extent also under the endothelium of the capillary wall and occasionally under the epithelium. In the last location they resemble the humps of post-infectious glomerulonephritis. Focal disruption of capillary basement membrane is not uncommon. Fibrin may be identified in the capillary lumina and in the crescents.

Immunofluorescence Microscopy: The characteristic feature is the presence of IgA in the deposits together with lesser amounts of IgG and occasionally IgM, even in the glomeruli that show only minor changes by light microscopy. C3 is also a constant feature, but early complement components are seldom seen. Fibrin is regularly found in the mesangium in addition to the capillary lumina and the crescents. IgA deposits and less frequently IgG and IgM are also found in the skin involving the capillary walls.

Berger's Disease

Definition: Chronic glomerular disease characterized by mild proliferative and sclerosing changes which may be diffuse or focal, and by invariable presence of IgA gamma globulin in the mesangium. C3, IgG and rarely IgM may also be present.

Clinical Manifestations: The disease is most often discovered in young adults and occurs more often in males than in females. It manifests as either recurrent gross hematuria or microscopic hematuria and proteinuria. Rarely nephrotic syndrome is seen. An attack is often precipitated by a mild intercurrent infection. On occasion it may simulate acute post-infectious glomerulonephritis. Serum IgA is moderately elevated in a considerable proportion of patients. Over a period of years hypertension and renal insufficiency may develop. In countries where Berger's disease is frequent, it is an important cause of chronic renal failure. IgA deposits tend to recur in transplants and be accompanied by microscopic hematuria and mild proteinuria. However graft function remains unimpaired for many years.

Light Microscopy: The characteristic pattern is that of mild diffuse mesangial change accompanied by focal segmental lesions. The mesangium is widened by deposits, increased number of cells and increased mesangial matrix. The deposits can often be seen by light microscopy in good preparations stained with trichrome or silver methenamine — chromotrope R. If no segmental lesions are present in the specimen, the appearance is that of mesangial glomerulonephritis, or in mild cases that of a minor change. The focal lesions are found in the majority of cases. They consist of segmental mesangial increase with cellularity, sclerosis and occasionally necrosis, accompanied by adhesions to Bowman's capsule. In a few patients crescents may be seen. On rare occasion the glomeruli show diffuse cellular proliferation.

Electron Microscopy: Electron microscopy confirms the light microscopic changes. The mesangial deposits lie mainly under the basement membrane but also elsewhere along the mesangial matrix. Occasionally they also extend under the endothelium of the capillary wall, or as "humps" between the capillary basement membrane and the epithelium.

Immunofluorescence Microscopy: IgA is invariably present irrespective of the type of histology. However the deposits vary in size and extent from very mild to massive. In many patients lesser amounts of other immunoglobulins may be found, particularly IgG, occasionally IgM. C3 is a constant accompaniment, but C1q and C4 are absent. Similar deposits, particularly of IgA and C3 are often found in skin and muscle biopsies, at the dermo-epidermal junction or around the small vessels.

Goodpasture's Syndrome

Definition: A syndrome consisting of pulmonary hemorrhages and glomerulonephritis of primary crescentic type. A third requirement is often added, namely the presence of anti-basement membrane antibodies, manifested by linear deposits in the glomeruli. This definition excludes cases in which crescents are superimposed upon another type of glomerulonephritis, and cases where pulmonary hemorrhage is due to uremic pneumonia, embolism or vasculitis. However the exact limits of Goodpasture's syndrome have not been definitively established. A suggestion has been made to use the term Goodpasture's syndrome in a purely clinical sense, without reference to pathology or immunopathology, and the term Goodpasture's disease for the combination of clinical, histological and immunological changes listed at the beginning of this paragraph. This division has not been widely used.

Clinical Manifestations: The disease is most common in young adult males, but occurs at any age. Its onset is sometimes preceded by a "flu-like" syndrome. In some cases there is a history of exposure to volatile hydrocarbons. Pulmonary hemorrhage is the leading manifestation and may be severe enough to cause exsanguination or severe ventilatory defect with asphyxia. Milder cases may show only blood-streaked sputum or variable densities on chest x-ray. Anemia is almost always present. In some cases renal symptoms such as gross hematuria precede the pulmonary changes. Rapidly progressing renal failure is the leading cause of death preventable only by dialysis, but some patients recover, temporarily or permanently.

In addition to hematuria, urinalysis discloses proteinuria, occasionally severe enough to cause nephrotic syndrome. Hypertension is usually mild or absent. Azotemia is often present at the first examination. However, in some patients renal manifestations are mild or even completely absent. Serum complement levels are usually in the normal range and immune complexes are absent. The characteristic feature is the presence of anti-glomerular basement membrane antibody in the serum, particularly at the onset of the disease.

Light Microscopy: The typical finding is the presence of large occlusive crescents in the glomeruli with little or no change of the tuft other than collapse of the capillaries. These changes are identical with those of diffuse crescentic glomerulonephritis (Table I). In milder or earlier cases only focal lesions may be seen, consisting of segmental tuft thrombosis and necrosis and small crescents containing fibrin. Occasionally no changes are found on light microscopy and the only evidence of renal involvement is demonstrated by immunofluorescence microscopy. Necrotizing vasculitis is seen on rare occasion.

Examination of the lung shows recent and old intra-alveolar hemorrhages, the latter manifested by numerous iron-containing macrophages. Necrosis of alveolar walls may be recognized, accompanied by polymorphonuclear infiltration.

Electron Microscopy: The glomerular findings are essentially those of idiopathic crescentic glomerulonephritis. This includes frequent breaks of the capillary walls and occasional presence of small subendothelial deposits. A pale zone may be seen between the endothelium and the basement membrane. Linear deposits in the basement membrane can rarely be recognized, probably because their density is equal to that of the lamina densa.

Immunofluorescence Microscopy: Linear deposits of IgG and less constantly of C3 along the glomerular basement membranes are practically diagnostic of Goodpasture's syndrome, if they are seen against the typical background of pulmonary hemorrhage and glomerular crescents. The diagnosis is also acceptable in those rare cases in which pulmonary hemorrhages are accompanied by linear deposits in glomeruli that are otherwise normal by light microscopy and electron microscopy. Since linear deposits occur in a number of diseases other than Goodpasture's syndrome, such as systemic lupus erythematosus, diabetes and periarteritis nodosa, it may be necessary in doubtful cases, to rely on the presence of anti-glomerular basement membrane antibodies in the serum, or, where possible, on elution of antibodies from the kidney tissue and demonstration of their affinity for normal glomerular basement membrane by indirect immunofluorescence. It has not been clearly established whether linear staining in cases of periarteritis nodosa is ever due to anti-glomerular basement membrane antibodies.

In some cases of pulmonary hemorrhages and crescentic glomerulonephritis, granular instead of linear deposits of IgG and C3 are found in the glomeruli, probably corresponding to the subendothelial deposits seen by electron microscopy. Such cases are excluded by those who consider linear deposits an essential part of Goodpasture's syndrome. However, clinically and anatomically they behave in a typical manner and demonstrate no other cause for pulmonary hemorrhages. Moreover, there are cases of diffuse crescentic glomerulonephritis without pulmonary hemorrhages which show linear deposits in the glomeruli.

Immunofluorescence microscopy of the lung demonstrates linear deposits along the alveolar basement membranes in a considerable proportion of cases. Such deposits can be eluted and shown to contain anti-basement membrane antibody which reacts with normal lung as well as with normal glomeruli.

GLOMERULONEPHRITIS OF SYSTEMIC DISEASES

NEPHRITIS OF HENOCH-SCHÖNLEIN PURPURA

Fig. 8-1 Henoch-Schönlein nephritis. Segmental thrombosis and beginning necrosis with accompanying small crescent. The remainder of the glomerular tuft shows practically no changes.
PAS stain. × 310.

Fig. 8-2 Same case as Fig. 8-1 one month later. Necrotic material has disappeared. There is segmental collapse of the capillaries and a fairly prominent fibroepithelial crescent.
PAS stain. × 310.

Fig. 8-3 Another case of Henoch-Schönlein purpura. There is diffuse endocapillary glomerulonephritis but no segmental lesions.
H&E stain. × 410.

Fig. 8-4 Same case as Fig. 8-3 one and a half years later. There is mild mesangial proliferation and sclerosis as well as a large scar adherent to the Bowman's capsule (top of the picture).
H&E stain. × 410.

Fig. 8-5 Immunofluorescence microscopy. Deposits of IgA mainly along the capillary basement membranes. × 260.

Fig. 8-6 Immunofluorescence microscopy. Segmental deposits of fibrinogen.
× 410.

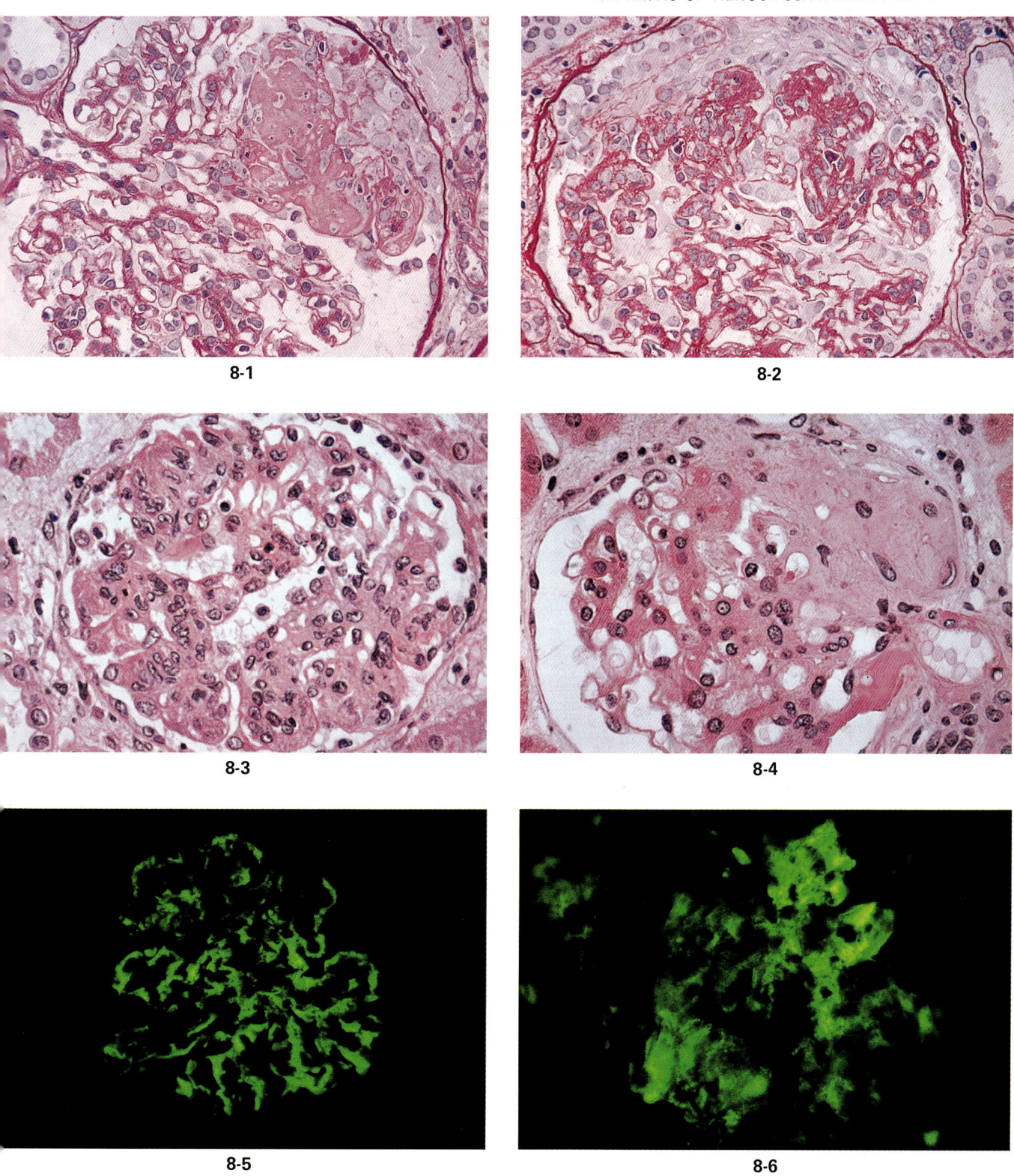

GLOMERULONEPHRITIS OF SYSTEMIC DISEASES

BERGER'S DISEASE (IgA NEPHROPATHY)

Fig. 8-7 Berger's disease. Glomerulus showing mesangial widening and mild cell proliferation. A few atrophic tubules are seen next to the glomerulus.
PAS stain.

Fig. 8-8 Segmental cell proliferation and sclerosis with adhesion to Bowman's capsule. Note also some mesangial proliferation.
PAS stain. x 260.

Fig. 8-9 Immunofluorescence microscopy. Deposits of IgA along the capillary loops and in the mesangium. x 410.

Fig. 8-10 Immunofluorescence microscopy. Deposits of IgG mainly along the capillary loops. x 410.

Fig. 8-11 Immunofluorescence microscopy. Deposits of C3 in the mesangium and along the capillary loops. x 260.

GOODPASTURE'S SYNDROME

Fig. 8-12 Goodpasture's syndrome. Early glomerular change consisting of capillary thrombosis and beginning necrosis, and hyperplasia of overlying epithelial cells. Polymorphonuclear leukocytes are present in a nearby capillary.
PAS stain. x 310.

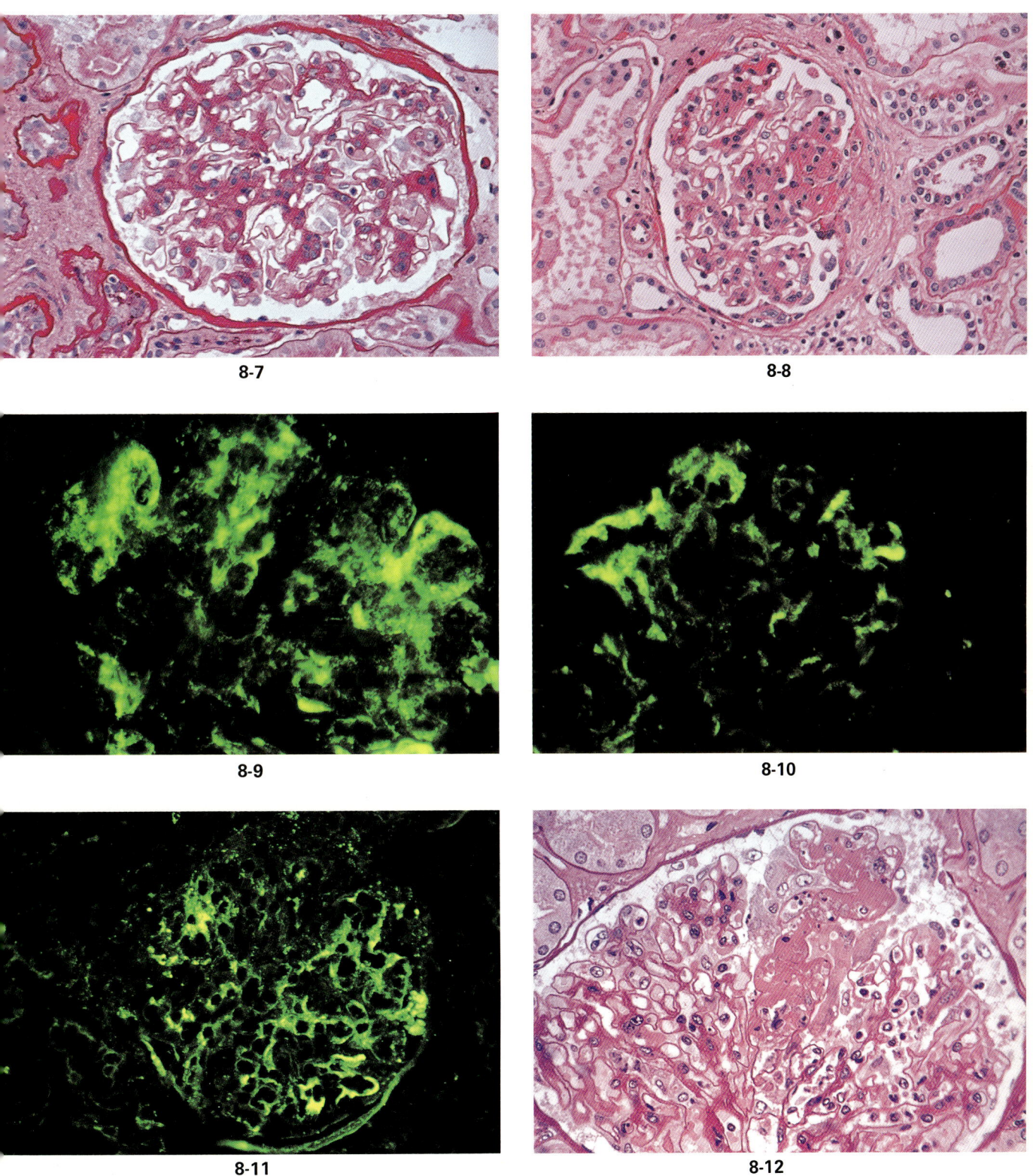
8-7
8-8
8-9
8-10
8-11
8-12

GLOMERULONEPHRITIS OF SYSTEMIC DISEASES

GOODPASTURE'S SYNDROME

Fig. 8-13 Goodpasture's syndrome. A more advanced stage. Fairly large area of thrombosis and necrosis.
PAS stain. x 260.

Fig. 8-14 A more advanced stage showing fibrin in the glomerular tuft and a crescent in the Bowman's space.
H&E stain. x 260.

Fig. 8-15 Same case as Fig. 8-12. Fibrin and crescent in the urinary space. Beginning collapse of the capillary tuft.
PAS stain. x 310.

Fig. 8-16 Immunofluorescence microscopy. Linear deposits of IgG along the glomerular capillary walls. x 260.

Fig. 8-17 Immunofluorescence microscopy. Large fibrin deposits in the crescent. x 260.

Fig. 8-18 Section of the lung showing hemorrhages in the alveoili. x 100.

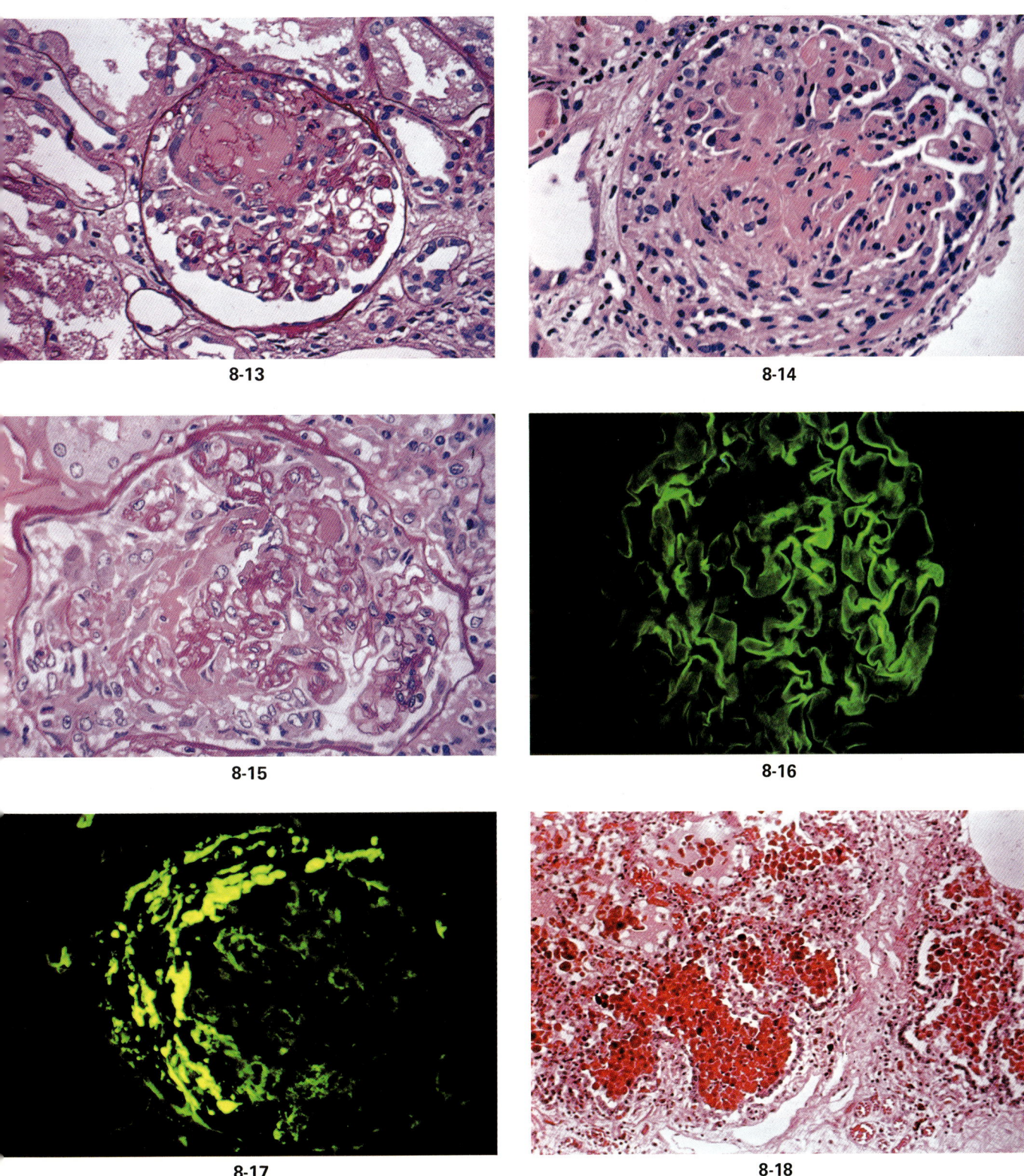

GLOMERULONEPHRITIS OF SYSTEMIC DISEASES

NEPHRITIS OF HENOCH-SCHÖNLEIN PURPURA

Fig. 8-19 Electron micrograph. Henoch-Schönlein nephritis. Same case as Fig. 8-1 showing an early thrombus in a glomerular capillary. The thrombus consists of agglutinated red blood cells (RBC). Note small electron dense deposits (D) in the mesangium. ×11,000.

Fig. 8-20 Electron micrograph. Large electron dense deposits (D) in the glomerular mesangium. ×11,000.

U: urinary space, BM: basement membrane, L: capillary lumen, MC: mesangial cell.

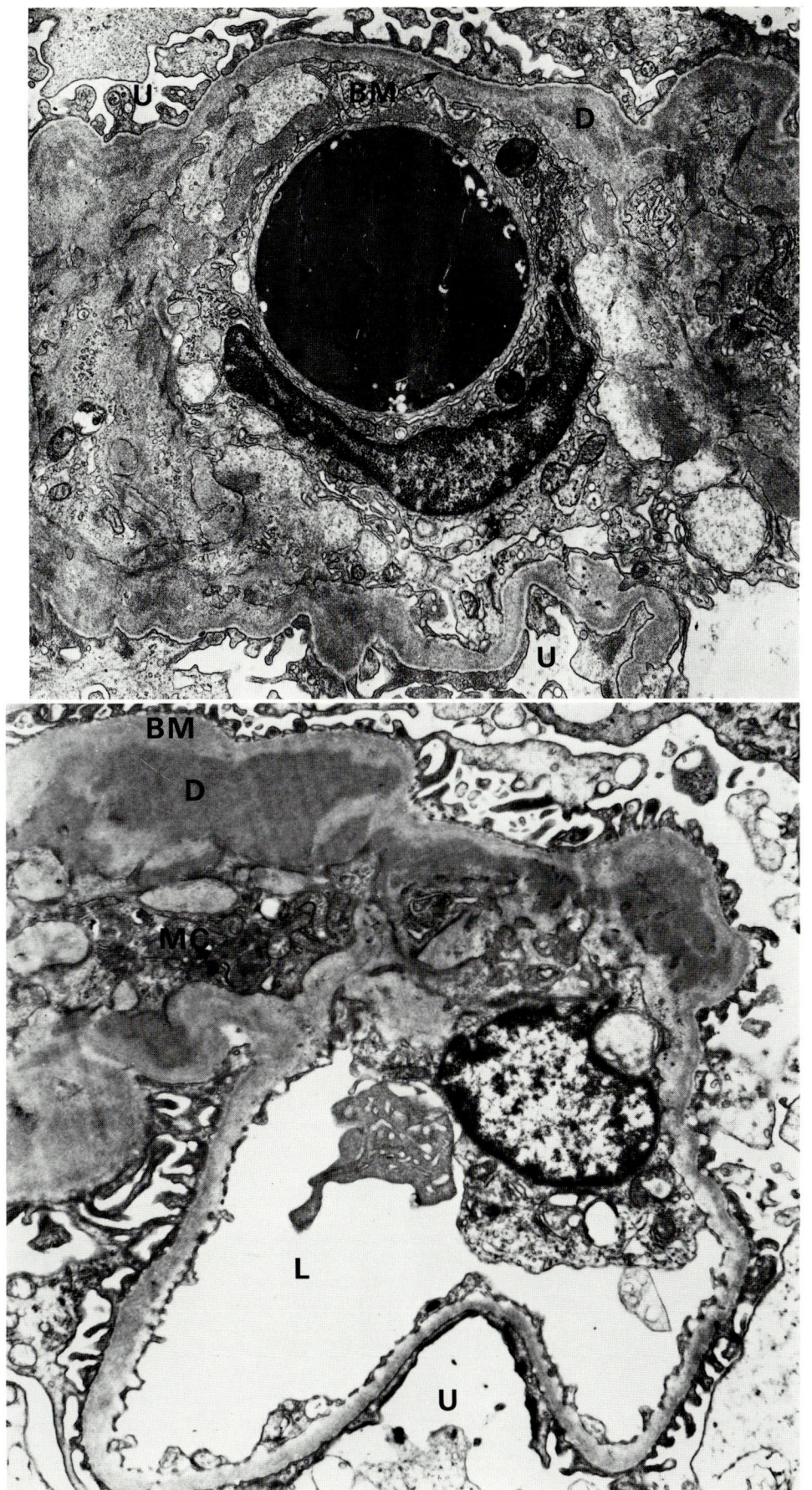

GLOMERULONEPHRITIS OF SYSTEMIC DISEASES

NEPHRITIS OF HENOCH-SCHÖNLEIN PURPURA

Fig. 8-21 Electron micrograph. Same case as Fig. 8-19. Subendothelial deposit (D).
x 7,000.

Fig. 8-22 Electron micrograph. Henoch-Schönlein nephritis. Subepithelial deposits (D) resembling humps. x 16,000.

BERGER'S DISEASE

Fig. 8-23 Electron micrograph. Mesangial area showing cell proliferation, matrix and small electron dense deposits. x 8,600.

U: urinary space, BM: basement membrane, L: capillary lumen, En: endothelial cell, P: podocyte, MC: mesangial cell.

GOODPASTURE'S SYNDROME

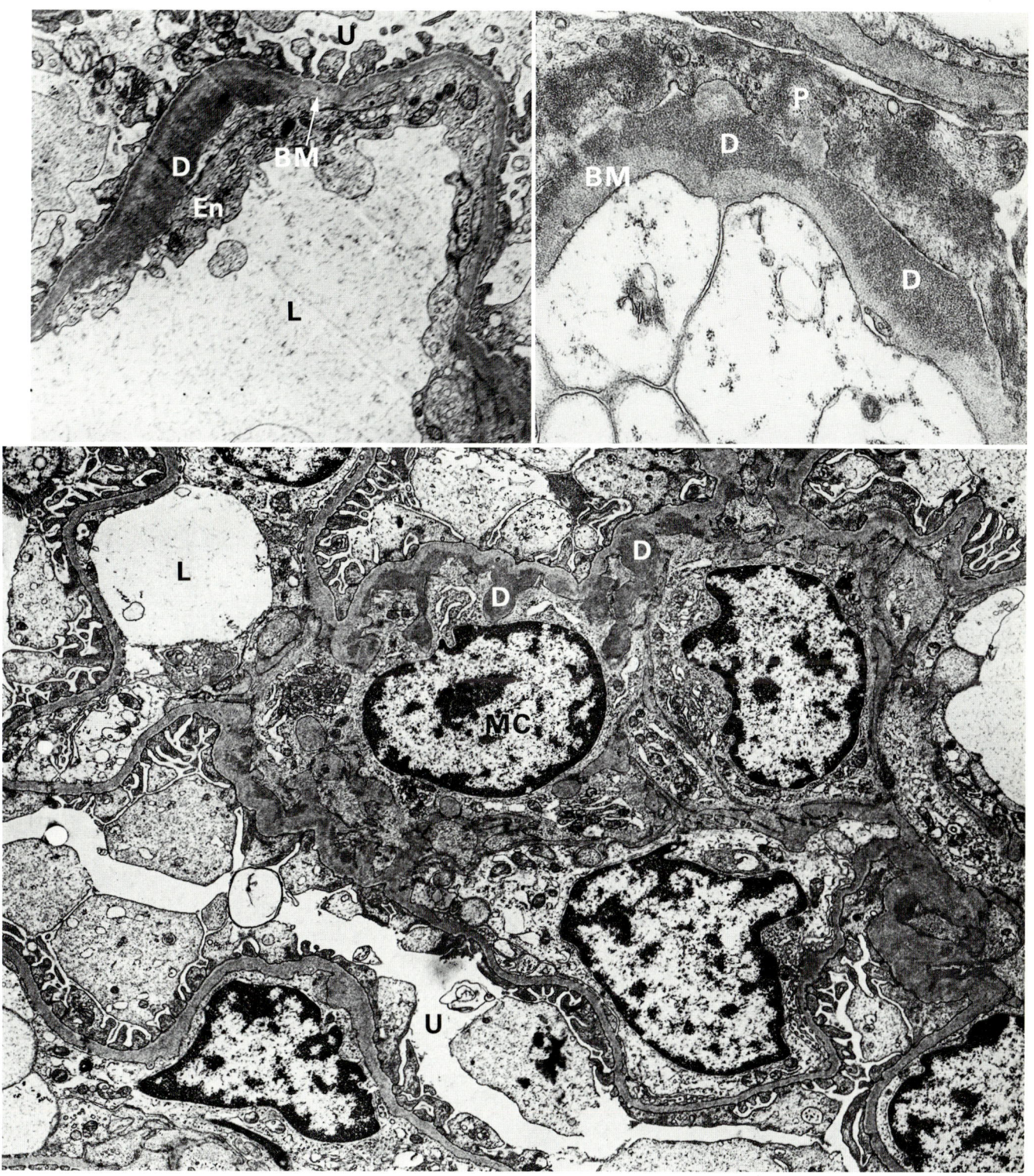

163

BERGER'S DISEASE

Fig. 8-24 Electron micrograph. Massive electron dense deposits (D) in the mesangium. ×25,000.

GOODPASTURE'S SYNDROME

Fig. 8-25 Electron micrograph. Goodpasture's syndrome, early stage, showing fibrin thrombus (F) in the capillary lumen (L) and hyperplasia of the mesangial cells (MC). ×7,000.

BM: basement membrane, U: urinary space.

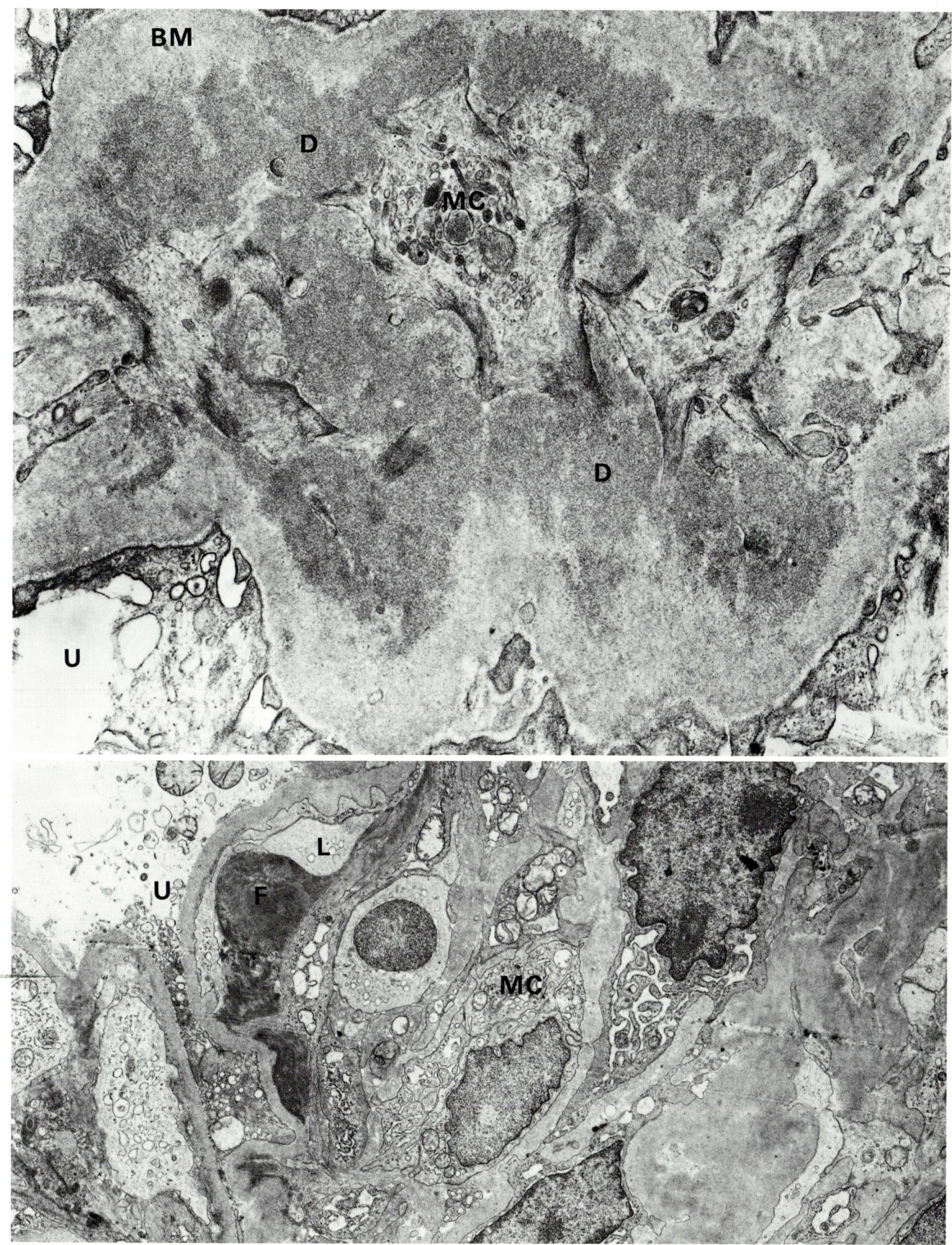

CHAPTER 9

Glomerular Lesions in Systemic Infections
    Septicemia
        (Figs. 9-1 to 9-3 and Fig. 9-11)
    Infective Endocardities
        (Figs. 9-4 to 9-6 and Fig. 9-12)
    Shunt Nephritis
        (Figs. 9-7 to 9-9 and Fig. 9-13)
    Syphilis
        (Fig. 9-10 and Figs. 9-14 to 9-15)

Glomerular Lesions in Systemic Infections

Definition: Glomerular disease accompanying acute and chronic infections. The changes vary depending upon the type of the infective agent and the type and severity of the disease. Only more striking or more common forms are described below.

Septicemia

Clinical Manifestations: Septicemia with gram-negative or gram-positive bacteria produces a variety of renal lesions and clinical manifestations. These range from acute renal failure to symptoms of glomerulonephritis.

Light Microscopy: The glomeruli may be the seat of bacterial localization with consequent purulent inflammation and even abscess formation. More common is focal necrotizing and crescentic glomerulonephritis, perhaps due to local thrombosis and induced either by bacterial toxins or by deposition of immune complexes. Sometimes a diffuse endocapillary glomerulonephritis is seen, with mesangial proliferation and immune deposits in the mesangium and under the epithelium ("humps"). This last entity has been described in greater detail under the heading of Endocapillary Glomerulonephritis.

Glomerulonephritis in Infective Endocarditis

Clinical Manifestations: Infective endocarditis may be of either acute or subacute type and involve any of the cardiac valves. Cardiovascular and other systemic signs and symptoms may suggest the diagnosis, but sometimes, particularly with right-sided infection, the disease remains silent. This is a fairly common finding in drug addicts. Confirmation is obtained by blood culture, but again false negative results may be obtained with the right-sided infection. A variety of bacterial species is found from Staphylococcus aureus to gram-negative rods. In the subacute form alpha hemolytic Streptococcus is the common pathogen. Infection of a traumatic arterio-venous shunt may be suggested by a local bruit.

Mild renal involvement may be overshadowed by systemic manifestations and be discovered only on routine urinalysis, which reveals hematuria and proteinuria. In an occasional patient there are no renal manifestations despite the presence of glomerular lesions. An acute nephritic syndrome is also seen and is sometimes of rapidly progressive variety. Nephrotic syndrome is uncommon. Serum complement (C_3, $C1q$) is often reduced. Appropriate treatment (antibiotics, removal of the shunt) will usually reverse or heal the renal disease, but some of the more severe cases will progress to irreversible renal failure despite therapy.

Light Microscopy: The most common lesion in infective endocarditis is focal glomerulonephritis with thrombosis, necrosis, cellular proliferation and segmental crescent formation. This was originally called focal "embolic" glomerulonephritis, but more likely represents local thrombosis perhaps provoked by immune complex deposition. Healing leads to segmental scars and capsular adhesions. When numerous, focal lesions may lead to renal insufficiency. Large crescents are usually associated with rapidly progressive course. Mesangial proliferative glomerulonephritis often co-exists with focal lesions and may be the dominant or the only feature. In some cases typical acute diffuse endocapillary glomerulonephritis develops; while in more chronic cases the picture may be reminiscent of mesangiocapillary glomerulonephritis. Periglomerular and interstitial inflammatory infiltrates are frequently present.

Electron Microscopy: Electron microscopy shows mesangial proliferation, crescent formation and electron dense mesangial, subendothelial and subepithelial deposits.

Immunofluorescence Microscopy demonstrates granular deposits of IgG and C3 and sometimes of other immune globulins. Not infrequently, these are accompanied by bacterial antigens, indicating that glomerular disease is due to immune-complex formation. Fibrinogen or fibrin are seen in the necrotic areas and in the crescents.

Shunt Nephritis

Clinical Manifestations: In infants in whom a shunt has been surgically established between a ventricular hydrocephalus and the circulatory system, infection of the shunt may occur. The most common infecting organism is Staphylococcus epidermidis but other bacteria occur on occasion and can be demonstrated by blood culture. The patients usually have fever, anemia and arthralgias but sometimes renal manifestations precede other symptoms. Nephrotic syndrome is very common and is usually accompanied by hematuria. Some patients have only proteinuria and hematuria.

Light Microscopy: The glomerulonephritis is usually of a diffuse type and assumes the form of mesangial or mesangiocapillary disease. Crescents may be present.

Electron Microscopy shows mesangial proliferation, double outlines, crescent formation and electron dense mesangial, subendothelial or subepithelial deposits.

Immunofluorescence Microscopy: The most common findings are granular deposits of IgM and sometimes also of IgG and C3 along the capillary walls. Bacterial antigens have been demonstrated in some cases.

Syphilis

Clinical Manifestations: The most common renal manifestation of syphilis, either acquired (secondary stage) or congenital, is proteinuria and nephrotic syndrome. Microscopic hematuria may be occasionally present. Anti-syphilitic therapy is the treatment of choice with excellent results, though on occasion the resolution of nephrotic syndrome may take months.

Light Microscopy: The glomeruli are uniformly affected and show slight to moderate mesangial proliferation and sometimes obvious thickening of the capillary walls.

Electron Microscopy: The typical changes are those of membranous glomerulonephritis combined with variable mesangial proliferation. With therapy the deposits disappear quite rapidly though subepithelial "spikes" may persist for some time.

Immunofluorescence Microscopy: The usual pattern is that of granular peripheral deposits of IgG and C3. IgM and IgA are seen on occasion, more often in the mesangium than along the periphery.

GLOMERULONEPHRITIS OF SYSTEMIC DISEASES

GLOMERULAR LESIONS IN SYSTEMIC INFECTIONS

Septicemia

Fig. 9-1 Staphylococcus aureus septicemia. Glomerular and periglomerular infiltration by polymorphonuclear leukocytes.
H&E stain.   x 260.

Fig. 9-2 Staphylococcus aureus septicemia in a heroin addict. Proliferative glomerulonephritis with many polymorphonuclear leukocytes.
PAS stain.   x 260.

Fig. 9-3 Same case as Fig. 9-2 six weeks later after treatment of infection. Clearing of proliferation with some residual mesangial changes.
PAS stain.   x 260.

Infective Endocarditis

Fig. 9-4 Acute Salmonella endocarditis. Glomerulus showing a segmental area of necrosis.
PAS stain.   x 260.

Fig. 9-5 Infective endocarditis. Glomerulus showing mesangial proliferation and a small segmental lesion at nine o'clock. There is interstitial periglomerular inflammation.
Trichrome stain.   x 260.

Fig. 9-6 Subacute bacterial endocarditis. Glomerulus showing a healed segmental lesion with partial preservation of the tuft.
PAS stain.   x 260.

GLOMERULAR LESIONS IN SYSTEMIC INFECTIONS

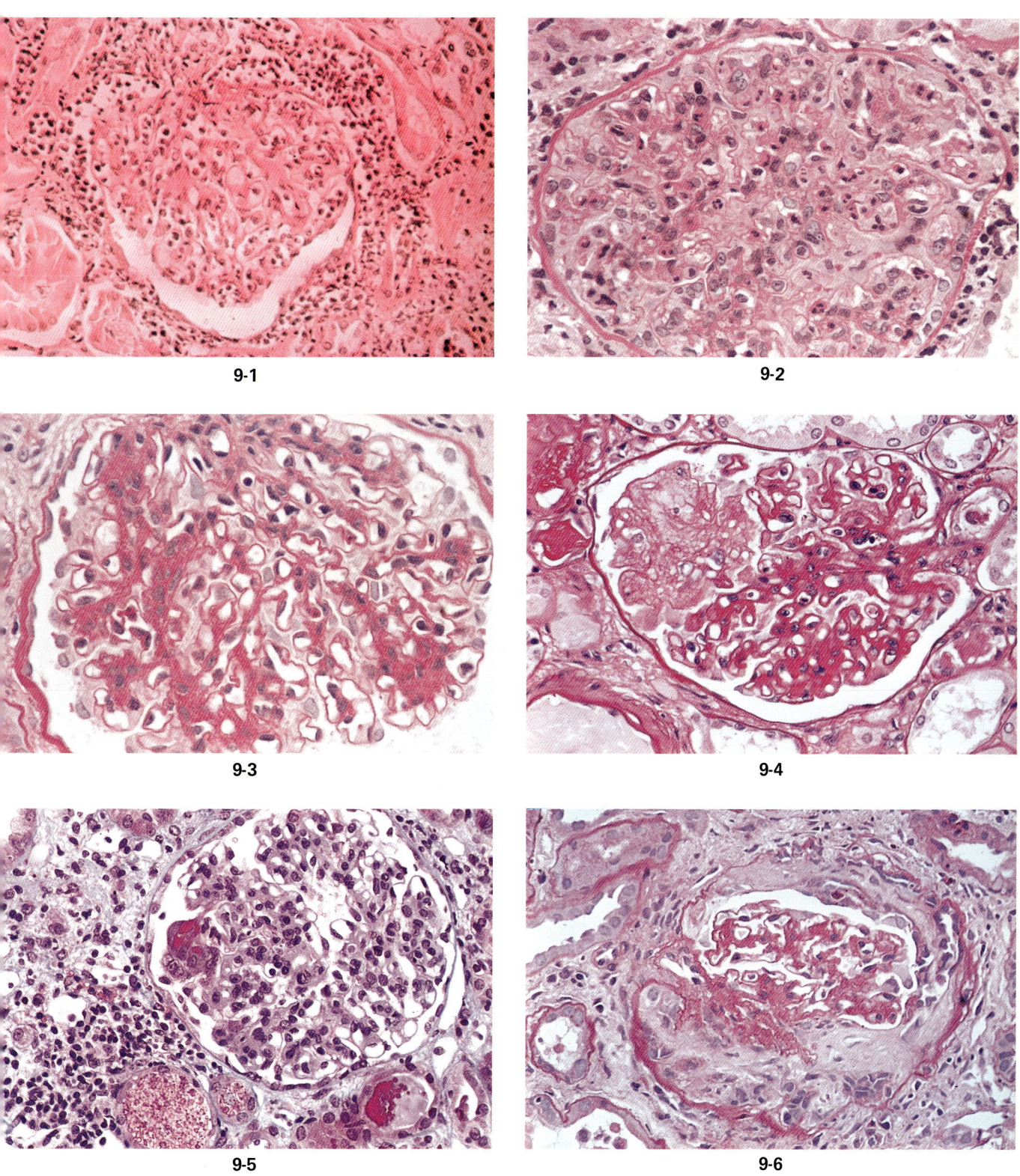

9-1

9-2

9-3

9-4

9-5

9-6

169

GLOMERULAR LESIONS IN SYSTEMIC INFECTIONS

Shunt Nephritis

Fig. 9-7 Shunt nephritis. Staphylococcus epidermidis infection. Glomeruli showing marked mesangial proliferation and lobulation.
2 micron section, Toluidine blue stain.   x 260.

Fig. 9-8 Immunofluorescence microscopy. Another case of shunt nephritis showing 3+ granular and nodular deposits of complement (C3) predominantly along the capillary loops of the glomerulus. The distribution of immune globulins was similar.   x 410.

Fig. 9-9 Immunofluorescence microscopy. Same case as in Fig. 9-8 showing 2+ granular deposits of Staphylococcus epidermidis antigen(s) along and in the capillary loops.   x 260.

Syphilis

Fig. 9-10 Nephrotic syndrome in a patient with congenital syphilis. The glomerulus shows very slight increase in the number of mesangial cells. The podocytes are prominent but perhaps no more so than in an infant of similar age.
   x 410.

GLOMERULAR LESIONS IN SYSTEMIC INFECTIONS

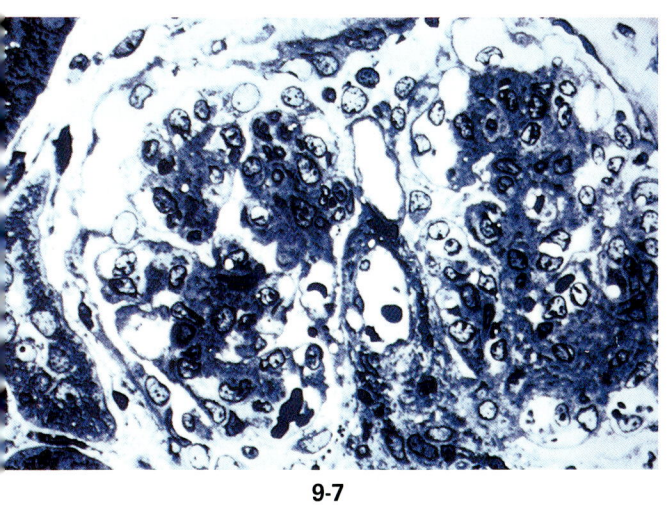
9-7

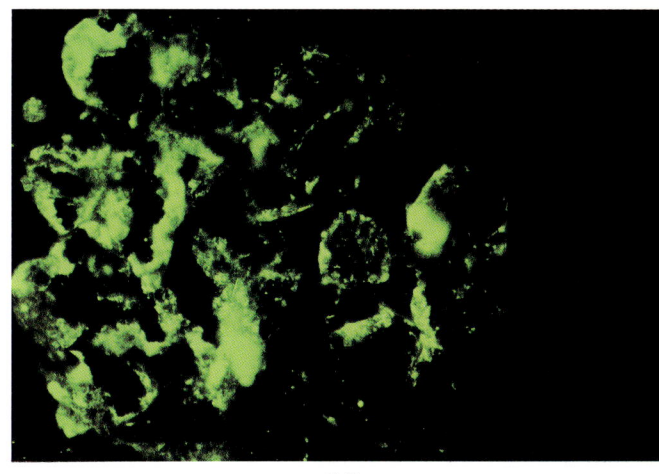
9-8

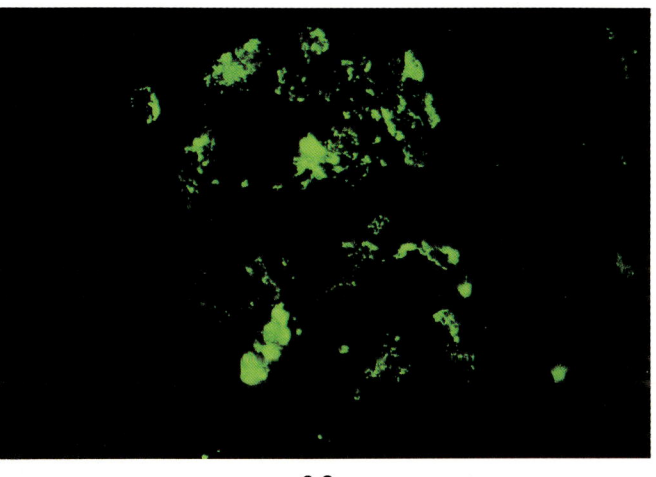
9-9

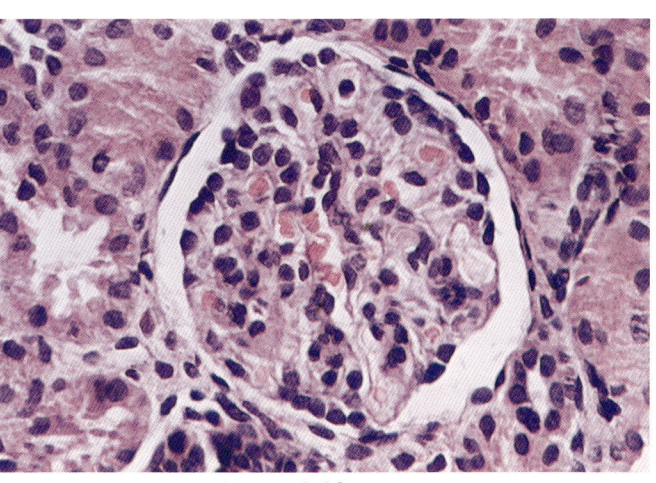
9-10

171

GLOMERULONEPHRITIS OF SYSTEMIC DISEASES

GLOMERULAR LESIONS IN SYSTEMIC INFECTIONS

Septicemia

Fig. 9-11 Electron micrograph. Same case as Fig. 9-3. A single large subepithelial deposit ("hump") (D) is seen in the center of the picture. x 3,200.

Infective Endocarditis

Fig. 9-12 Electron micrograph. Same case as Fig. 9-6. Residual mesangial proliferation and interlacing strands of matrix   x 7,000..

U: urinary space, L: capillary lumen, MC: mesangial cell, MM: mesangial matrix.

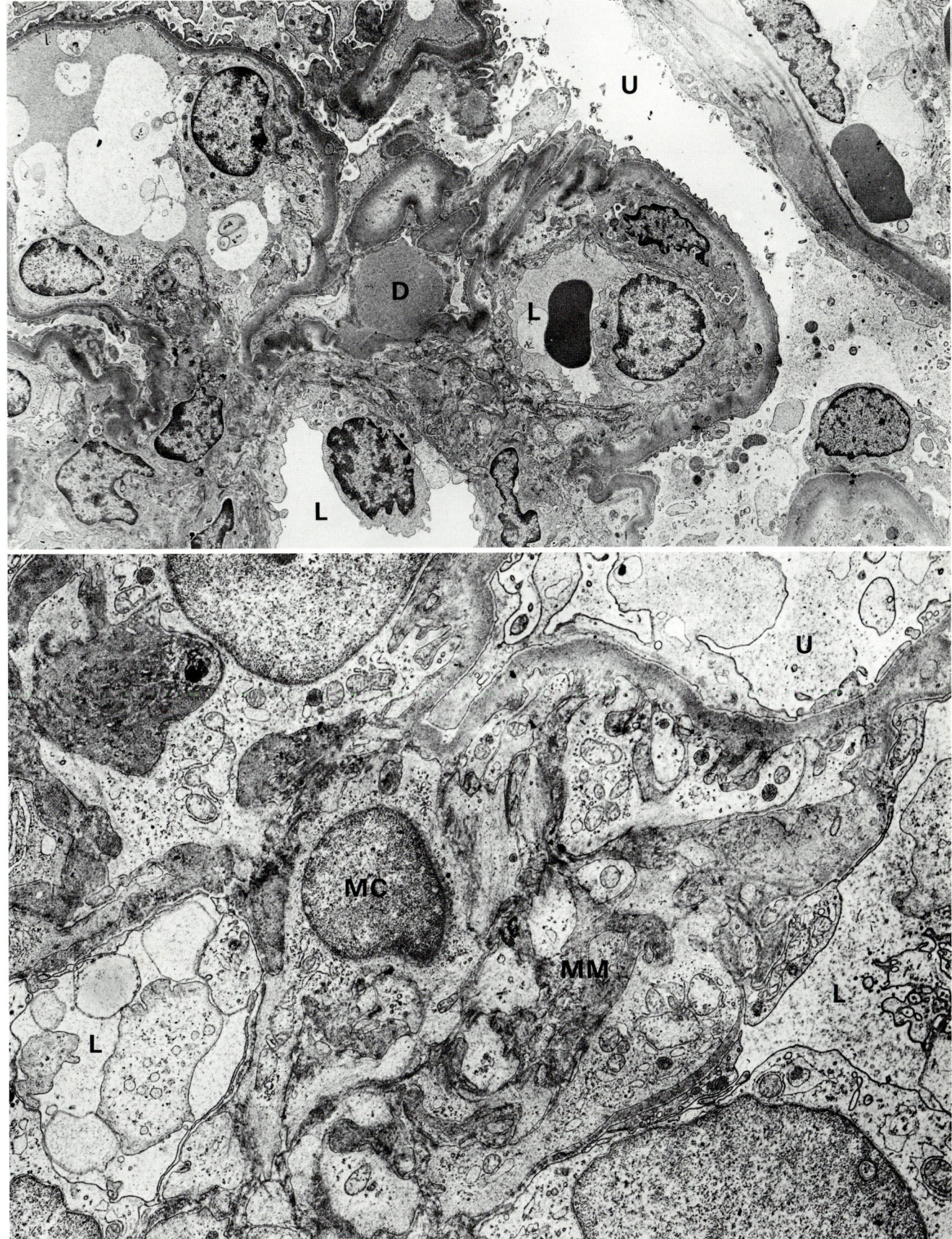

GLOMERULAR LESIONS IN SYSTEMIC INFECTIONS

Shunt Nephritis

Fig. 9-13 Electron micrograph. Same case as Fig. 9-7. Part of a glomerulus showing mesangial proliferation and mesangial interposition in the capillary walls. Electron dense deposits (D) are present in the mesangium and in the capillary wall, apprently in the interposed mesangium. × 7,000.

Ep: epithelial cell, RBC: red blood cell, BM: basement membrane, MC: mesangial cell, MM: mesangial matrix.

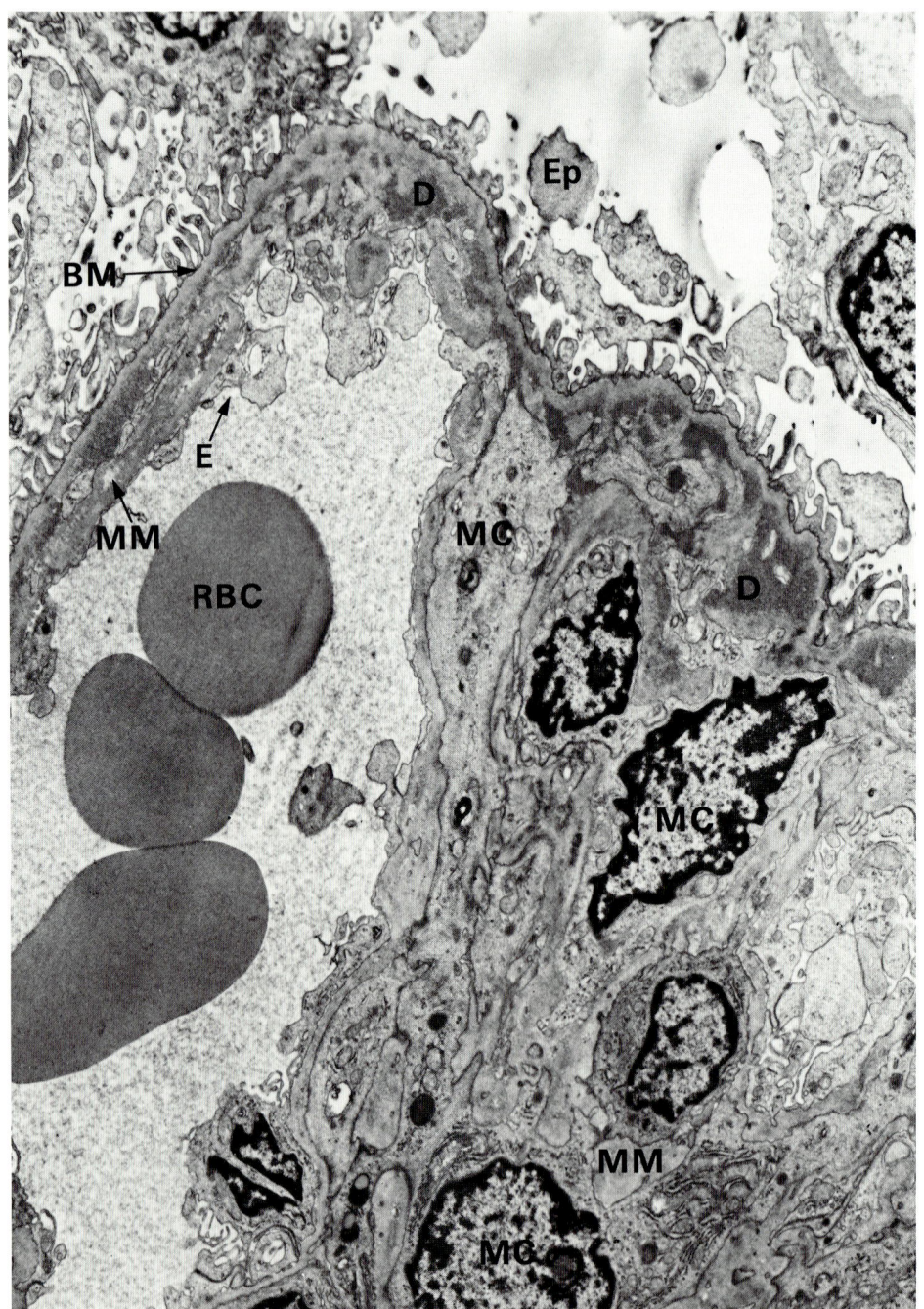

GLOMERULAR LESIONS IN SYSTEMIC INFECTIONS

Syphilis

Fig. 9-14   Electron micrograph. Same case as Fig. 9-10 showing a focal area of membranous transformation with subepithelial deposits (D), spikes (S) and effacement of overlying foot processes (FP). There are microvilli in the urinary space (U). × 15,000.

Fig. 9-15   Electron micrograph. Same patient as in Fig. 9-14 after treatment with penicillin. The deposits have disappeared but spikes (S) and some general distortion of the basement membrane persist. Foot processes have partly recovered but microvilli are still present in the urinary space (U). × 20,000.

L: capillary lumen.

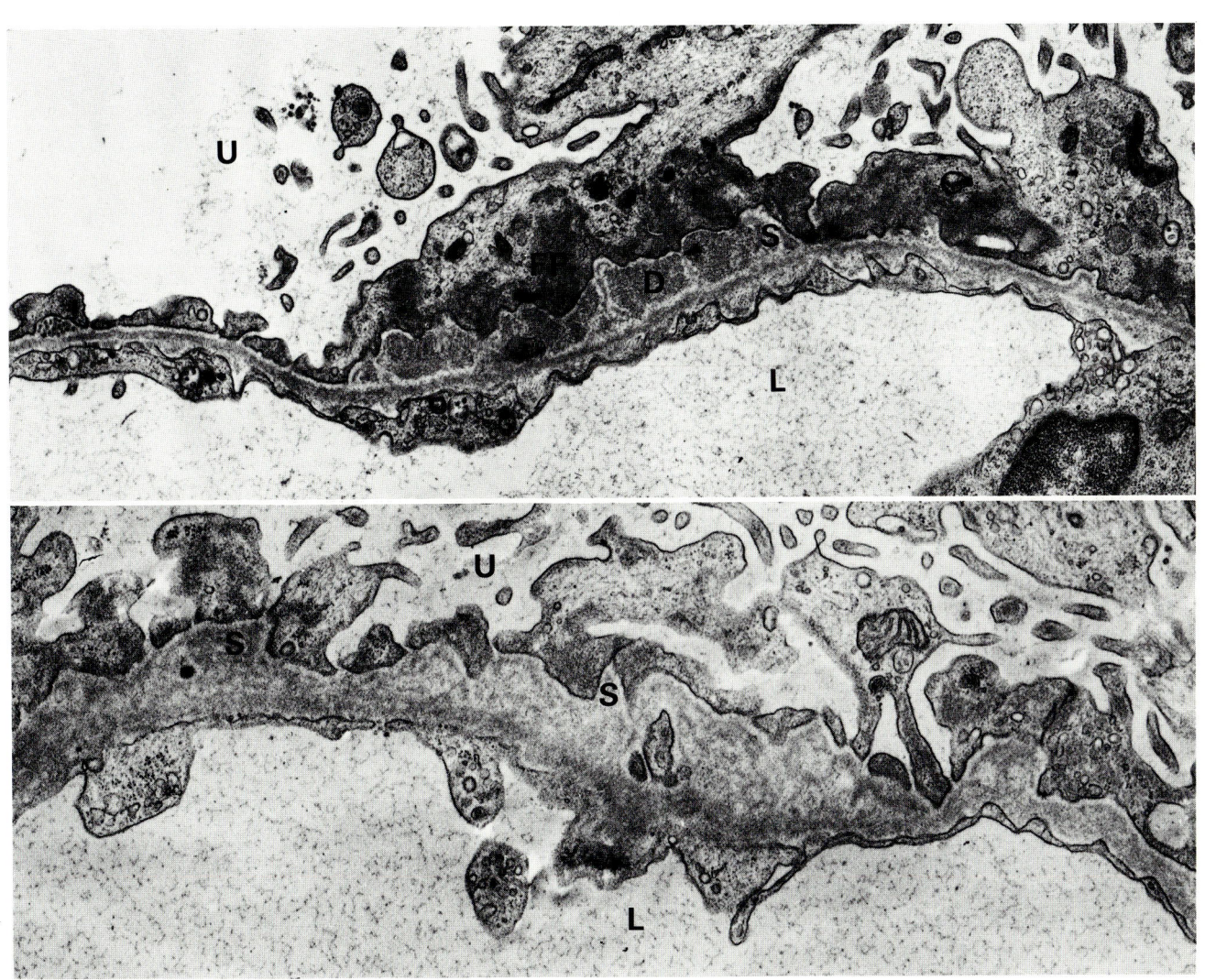

CHAPTER 10

Parasitic Nephropathies
   Malaria
      (Figs. 10-1 to 10-4 and Figs. 10-13 to 10-14)
   Schistosomiasis
      (Figs. 10-5 to 10-10 and Figs. 10-15 to 10-16)
   Strongyloidosis
      (Figs. 10-11 to 10-12 and Fig. 10-17)

Parasitic Nephropathies

Glomerular changes have been described in several parasitic diseases such as malaria, schistosomiasis and trypanosomiasis. On rare occasion it may also be seen in association with other parasites.

Malarial Nephropathy*

Definition: Glomerular disease associated with malarial infection. Two forms are recognized: (1) Acute and transient proliferative glomerulonephritis which occurs mainly with P. falciparum disease, and (2) Chronic and progressive glomerulonephritis which resembles membranous or mesangiocapillary forms and which is seen in patients with P. malariae (Quartan malaria). It is not certain whether renal disease of the second type is due to the infection per se, whether the infection predisposes to the development of nephrotic syndrome which is caused by other factors, or whether the disease is unrelated to malaria and should be called *Tropical Nephropathy*. Some cases may be due to infection with virus of hepatitis B (compare illustrations under Nephropathy of Liver Disease).

Clinical Manifestations: In the acute form which is generally mild, the patients show hematuria, proteinuria and only occasionally the nephrotic syndrome. These symptoms abate following antimalarial treatment but nephrotic syndrome may persist. The chronic form is most often seen in children and usually begins as nephrotic syndrome. In time the edema disappears, but proteinuria persists and hypertension and renal failure gradually develop. This form does not respond to the antimalarial therapy.

Light Microscopy: In the acute form the appearance is that of proliferative glomerulonephritis, varying in severity and type, from mesangial or segmental to mild diffuse. In the chronic form, proliferative changes are common in some countries (Uganda) especially in adults, but rare in others (Nigeria). Most patients show capillary wall thickening, sometimes "plexiform" in appearance. Gradual development of focal segmental sclerosis leads to progressive glomerular obsolescence and tubular atrophy.

Electron Microscopy: Variable degrees of cellular proliferation, mesangial matrix formation and mesangial electron dense deposits are the common findings. Capillary wall changes consist of subepithelial and intramembranous deposits and basement membrane thickening. Subendothelial deposits are seen occasionally. In some reports, mesangial proliferation and capillary wall deposits were not found, but the basement membrane was irregularly thickened by a plexiform layer of fibrillar basement membrane-like material in the subendothelial zone. This plexiform layer accounted for the

---

* Appreciation is expressed to Dr. Liliane Morel-Maroger for critical comments.

"lacunae" seen on light microscopy.

The combination of mesangial proliferation and deposits with subepithelial and intramembranous deposits suggests the diagnosis of membranous *and* proliferative glomerulonephritis, similar to that seen in some cases of systemic lupus erythematosus. In other cases the histological picture is more consistent with mesangiocapillary (membranoproliferative) glomerulonephritis.

Immunofluorescence Microscopy: In both, the acute and the chronic form, immunoglobulins (IgM, IgG), C3, occasionally C1q, C4 and in about 1/4–1/3 of cases also malarial antigens are found in the glomeruli, suggesting deposition of immune complexes. In the acute disease the deposits are predominantly mesangial; in the chronic — mainly along the capillary wall as fine or coarse granules or short linear stretches. However these changes are not constant.

Schistosomal Nephropathy

Definition: Glomerular disease accompanying infection by several species of schistosoma especially that by S. Mansoni and S. Japonicum. Prominent glomerular involvement is relatively uncommon, being most evident in the hepato-splenic form, which is the most severe but infrequent manifestation of schistosomiasis.

Clinical Manifestations: Renal disease is usually seen in young adults, especially males who come from endemic areas of schistosomiasis. Liver and spleen are almost invariably enlarged. Nephrotic syndrome or isolated non-selective proteinuria are the most common manifestations; microscopic hematuria or hypertension occur in a proportion of patients, as does elevation of serum globulin. The disease appears to be slowly progressive and shows little if any response to steroid or immunosuppressive therapy. The long term effects of anti-schistosomal treatment are not yet known.

Light Microscopy: A whole gamut of lesions is observed in the glomeruli, from mesangial thickening to focal segmental sclerosis, to diffuse proliferative glomerulonephritis and crescentic glomerulonephritis. The most common combination is mesangial proliferation and thickening of capillary walls, often interpreted as mesangiocapillary (membranoproliferative) glomerulonephritis.

Electron Microscopy: Mesangial proliferation and matrix deposition are observed very frequently. Electron dense deposits are found under the epithelium, in the basement membrane, under the endothelium and in the mesangium. This constellation of findings is more suggestive of combined membranous *and* proliferative glomerulonephritis than of true mesangiocapillary glomerulonephritis, but the latter probably occurs in some patients (see Malarial Nephropathy).

Immunofluorescence Microscopy demonstrated deposits in the mesangium and along the capillary walls. The deposits contain immunoglobulins (IgG, IgM, occasionally IgA and interestingly, IgE) and C3. Demonstration of schistosomal antigens and elution of anti-schistosomal antibodies has been accomplished in some cases. These findings suggest the presence of immune complexes.

Strongyloides Nephropathy

Intestinal parasites are not known to be associated with renal disease. However, systemic invasion, particularly in debilitated patients, may lead to renal involvement as in a case of Strongyloides infestation. The clinical manifestations in that case were those of nephrotic syndrome and the morphological changes those of membranous glomerulonephritis. In one case (*) extraction of kidney tissue obtained by open biopsy yielded Strongyloides antibodies.

---

* This case was provided by Dr. M. Needle.

PARASITIC NEPHROPATHIES

Malarial Nephropathy

Fig. 10-1 Quartan malarial nephropathy. Glomerulus showing mesangial widening with some increase in cells, and thickening of the capillary walls.
PAS stain. × 410.

Fig. 10-2 Same case as Fig. 10-1 showing double outline of glomerular capillary walls and narrowing of the lumina.
PASM stain. × 1,000.

Fig. 10-3 Immunofluorescence microscopy. Granular deposits of immunoglobulin along the glomerular capillary wall. × 410.

Fig. 10-4 Advanced stage of malarial nephropathy showing partly or completely sclerosed glomeruli, focal tubular atrophy and dilatation, and interstitial fibrosis with inflammatory infiltration.
PAS stain. × 100.

Schistosomal Nephropathy

Fig. 10-5 Hepatosplenic schistosomiasis. Glomerulus showing mild mesangial widening.
PAS stain. × 260.

Fig. 10-6 Immunofluorescence microscopy. Same case as Fig. 10-5. Peripheral and mesangial irregularly distributed deposits of IgM. × 260.

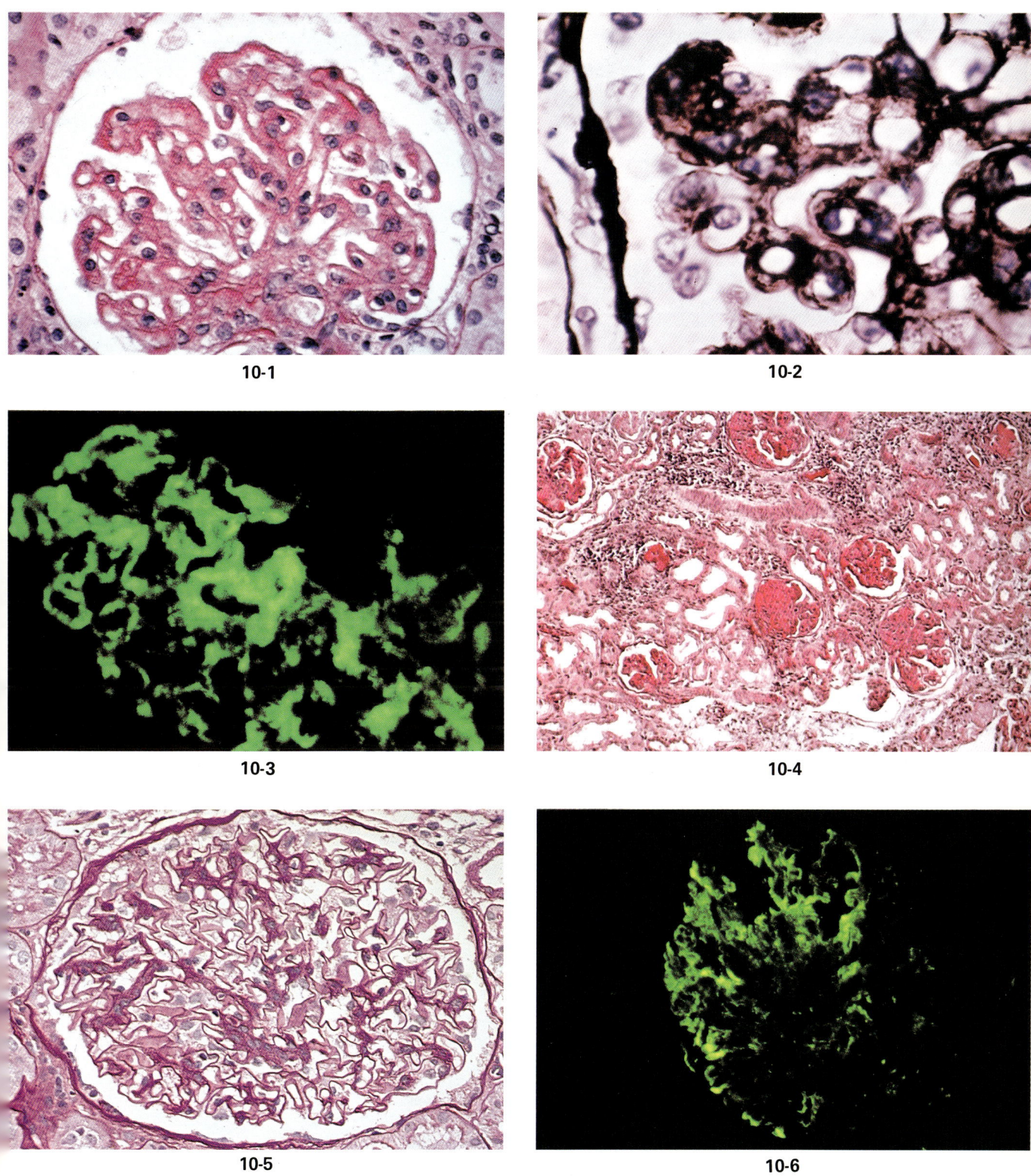

GLOMERULONEPHRITIS OF SYSTEMIC DISEASES

PARASITIC NEPHROPATHIES

Schistosomal Nephropathy

Fig. 10-7 Immunofluorescence microscopy. Same case as Fig. 10-5. Small mesangial deposits of IgA.   × 260.

Fig. 10-8 Immunofluorescence microscopy. Same case as Fig. 10-5. Coarse granules of complement (C3).   × 260.

Fig. 10-9 Another case of hepatosplenic schistosomiasis. Glomerulus showing thickening of capillary walls and focal mesangial widening.
PAS stain.   × 410.

Fig. 10-10 Same case as Fig. 10-9 showing mesangial widening and sclerosis and thickening of capillary walls, with suggestion of double outlines.
PAS stain.   × 410.

Strongyloides Nephropathy

Fig. 10-11 Disseminated strongyloidosis. Glomerulus showing diffuse thickening of capillary walls.
PAS stain.   × 260.

Fig. 10-12 Same case as Fig. 10-11. Glomerulus under high magnification. Membranous change with spike formation is evident.
PAS stain.   × 1,000.

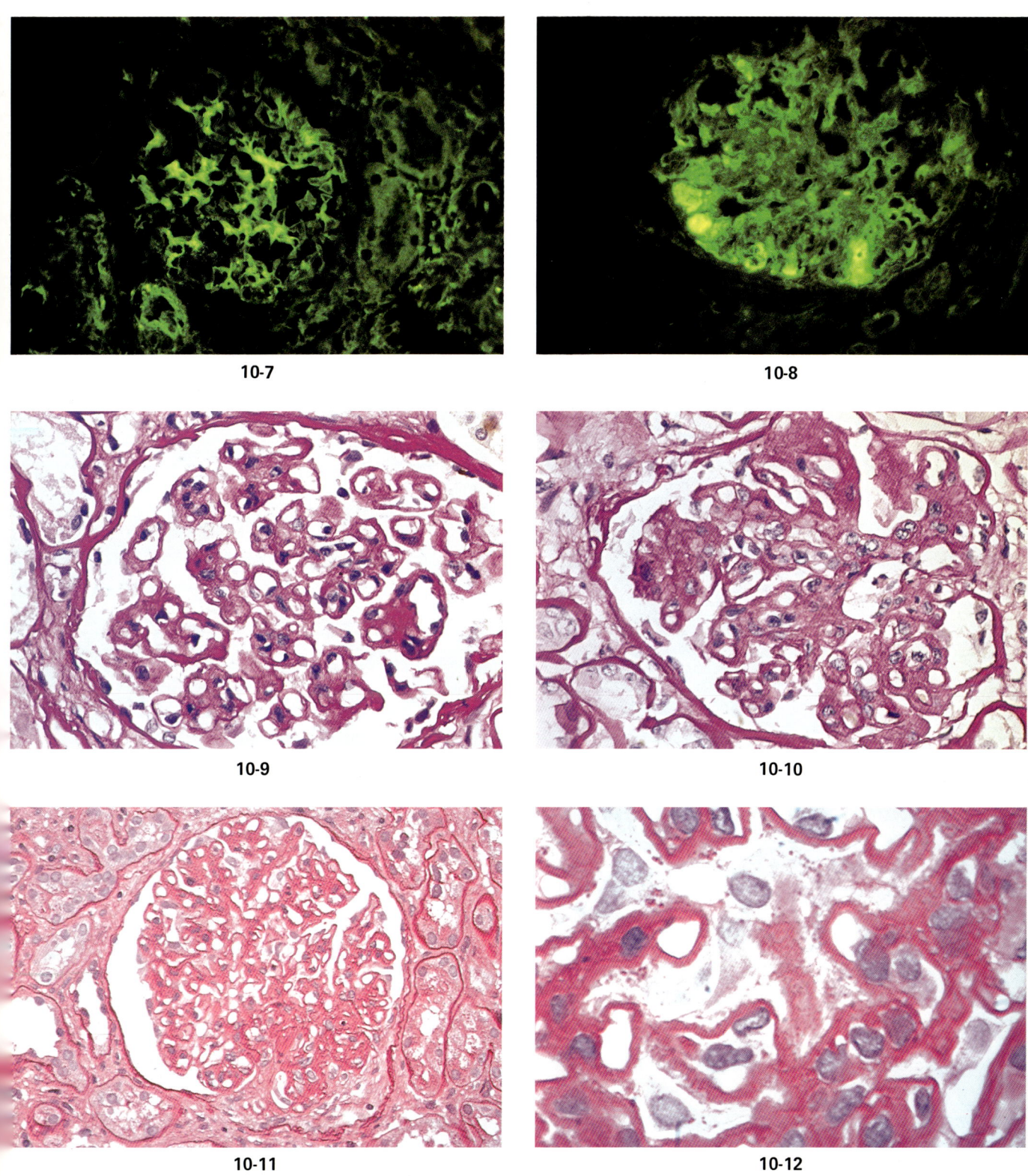

PARASITIC NEPHROPATHIES

Malarial Nephropathy

Fig. 10-13 Electron micrograph. Glomerular capillary loop showing "double outline" with cell cytoplasm between the original basement membrane (BM) and the inner layer of mesangial matrix. × 6,300.

Fig. 10-14 Electron micrograph. Diffuse thickening of the glomerular capillary basement membrane (BM) with small lacunae (l) imparting a plexiform appearance to the basement membrane. × 33,000.

P: podocyte, L: capillary lumen, U: urinary space.

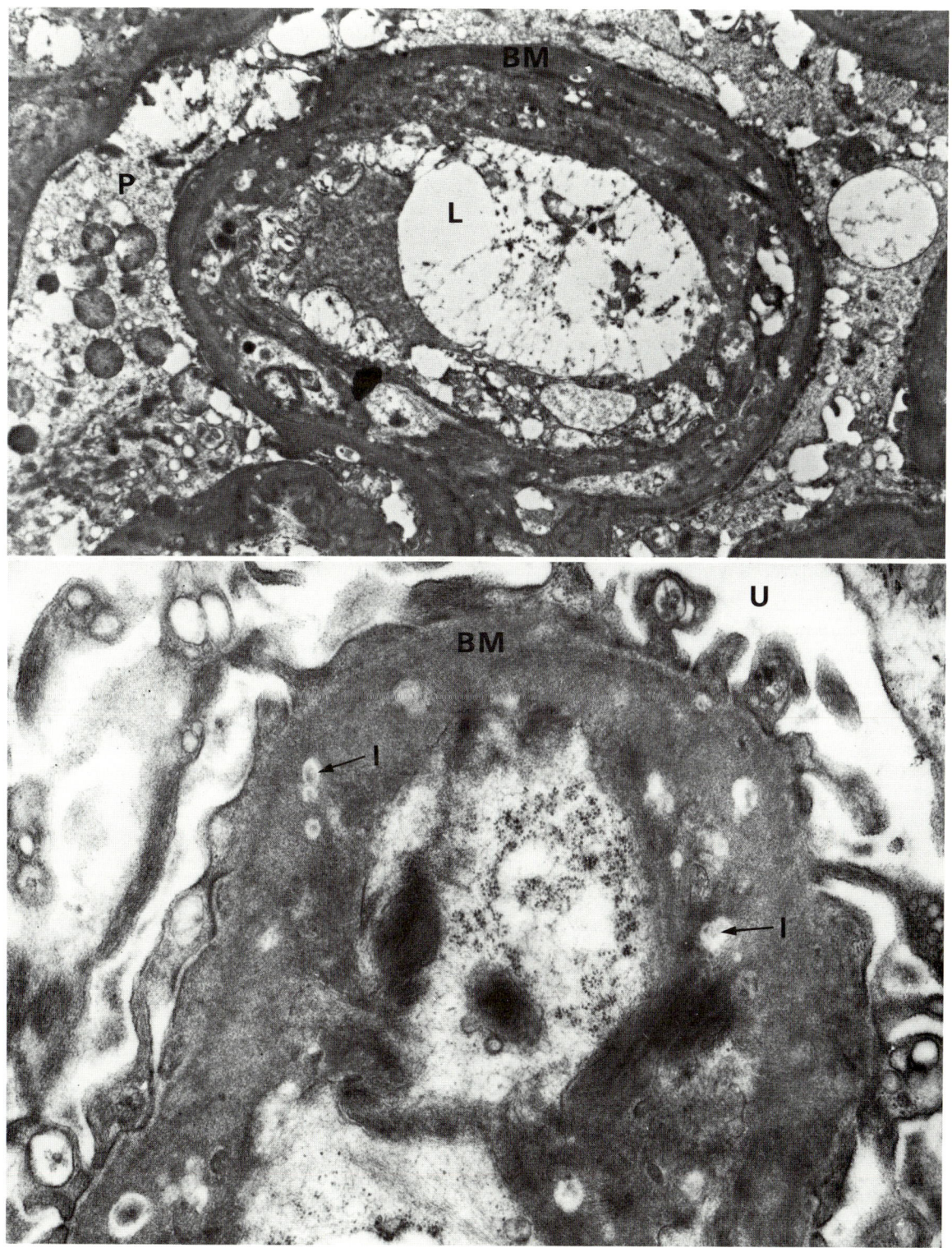

GLOMERULONEPHRITIS OF SYSTEMIC DISEASES

PARASITIC NEPHROPATHIES

Schistosomal Nephropathy

Fig. 10-15 Electron micrograph. Same case as Fig. 10-5. Part of glomerular mesangium showing small electron dense deposits (D) under the basement membrane (BM). x 21,000.

Fig. 10-16 Electron micrograph. Same case as Fig. 10-5. Small rarefaction (arrow) of basement membrane (BM) suggests the presence of subepithelial deposits. x 19,000.

MC: mesangial cell, U: urinary space.

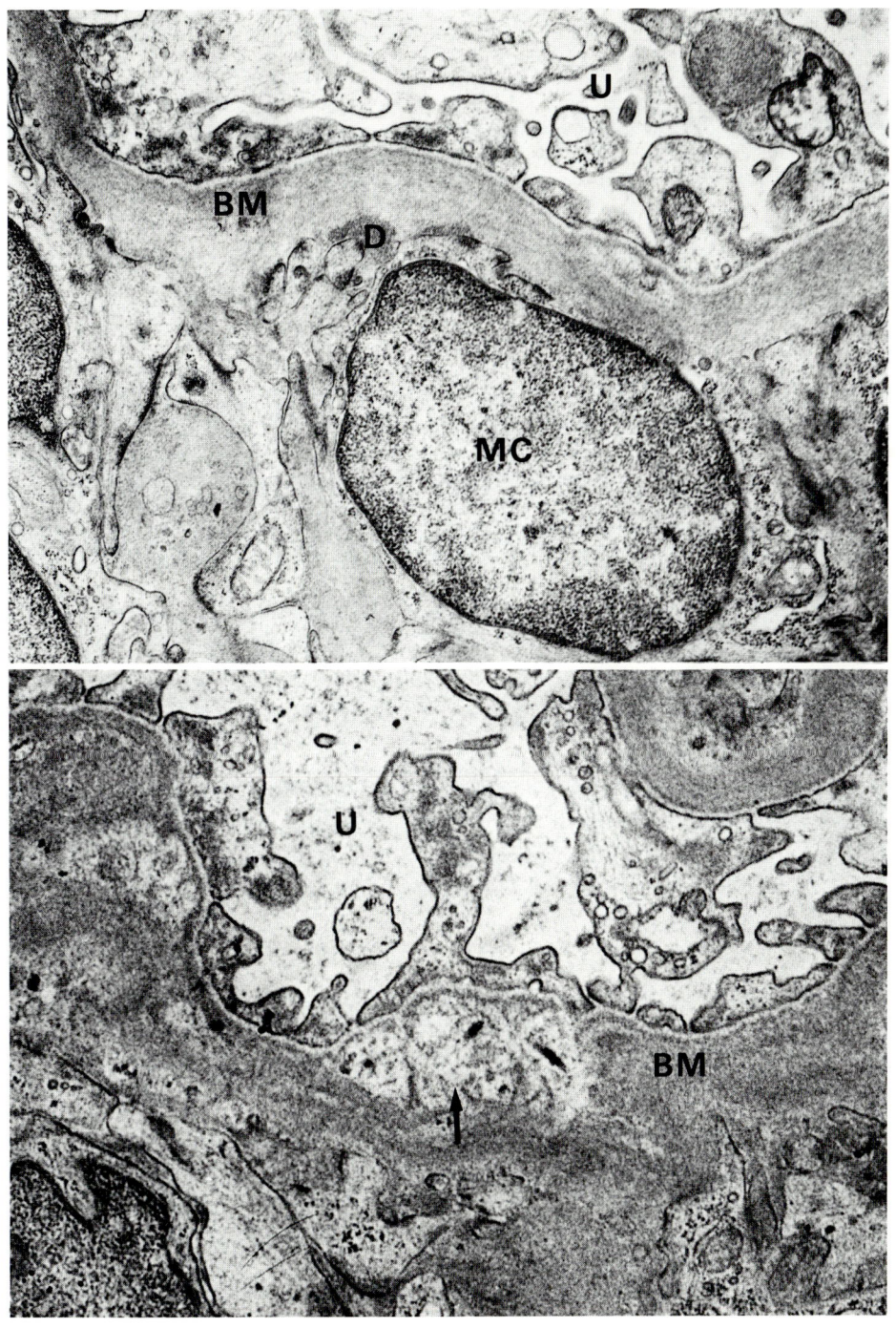

PARASITIC NEPHROPATHIES

Strongyloides Nephropathy

Fig. 10-17 Electron micrograph. Part of a glomerular capillary with "washed out" areas under the epithelium, suggestive of previous deposits. Projections of basement membrane (BM) (spikes) (S) are seen between the washed out areas. Same case as Fig. 10-11. × 20,000.

P: podocyte, L: capillary lumen.

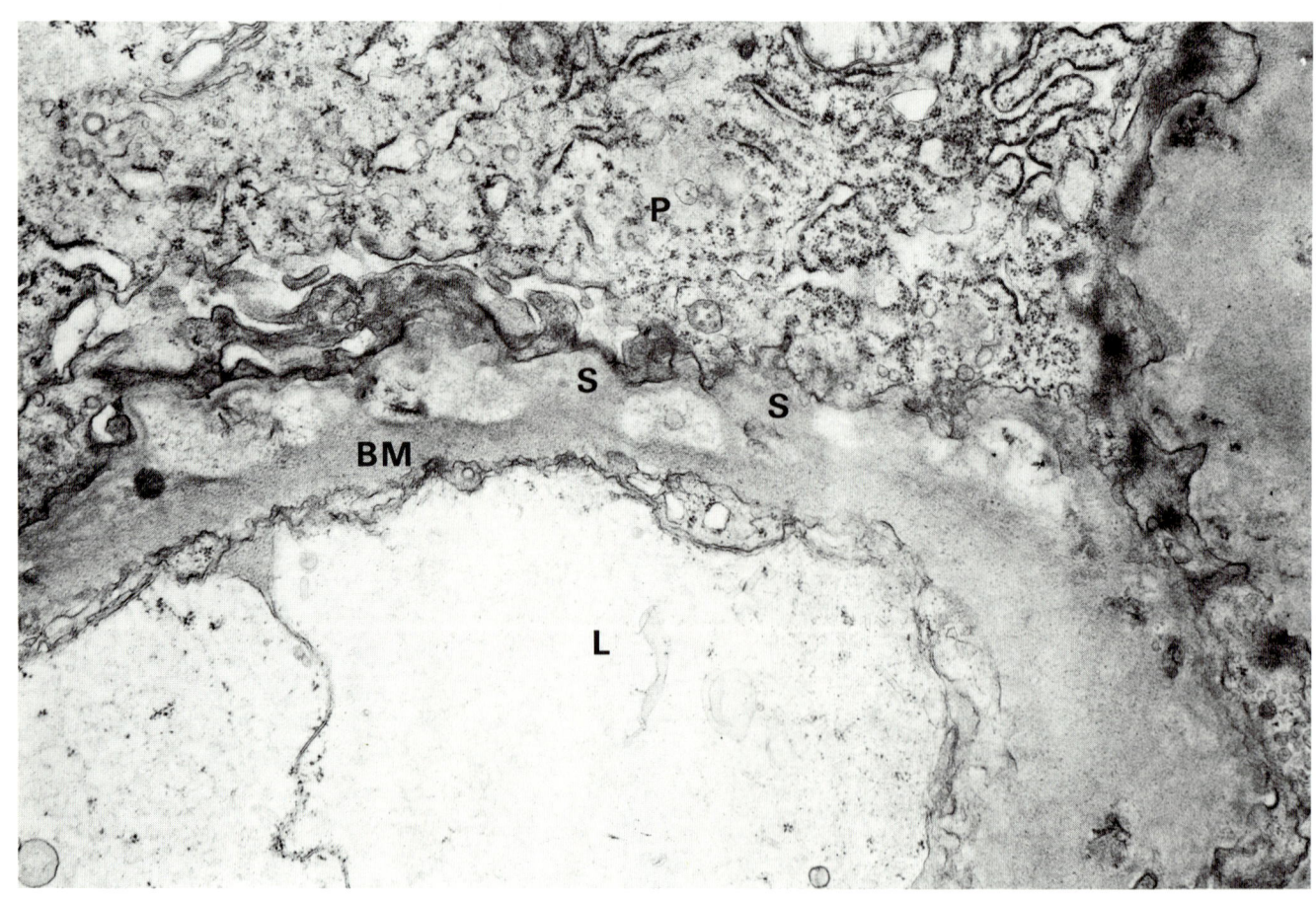

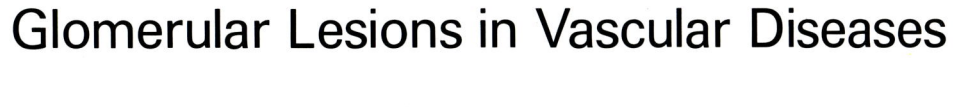

CHAPTER 11

Periarteritis Nodosa
 (Figs. 11-1 to 11-4 and Figs. 11-10 to 11-11)
Wegener's Granulomatosis
 (Figs. 11-5 to 11-9 and Figs. 11-12 to 11-13)

Periarteritis Nodosa and Wegener's Granulomatosis

Definition: Glomerular disease associated with various forms of idiopathic necrotizing angiitis, including the classical periarteritis nodosa (Kussmaul-Maier), hypersensitivity angiitis (microscopic periarteritis nodosa), Wegener's granulomatosis and allergic granulomatosis. This definition excludes angiitis of various systemic and renal diseases — systemic lupus erythematosus, scleroderma, cryoglobulinemia, Henoch-Schönlein purpura, Goodpasture's syndrome, post-infectious glomerulonephritis, etc. — which are discussed in other chapters of this book. Renal involvement in giant cell arteritis and Takayasu arteritis occurs very rarely, if at all, though Takayasu arteritis may lead to renal artery stenosis.

Clinical Manifestations: Multisystem involvement with fever, anemia, sometimes of microangiopathic type, arthralgias and neuritis occur in all forms of periarteritis nodosa. Allergic reaction to drugs with various cutaneous manifestations are common in the microscopic form. Necrotizing lesions of the upper respiratory tract including the mouth and middle ear, and pulmonary infiltrates with cavitation are characteristic of Wegener's granulomatosis. History of asthma or other allergies, striking blood eosinophilia and transient pulmonary infiltrates are typically seen in allergic granulomatosis.

Renal manifestations vary from none to rapidly progressive failure and anuria. In the past renal failure accounted for most of the deaths in Wegener's granulomatosis. Pain in the lumbar region is usually a sign of renal infarction. Gross or microscopic hematuria and proteinuria are most common symptoms. Occasionally a nephrotic syndrome develops. Hypertension, occasionally of the malignant type, is usually a late manifestation, most often complicating the classical periarteritis nodosa, and probably related to the narrowing of larger renal vessels by inflammation and thrombosis. Urinary sediment contains red cells and white blood cells as well as red cell casts, hyaline casts and occasionally also broad casts ("telescoped" urinary sediment).

Treatment with steroids, immunosuppressive drugs and with antihypertensives when indicated have been successful in many cases. In Wegener's granulomatosis prognosis has been radically improved by cyclophosphamide therapy, which also reverses many of the renal lesions.

Gross Appearance and Light Microscopy: Infarcts of various sizes are secondary to vascular obstruction, and eventually are converted into depressed scars. Actual vascular lesions are often absent from needle biopsy specimen, especially when larger arteries are involved. Glomerular lesions vary from capillary collapse due to ischemia, to focal or diffuse glomerulonephritis. Ischemia is more often associated with the classical periarteritis nodosa. In the other forms of arteritis the typical glomerular lesions are focal segmental thrombosis and necrosis with cellular proliferation and crescent formation. The latter may lead to diffuse crescentic glomerulonephritis, histologically indistinguishable from the idiopathic form of this disease. Granulomatous glomerulitis and interstitial granulomata are occasionally seen in Wegener's granulomatosis. Healing of segmental lesions leads to partial scarring of glomeruli and capsular adhesions, while diffuse crescentic glomerulonephritis ends in extensive glomerular obliteration. Mild to moderate mesangial proliferation may accompany the segmental lesions, and on occasion, true diffuse endocapillary or mesangiocapillary glomerulonephritis occurs.

Electron Microscopy generally amplifies the light microscopic findings in the mesangium, the capillary wall and the Bowman's space. Breaks in the basement membrane may be present. Small electron dense deposits are occasionally seen in the mesangium.

Immunofluorescence Microscopy is generally not characteristic. Deposits are either absent or are present segmentally as scattered granular deposits, particularly of IgG and C3, in the mesangium. Fibrin may be present in the capillaries or in the crescents. Rarely, granular and on occasion linear peripheral deposits may be noted.

PERIARTERITIS NODOSA

Fig. 11-1   Periarteritis nodosa in the kidney. Fibrinoid necrosis of an arteriole at the glomerular hilus, but only slight changes in the glomerules.
H&E stain.   x 260.

Fig. 11-2   Same case as Fig. 11-1. Glomerulus showing fibrin exudation and beginning crescent formation.
PAS stain.   x 260.

Fig. 11-3   Proliferative glomerulonephritis with moderate mesangial sclerosis.
PAS stain.   x 260.

Fig. 11-4   Same case as Fig. 11-3. Arteritis in subcutaneous tissue.
H&E stain.   x 410.

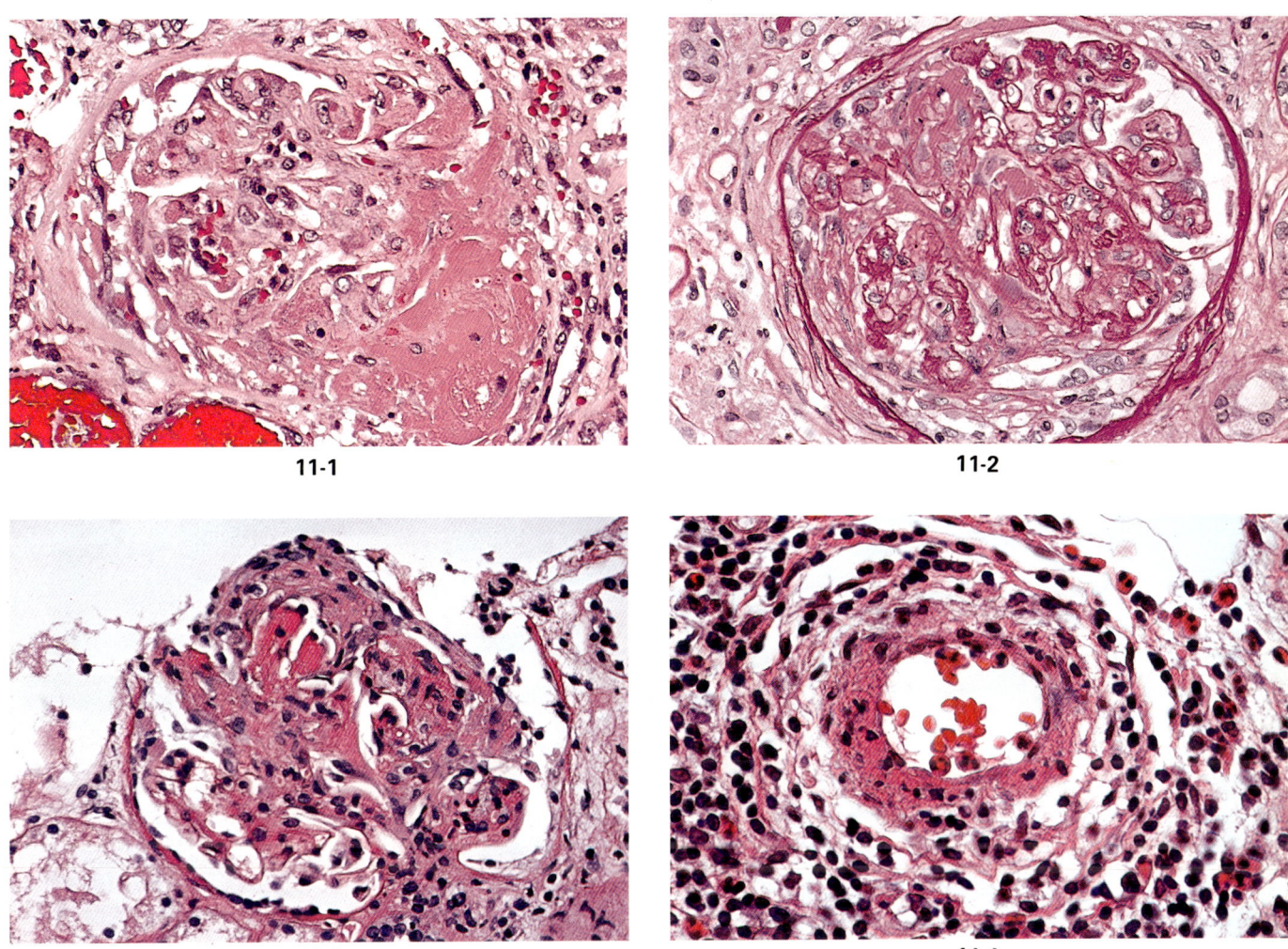

GLOMERULAR LESIONS IN VASCULAR DISEASES

WEGENER'S GRANULOMATOSIS

Fig. 11-5 Wegener's granulomatosis. Glomerulus showing segmental areas of necrosis.
H&E stain. × 260.

Fig. 11-6 Large crescent in the urinary space with partial collapse of the glomerular tuft.
PASM stain. × 260.

Fig. 11-7 Immunofluorescence microscopy. Mesangial deposits of C3.
× 410.

Fig. 11-8 Immunofluorescence microscopy. Extensive deposits of fibrin in the urinary space. × 260.

Fig. 11-9 Healed glomerulitis in Wegener's granulomatosis. Segmental areas of sclerosis adherent to the Bowman's capsule.
H&E stain. × 260.

WEGNER'S GRANULOMATOSIS

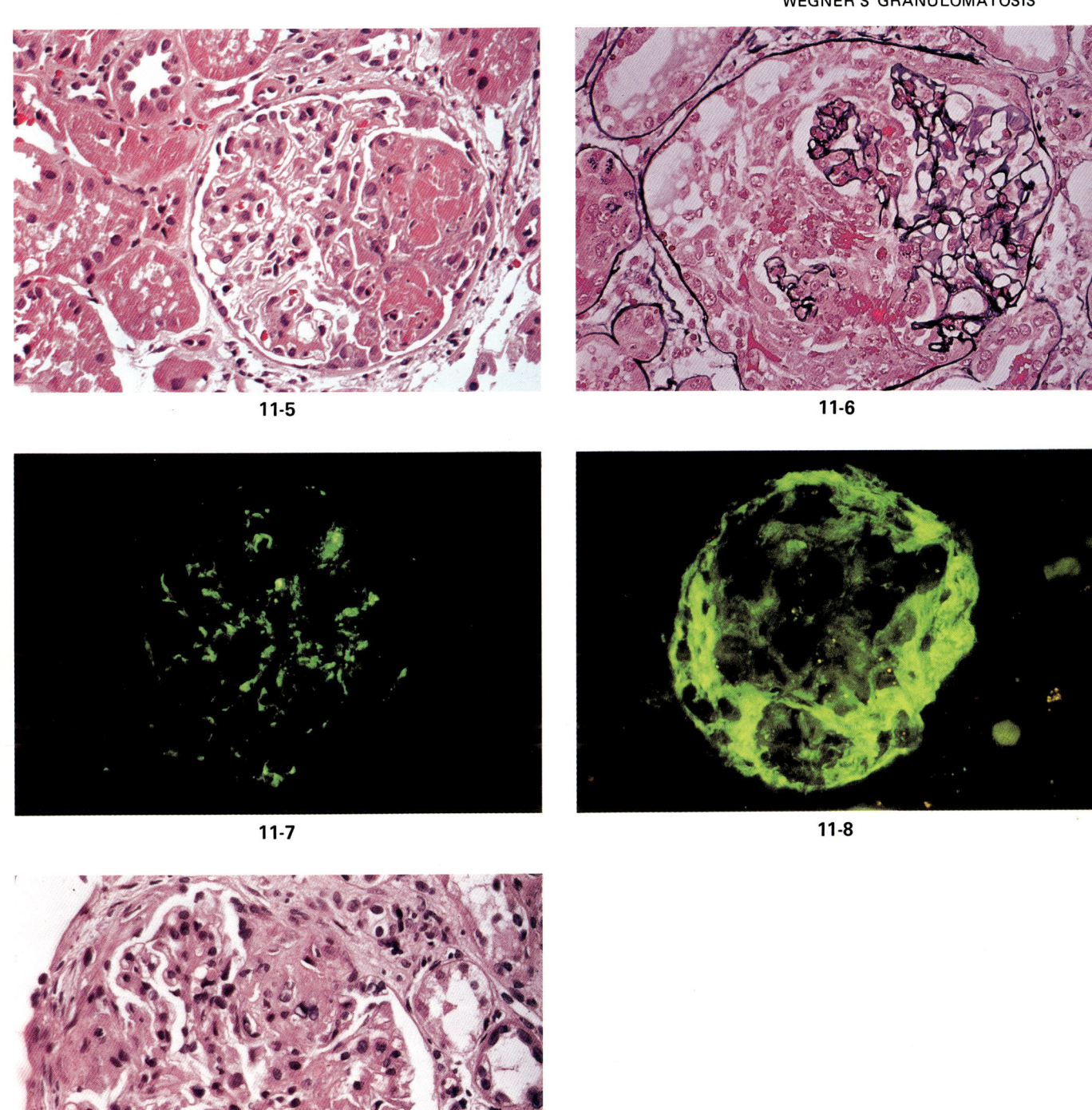

11-5

11-6

11-7

11-8

11-9

GLOMERULAR LESIONS IN VASCULAR DISEASES

PERIARTERITIS NODOSA

Fig. 11-10 Electron micrograph. Same case as Fig. 11-3. Part of a glomerulus showing subendothelial electron dense deposits (D), probably fibrin, in the capillary loop, as well as mononuclear cells in the capillary lumen and the urinary space (U) x 4,600.

Fig. 11-11 Electron micrograph. Same case as Fig. 11-3. Fibrinoid necrosis of a small renal artery. x 9,600.

BM: basement membrane, L: vascular lumen.

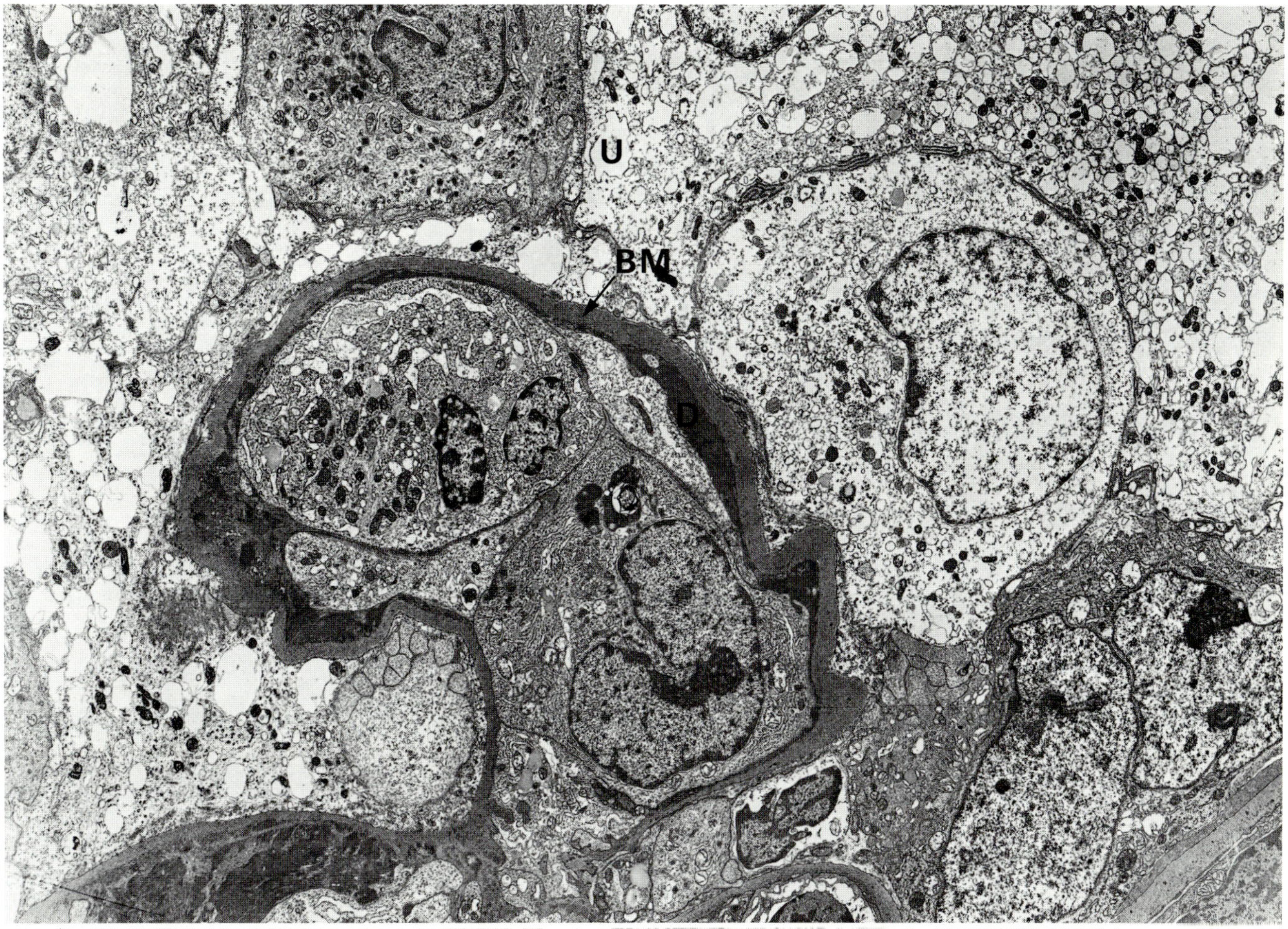

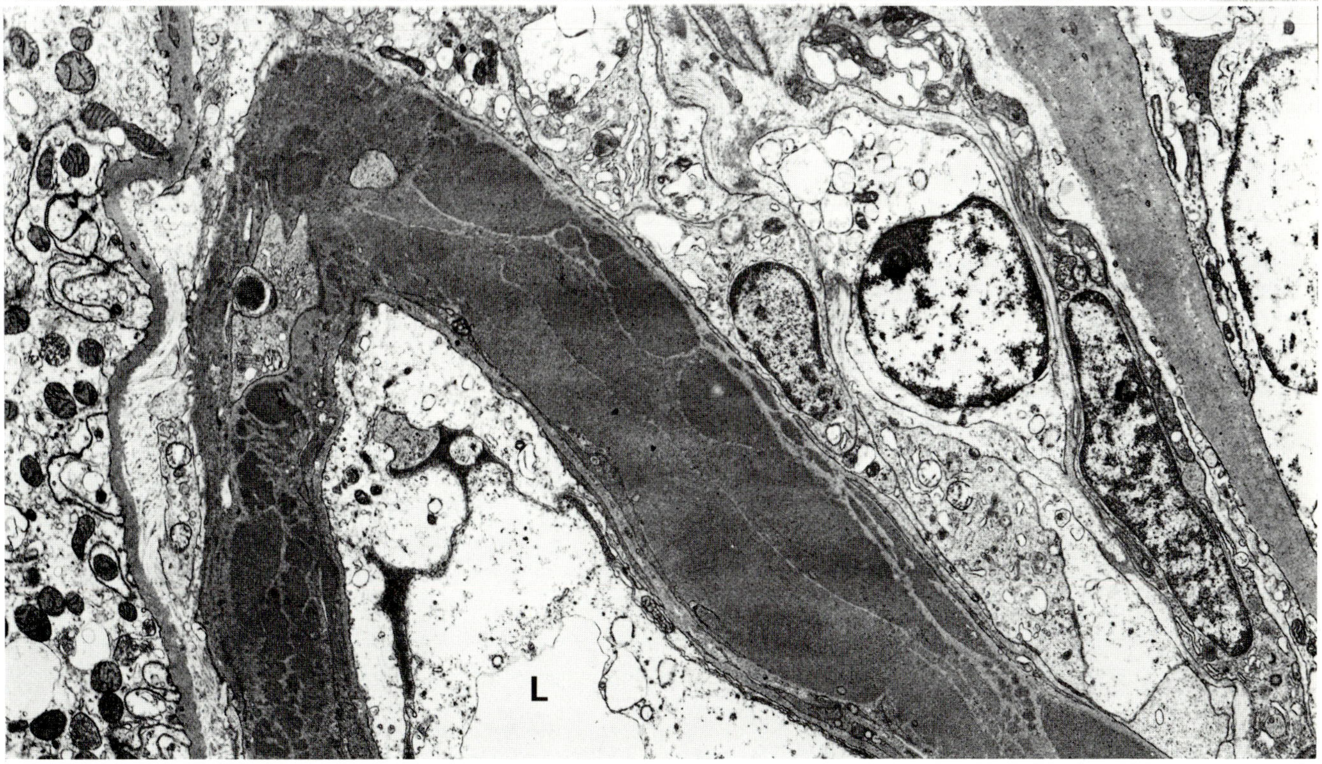

WEGENER'S GRANULOMATOSIS

Fig. 11-12 Electron micrograph. Same case as Fig. 11-5. Part of a glomerular tuft showing mesangial proliferation. Fibrin (F) is present in the left upper corner of the picture, overlaying the basement membrane (BM). Under the basement membrane there is accumulation of granular material (GrD).
x 6,600.

Fig. 11-13 Electron micrograph. Part of a glomerulus showing disruption of the basement membrane (BM) and spilling of fibrin (F) into the urinary space. Note small dense areas in the lamina densa of the basement membrane (fibrin ?, immune deposits ?). x 8,000.

MC: mesangial cell. MM: mesangial matrix.

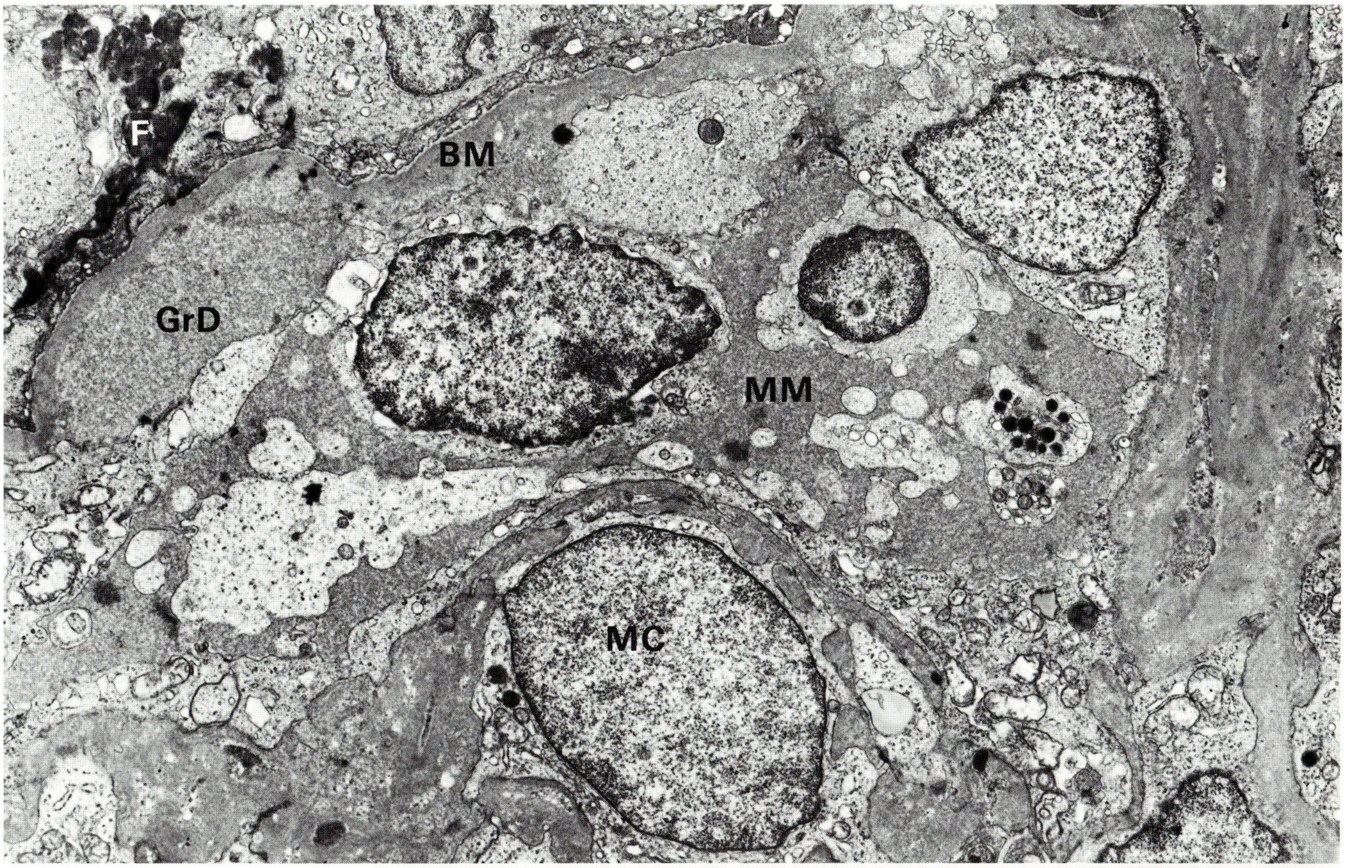

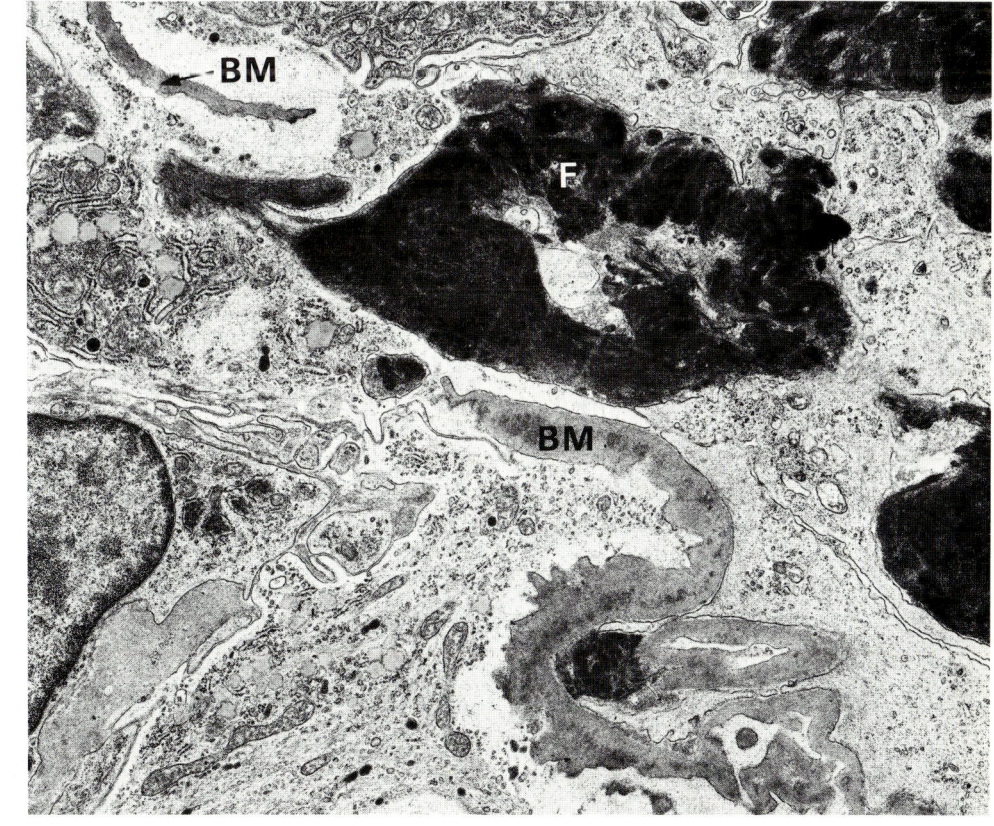

CHAPTER 12

Hemolytic-Uremic Syndrome
  (Figs. 12-1 to 12-13 and Figs. 12-20 to 12-23)
Thrombotic Thrombocytopenic Purpura
  (Figs. 12-14 to 12-16)
Glomerular Thrombosis
  (Figs. 12-17 to 12-19)

Thrombotic Microangiopathy
(Hemolytic-Uremic Syndrome and Thrombotic Thrombocytopenic Purpura)

Definition: Glomerular and arteriolar disease associated with changes in the vascular walls and intraluminal thrombosis, and accompanied by a clinical syndrome of hemolytic anemia, fragmentation of red blood cells and thrombocytopenia. In one form, known as hemolytic-uremic syndrome, there is severe renal disease with oliguria and uremia, but few extrarenal manifestations. In the second form, thrombotic thrombocytopenic purpura, the renal changes are similar but considerably milder, but widespread systemic manifestations are common.

Clinical Manifestations: Hemolytic-uremic syndrome is most common in children, especially in boys under the age of four years, but also occurs in adults. It often follows a gastrointestinal or an upper respiratory illness. There is usually a latent interval of a few days or 1–2 weeks before the onset of weakness, vomiting, pallor, purpura, hematemesis and bloody diarrhea. Anemia is of the hemolytic type with elevation of reticulocyte count. Fragmented erythrocytes appear as "burr", "helmet" or "arrow" cells in smears. Thrombocytopenia is often profound, but other coagulation factors are affected little if at all.

Renal symptoms include hematuria, proteinuria and rapidly developing oliguria with uremia. With proper supportive treatment including dialysis, mortality or irreversible renal failure is of the order of 5% in children, but much higher in adults. In the latter age group, hemolytic-uremic syndrome is often a complication of an immunologic disease such as systemic lupus erythematosus; hormonal imbalance (pregnancy, contraceptive medication), puerperium (postpartum renal failure); malignant hypertension, or transplant rejection. Patients who recover may have recurrent attacks, develop malignant hypertension or chronic renal disease ("chronic sclerosing glomerulonephritis").

Thrombotic thrombocytopenic purpura usually develops without a prodromal syndrome. It occurs mainly in adults and is more frequent in females. It may be idiopathic or secondary, in the same manner as hemolytic-uremic syndrome. Systemic manifestations, especially the involvement of central nervous system, predominate over renal abnormalities, which are moderate or mild. Prognosis is generally poor and death is due to cerebral damage, cardiac failure or hemorrhage.

Light Microscopy: Renal involvement varies from case to case and from glomerulus to glomerulus. The latter show many non-specific changes such as striking congestion, or on the contrary, capillary collapse, mild cellular proliferation, rare crescents, and occasionally total infarction. More specific is thickening of the capillary walls with formation of double outlines, thrombosis of lumina and the presence of red cell fragments. Mild lesions apparently resolve completely. Severe lesions lead to bland glomerular sclerosis with preservation of lobular architecture, but few if any capsular adhesions.

Arterioles and small arteries, occasionally up to the size of arcuates are also affected by subendothelial swelling and luminal thrombosis. Medial hypertrophy may be seen in cases of longer duration. Some arterioles, particularly those at the hilus, develop aneurysms, which undergo partial thrombosis, organization and endothelialization (so-called "glomeruloid structures"). Narrowing of arterial lumina in hemolytic-uremic syndrome may lead to focal or more widespread infarction up to diffuse cortical necrosis. Malignant nephrosclerosis develops in some patients.

Electron Microscopy: The capillary wall changes are characterized by separation of endothelium from the basement membrane and accumulation of pale fluffy material in the newly formed space. Within this material lie scattered fine fibrils (microfibrils), occasional strands of fibrin, fragments of red blood cells and platelets, and cytoplasmic processes of endothelial and mesangial cells. Electron dense deposits are uncommon. A newly formed thin basement membrane often follows the outline of the endothelial cells. The mesangium is also affected by accumulation of pale material, edema, reticulation and disruption of the matrix, leading, in more severe cases, to mesangiolysis, degeneration of mesangial cells and deposition of fibrin. The more advanced mesangial lesions heal by sclerosis often leading to capillary obliteration.

Endothelial separation and fluffy material are also found in the walls of small arteries, producing "mucoid" or hyaline thickening of the intima.

Immunofluorescence Microscopy: Fibrinogen or fibrin-related antigen are usually present in the early stages in the capillary wall and the mesangium, but may be absent later on. Occasionally IgM, IgG and perhaps other immunoglobulins can be demonstrated, together with complement components (C3, C1q). Similar changes are seen in the walls of arteries and arterioles. Fibrin is invariably present in the thrombi.

Glomerular Thrombosis

Definition: This is defined by the presence within the glomerular capillaries of eosinophilic masses often containing fibrin. The endothelial cells are relatively normal.

The prototype of glomerular thrombosis is the experimental Generalized Shwartzman Phenomenon (GSP) where properly spaced injections of endotoxin lead to deposition of fibrin in the capillary lumina and sometimes also under the endothelium. The human analogue of GSP is the gram-negative sepsis, which may result in terminal shock and renal failure associated with glomerular capillary thrombi. Although glomerular involvement in hemolytic-uremic syndrome and thrombotic thrombocytopenic purpura (see there) bears a similarity to GSP, it is probably an expression of localized endothelial damage rather than of generalized intravascular coagulation. Endothelial damage is probably also responsible for thrombosis in transplant rejection, and for the instances of localized segmental thrombosis in diffuse or focal proliferative glomerulonephritis, Henoch-Schönlein purpura, Goodpasture's syndrome, malignant hypertension and scleroderma. In all of these thrombosis may be followed by necrosis and secondary crescent formation. Glomerular thrombi in cryoglobulinemia and in systemic lupus erythematosus are of different nature, being composed mainly of immune complexes. However fibrin thrombosis also occurs in lupus, leading to localized necrosis.

GLOMERULAR LESIONS IN VASCULAR DISEASES

THROMBOTIC MICROANGIOPATHY

Hemolytic-Uremic Syndrome

Fig. 12-1 Blood smear typical of microangiopathic hemolytic anemia. Note burr cells, helmet cells and an arrow cell.
Wright's stain.   x 1,000.

Fig. 12-2 Hemolytic-uremic syndrome. Glomerulus showing slight mesangial widening without significant cellular proliferation.
PAS stain.   x 260.

Fig. 12-3 Hemolytic-uremic syndrome. Glomerulus showing moderately diffuse cellular proliferation.
H&E stain.   x 260.

Fig. 12-4 Glomerulus showing slight cellular proliferation, lobulation of the tuft and a small crescent.
PAS stain.   x 260.

Fig. 12-5 Numerous thrombi in the glomerular capillaries.
H&E stain.   x 260.

Fig. 12-6 Glomerulus showing many fragmented Rbc's. Note thrombus in the arteriole at the glomerular hilus (right lower corner).
H&E stain.   x 410.

HEMOLYTIC-UREMIC SYNDROME

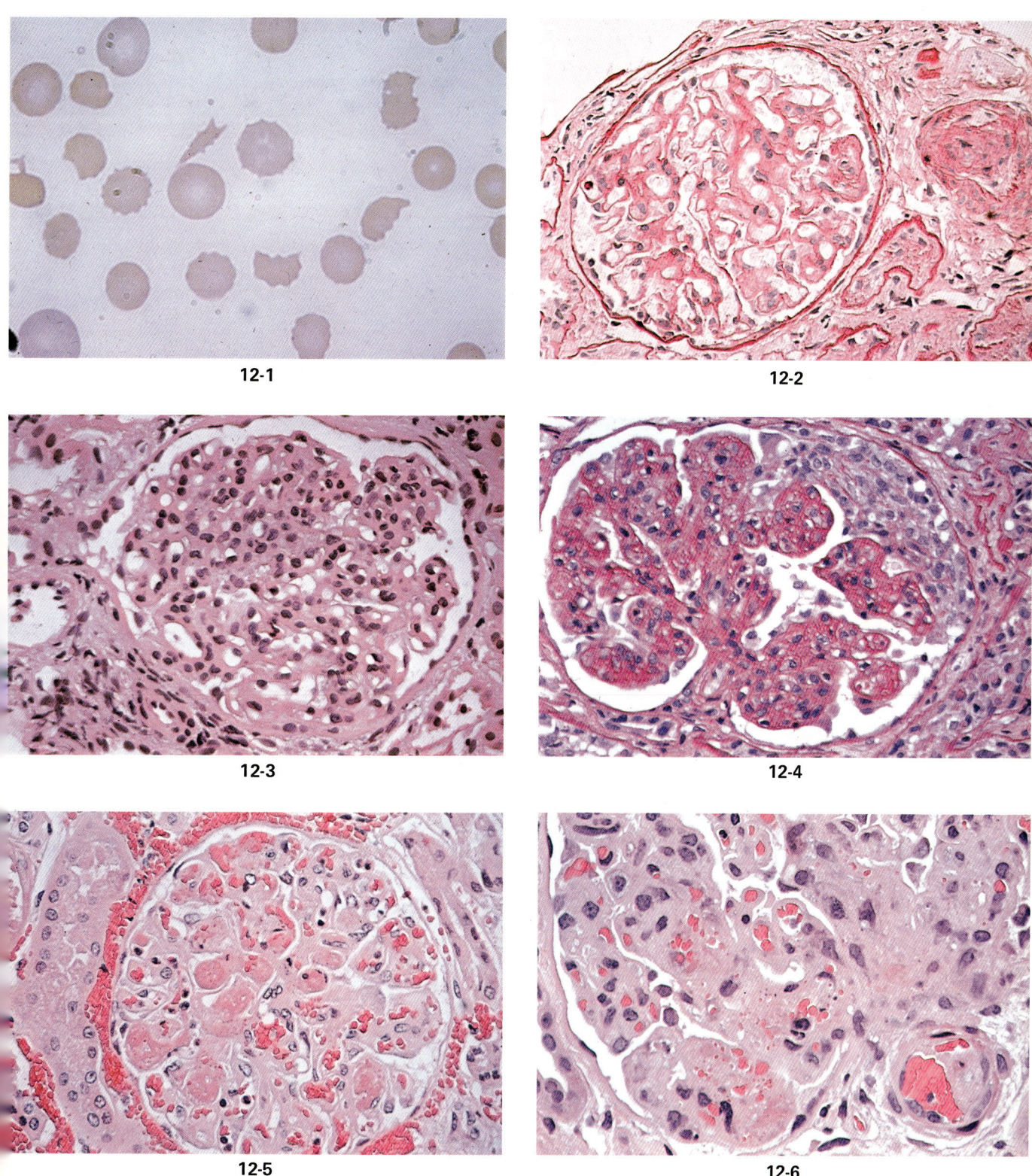

12-1

12-2

12-3

12-4

12-5

12-6

GLOMERULAR LESIONS IN VASCULAR DISEASES

Hemolytic-Uremic Syndrome

Fig. 12-7   Glomerulus showing thickening of capillary walls with prominent double outlines.
PAS stain.   x 410.

Fig. 12-8   Immunofluorescence microscopy. Extensive deposits of fibrinogen along the capillary walls.   x 260.

Fig. 12-9   Immunofluorescence microscopy. Deposits of IgG in the glomerular mesangium and along some capillary walls.   x 260.

Fig. 12-10   Advanced glomerular sclerosis. There is distinct lobulation of the tuft, lack of capsular adhesions and almost complete absence of cell.
PAS stain.   x 260.

Fig. 12-11   Area of tubular necrosis in the renal cortex.
H&E stain.   x 100.

Fig. 12-12   Same case as Fig. 12-3. "Hyaline" thickening of the walls of small arteries in the renal cortex.
PAS stain.   x 410.

HEMOLYTIC-UREMIC SYNDROME

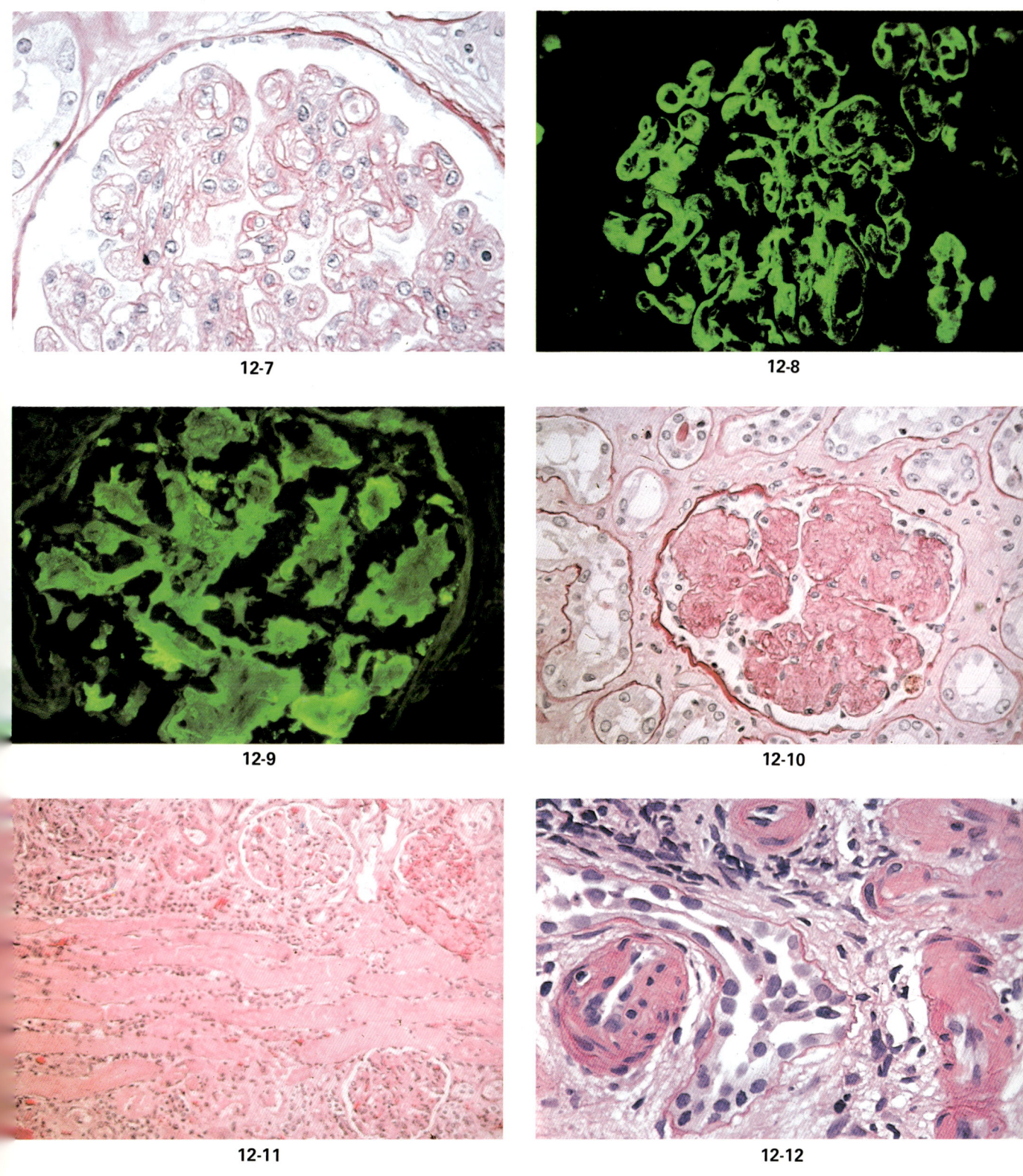

12-7

12-8

12-9

12-10

12-11

12-12

Hemolytic-Uremic Syndrome

Fig. 12-13 Small artery in the renal cortex showing marked mucoid thickening of the intima and severe narrowing of the lumen.
H&E stain.   x 260.

THROMBOTIC THROMBOCYTOPENIC PURPURA

Fig. 12-14 Thrombotic thrombocytopenic purpura. Small thrombi in the capillaries of a glomerlus.
PTAH stain.   x 260.

Fig. 12-15 Same case as Fig. 12-14. Fibrin thrombus in a small artery.
PTAH stain.   x 260.

Fig. 12-16 Same case as Fig. 12-14. Aneurysmal dilatation, thrombosis and organization of an arteriole at the glomerular hilus (so-called glomeruloid lesion).
PAS stain.   x 410.

GLOMERULAR THROMBOSIS (INTRAVASCULAR COAGULATION)

Fig. 12-17 Large glomerular thrombi in a patient with disseminated intravascular coagulation.
H&E stain.   x 260.

Fig. 12-18 Case of intravascular coagulation. Fibrin deposits in small arteries.
PAS stain.   x 260.

Fig. 12-19 Same case as Fig. 12-18. Fibrin filling the lumen of an arteriole.
PTAH stain.   x 410.

GLOMERULAR THROMBOSIS

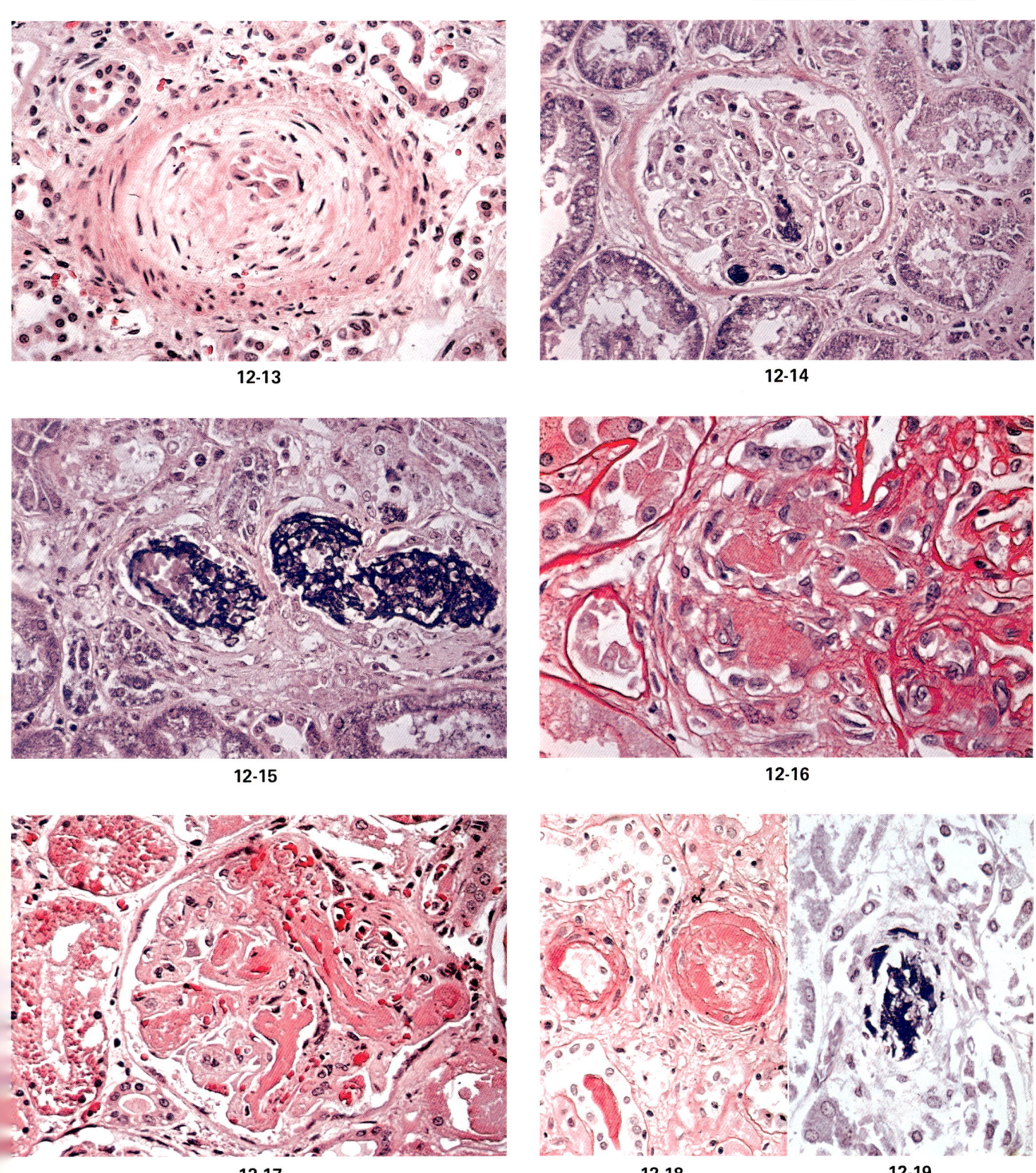

12-13

12-14

12-15

12-16

12-17

12-18

12-19

GLOMERULAR LESIONS IN VASCULAR DISEASES

Hemolytic-Uremic Syndrome

Fig. 12-20 Electron micrograph. Typical case of hemolytic-uremic syndrome. Mesangiolysis with much edema and reticulation of mesangial matrix (MM).
x 34,000.

Fig. 12-21 Electron micrograph. Glomerular capillary showing marked widening of the subendothelial space, which is filled with loose fibrillar and granular material and small remnants of cytoplasm. A thin irregular basement membrane (bm) separates the detached endothelium (En) from the subendothelial space. The foot processes (FP) are partly effaced.   x 25,000.

U: urinary space, BM: basement membrane.

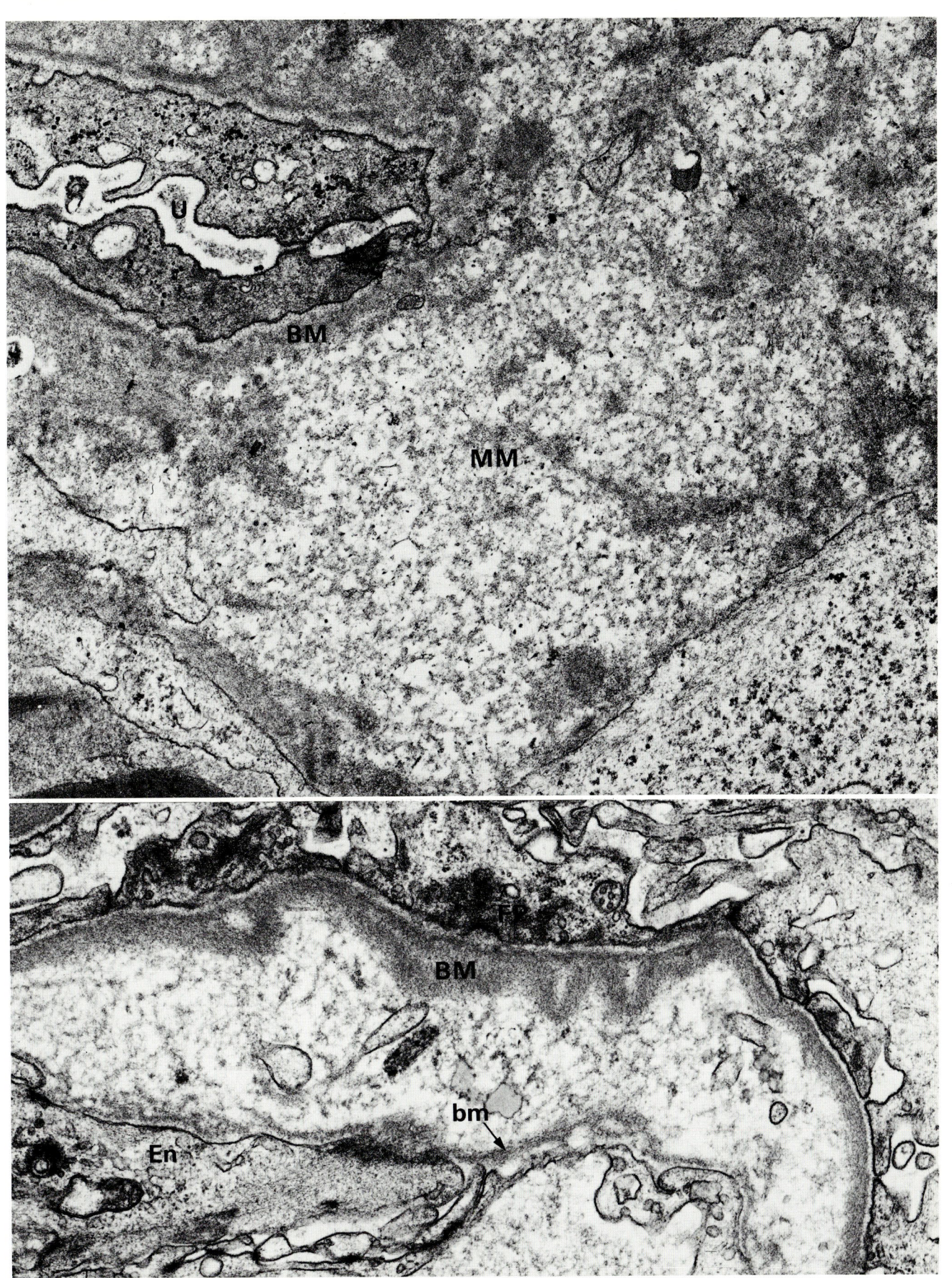

GLOMERULAR LESIONS IN VASCULAR DISEASES

Hemolytic-Uremic Syndrome

Fig. 12-22 Electron micrograph. Advanced lesion similar to that in Fig. 12-21. In addition to the granular material, two Rbc's are seen in the markedly widened subendothelial space. The foot processes (FP) are extensively effaced.   x 20,000.

Fig. 12-23 Electron micrograph. Same case as Fig. 12-3. Part of a wall of small artery. The vascular endothelium (En) (right upper corner) is separated from its basement membrane. The resulting space is filled with finely granular and fibrillar material and remnants of cell cytoplasm.   x 12,000.

U: urinary space, BM, bm: basement membrane, RBC: red blood cell, SM: smooth muscle.

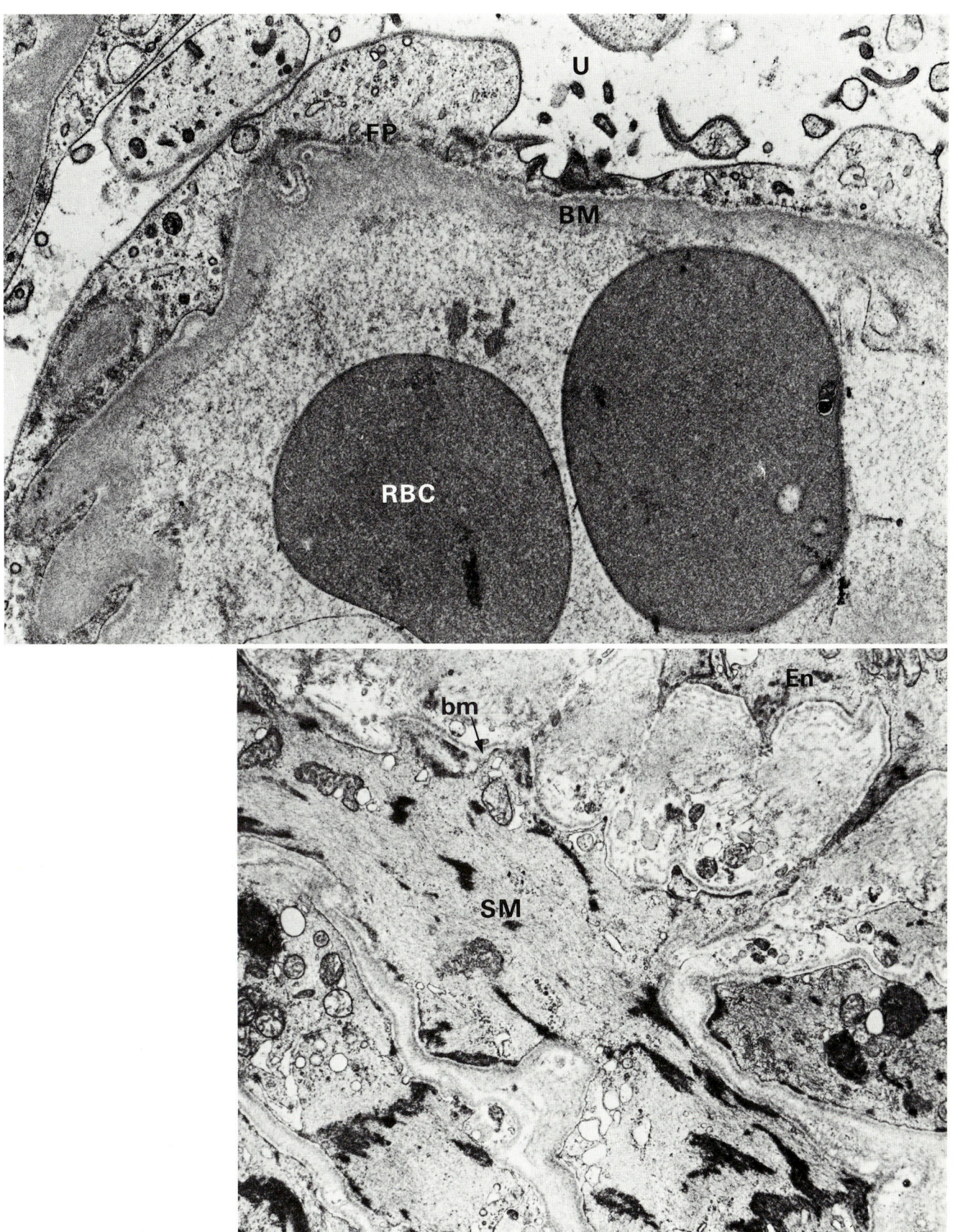

CHAPTER 13

Benign Nephrosclerosis
    (Figs. 13-1 to 13-4 and Fig. 13-17)
Malignant Nephrosclerosis
    (Figs. 13-5 to 13-8 and Fig. 13-18)
Scleroderma
    (Figs. 13-9 to 13-16 and Figs. 13-19 to 13-21)

Benign Nephrosclerosis

Definition: Glomerular lesions associated with benign hypertension and due to moderate ischemia caused by the narrowing of the arterial tree, especially of the arterioles. The glomeruli show various degrees of glomerular collapse with thickening and wrinkling of basement membranes. In advanced stages the collapsed tuft is accompanied by fibrous obliteration of Bowman's space. Hyalinization of arterioles and intimal thickening and fibrosis of arteries are always present.

Clinical Manifestations: Benign essential hypertension is characterized by moderate elevation of blood pressure (diastolic of 90 to 120 mm Hg but occasionally higher), cardiac enlargement and a tendency to coronary artery disease, cardiac failure and cerebral hemorrhage. Renal changes are generally mild and renal failure is rare. Minimal microscopic hematuria and trace proteinuria eventually develop in many patients and on occasion nephrotic syndrome supervenes.

Light Microscopy: The most typical vascular change is hyaline sclerosis of arterioles, especially afferent arterioles, best seen at the glomerular hilus. The arteriolar wall is thickened by homogeneous eosinophilic material which lies under the endothelium and infiltrates the media. The lumen is proportionately narrowed. Arteries may show medial hypertrophy and subsequent intimal sclerosis.

The glomeruli show wrinkling and apparent thickening of the capillary walls and frequently mild to moderate mesangial thickening. Diminution of the luminal cross-sections is generally proportional to the arteriolar narrowing, but is sometimes due to the narrowing of larger vessels. Progressive collapse of the capillary tuft is accompanied by accumulation of hyaline material in some of the remaining capillaries and by fibrous thickening of Bowman's capsule with splitting and reduplication of its basement membrane. Progressive deposition of fibrous tissue on its inner aspect (fibrous crescent) leads to obliteration of the urinary space. Vascular and glomerular lesions are not uniformly distributed. They are most prominent in the cortical scars, while adjacent areas may contain normal or nearly normal glomeruli. In many cases the glomerular mesangium is slightly widened. With more severe vascular disease approaching the levels of malignant hypertension, segmental areas of hyalinization, slight cellular proliferation and sclerosis may be seen, especially at the hilus but also elsewhere in the glomerulus. This process, sometimes known as alterative glomerulitis is generally due to ischemia, but on occasion to embolization by platelet microthrombi or atherosclerotic material from the aorta or main renal artery. The sclerotic lesions bear a good deal of resemblance to focal segmental sclerosis associated with nephrotic syndrome, or to healed focal glomerulonephritis.

Focal tubular atrophy with interstitial fibrosis and focal lymphocytic infiltration accompanies the glomerular disease. In cases where severe narrowing affects the large vessels, on the order of main and interlobar arteries, tubular atrophy is diffuse and disproportional to the degree of glomerular collapse.

Electron Microscopy: The glomerular basement membranes along the periphery of the capillaries are wrinkled but generally not thickened. Mesangial expansion is mainly due to increase of mesangial matrix. Occasionally small deposits may be seen in the mesangium. The fibrous crescents contain large amounts of collagen.

Malignant Nephrosclerosis

Definition: Glomerular changes secondary to malignant hypertension and severe renal ischemia. Malignant hypertension is defined by very high diastolic pressure (over 130 mm Hg), retinopathy with papilledema, hemorrhages and exudates, and renal failure. Malignant nephrosclerosis is usually secondary to another renal disease, such as benign nephrosclerosis, glomerulonephritis or pyelonephritis, but in a considerable proportion of cases, it is "primary". There is some evidence that some of the primary cases follow a recognized or unrecognized attack of hemolytic-uremic syndrome. On the other hand, hemolytic-uremic syndrome or microangiopathic anemia occasionally develop during the course of malignant hypertension. Some consider all cases associated with or preceded by hemolytic-uremic syndrome as true primary malignant hypertension.

Clinical Manifestations: Renal failure develops rapidly but in its earlier stages may be reversed by antihypertensive therapy. Gross or microscopic hematuria and proteinuria are almost invariably present. The latter occasionally falls in the nephrotic range.

Light Microscopy: The arterial lesions are of two types: "onion-peel" mucoid thickening of the intima in the arteries up to the size of arcuate, and fibrinoid necrosis of the arterioles. Neither lesion is accompanied by inflammatory reaction, but both lead to severe narrowing of the lumina, sometimes aggravated by thrombosis. Fibrinoid necrosis may be reversed by anti-hypertensive therapy, but mucoid intimal thickening is much more resistant to treatment.

If malignant hypertension is superimposed upon a pre-existing renal disease, glomeruli show appropriate changes, e.g. diffuse sclerosing glomerulonephritis or ischemic collapse. In primary malignant hypertension most glomeruli show only slight or moderate capillary wall wrinkling. However, fibrinoid necrosis of the arterial wall often extends into the glomerulus, and leads to segmental crescent formation. In contradistinction to crescentic glomerulonephritis such lesions involve only a few glomeruli, rarely more than one-third. In the early stages of idiopathic malignant hypertension, tubular atrophy is minimal but diffuse atrophy may eventually develop. The juxtaglomerular apparatus often shows hypertrophy and hypergranulation.

Electron Microscopy shows capillary wall wrinkling and, particularly in cases with microangiopathic anemia, widening of the subendothelial zone with translucent deposits. Mesangium shows edema of the matrix and rarely, true mesangiolysis.

Immunofluorescence Microscopy: Fibrin or fibrin-related antigens are present in the areas of fibrinoid necrosis, in the glomerular crescents and in the mucoid intimal thickening of the arteries. Necrotic areas may also contain immunoglobulins (IgM, IgG) and complement (C3) but the significance of these findings is unknown. They possibly represent a non-specific trapping.

Scleroderma
(Systemic Sclerosis)

Definition: Renal lesions associated with scleroderma, involving arteries and glomeruli. These lesions are very similar to those of Malignant Nephrosclerosis but occur even in the absence of hypertension.

Clinical Manifestations: Progressive sclerotic changes of skin and internal organs occur mostly in adults, particularly in females. The skin becomes smooth, thick and stiff, beginning in extremities and spreading to face and body. Vascular changes (Raynaud's phenomenon, trophic ulcers of fingers and toes) are frequent. Involvement of the gastrointestinal tract, lungs and heart leads to dysphagia, malabsorption, reduced vital capacity and cardiac failure. Renal disease is common and may run a slowly progressive course or an acute rapidly progressive course. The symptoms include proteinuria, azotemia and hypertension. Proteinuria is generally mild, but nephrotic syndrome is seen occasionally. Azotemia and hypertension, particularly of malignant type, usually but not always occur together and indicate severe involvement, ending in rapid renal failure. In some patients there is evidence of microangiopathic anemia. Renal angiography may show vasoconstrictive response to cold paralleling the Raynaud's phenomenon in the extremities. It has been suggested that vasoconstriction precipitates the severe arterial disease.

Light Microscopy: In the slowly progressive disease the vascular lesions resemble those of benign nephrosclerosis, but tend to be limited to the arcuate and interlobular arteries. In severe rapidly progressive disease arterial changes are similar to those of malignant hypertension, but occur also in patients who have normal blood pressure. Arcuate and interlobular arteries show marked "mucoid" intimal thickening while larger vessels often exhibit adventitial fibrosis. Fibrinoid necrosis, unaccompanied by inflammation, is seen in the arterioles. It tends to involve the glomeruli and leads to crescent formation. Glomeruli may also show capillary wall wrinkling and occasionally mild cellular proliferation. Hyperplasia of the juxtaglomerular apparatus is common. Severe narrowing of the arterial tree and superimposed thrombosis result in infarction of glomeruli and tubules and cortical infarcts of various sizes.

Electron Microscopy recapitulates changes seen on light microscopy. In the glomeruli mild mesangial thickening and segmental thickening of basement membranes are seen occasionally.

Immunofluorescence Microscopy: Fibrin or fibrinogen and occasionally immunoglobulins (IgM, IgG, IgA) and complement (C3, C1q) are seen in the areas of fibrinoid necrosis. Fibrin-related antigens are also present in the "mucoid" intimal thickening.

GLOMERULAR LESIONS IN VASCULAR DISEASES

BENIGN NEPHROSCLEROSIS

Fig. 13-1 Benign nephrosclerosis. There is contraction and sclerosis of glomerular tufts, tubular atrophy and marked thickening of the wall of a small artery (left upper corner).
PAS stain. x 100.

Fig. 13-2 Benign nephrosclerosis. Intimal fibrosis of a small artery with narrowing of the lumen.
H&E stain. x 180.

Fig. 13-3 Benign nephrosclerosis. Hyaline deposits in the wall of an arteriole.
PAS stain. x 410.

Fig. 13-4 Benign nephrosclerosis. Glomerulus showing almost complete collapse of the capillary tuft.
PAS stain. x 390.

BENIGN NEPHROSCLEROSIS

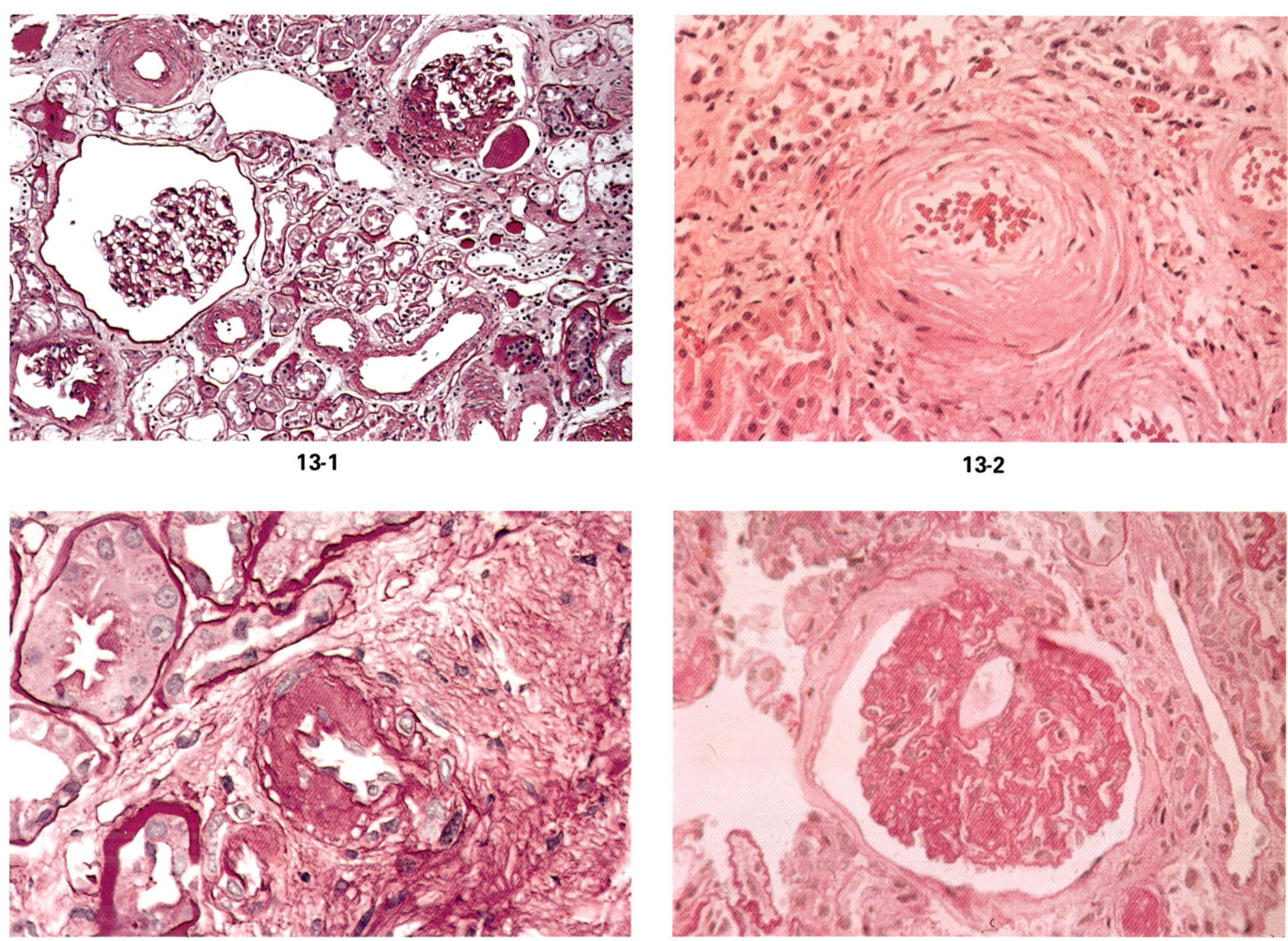

13-1

13-2

13-3

13-4

GLOMERULAR LESIONS IN VASCULAR DISEASES

MALIGNANT NEPHROSCLEROSIS

Fig. 13-5 Malignant nephrosclerosis. Striking "onion peel" thickening of the intima of a small artery with marked constriction of the lumen.
PAS stain. x 260.

Fig. 13-6 Fibrinoid necrosis of an arteriole at the glomerular hilus.
H&E stain. x 260.

Fig. 13-7 Partial collapse of a glomerular tuft.
PAS stain. x 410.

Fig. 13-8 Glomerulus showing partial collapse of the tuft and proliferation of cells in the urinary space suggestive of early crescent formation.
PAS stain. x 260.

SCLERODERMA

Fig. 13-9 Scleroderma. Small artery of a kidney showing loose intimal fibrosis and narrowing of the lumen. The internal elastica is well preserved.
Elastica-Van Gieson stain. x 100.

Fig. 13-10 Intimal thickening and thrombosis of a small renal artery.
Trichrome stain. x 260.

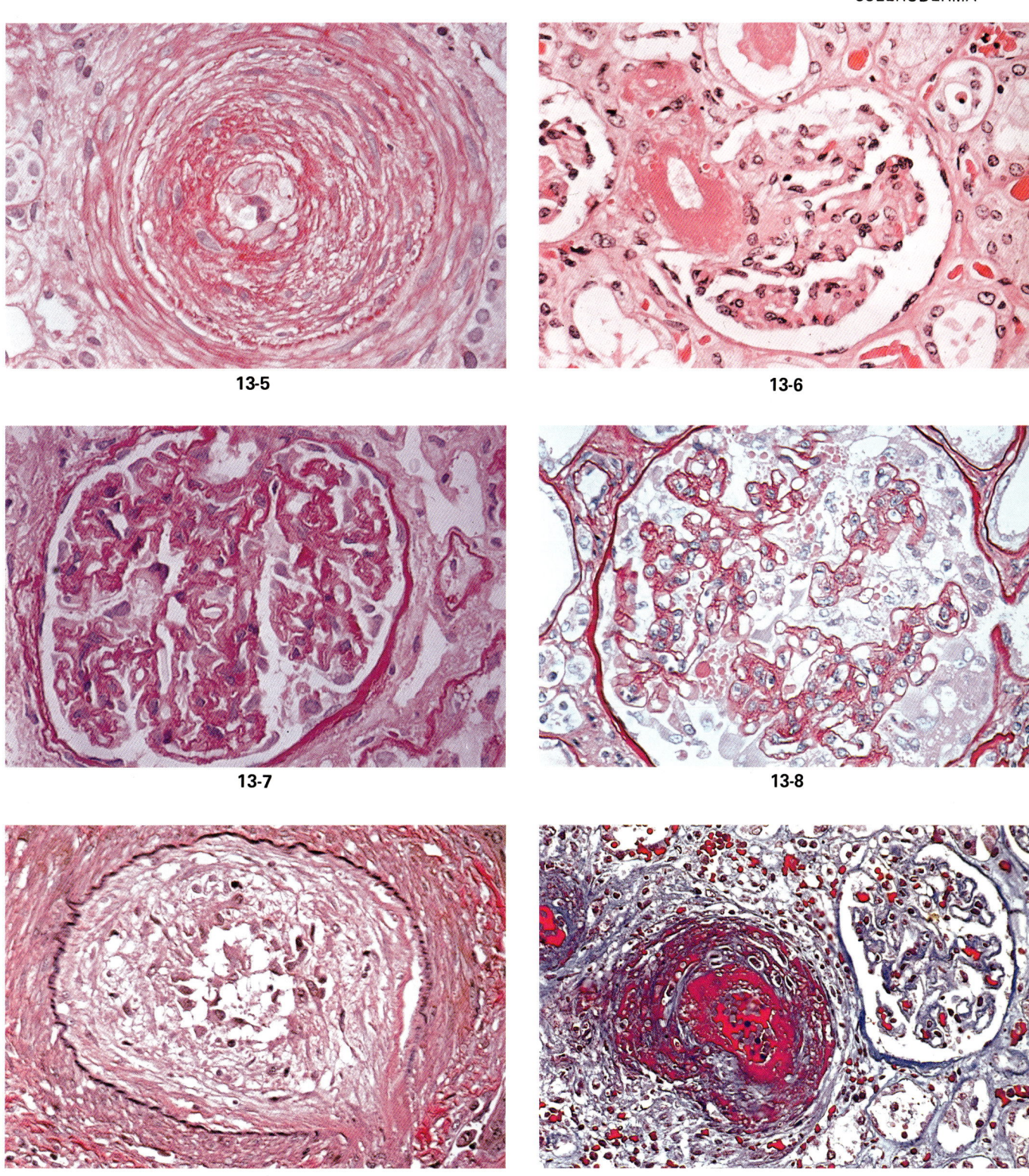

SCLERODERMA

Fig. 13-11 Same case as Fig. 13-10. True fibrinoid arteritis in scleroderma.
H&E stain. x 100

Fig. 13-12 Glomerulus showing thickening of capillary walls.
H&E stain. x 410.

Fig. 13-13 Same case as Fig. 13-12. With PAS stain capillary wall thickening is partly due to wrinkling.
PAS stain. x 410.

Fig. 13-14 Immunofluorescence microscopy. Same case as Fig. 13-12. Deposits of IgG mainly mesangial in distribution. x 260.

Fig. 13-15 Immunofluorescence microscopy. Same case as Fig. 13-10. Deposits of IgM in the glomerulus and in the wall of a hilar arteriole (left side of the picture). x 260.

Fig. 13-16 Immunofluorescence microscopy. Same case as Fig. 13-15. Fibrinogen deposits in the glomeruli and in the walls of small arteries. x 100.

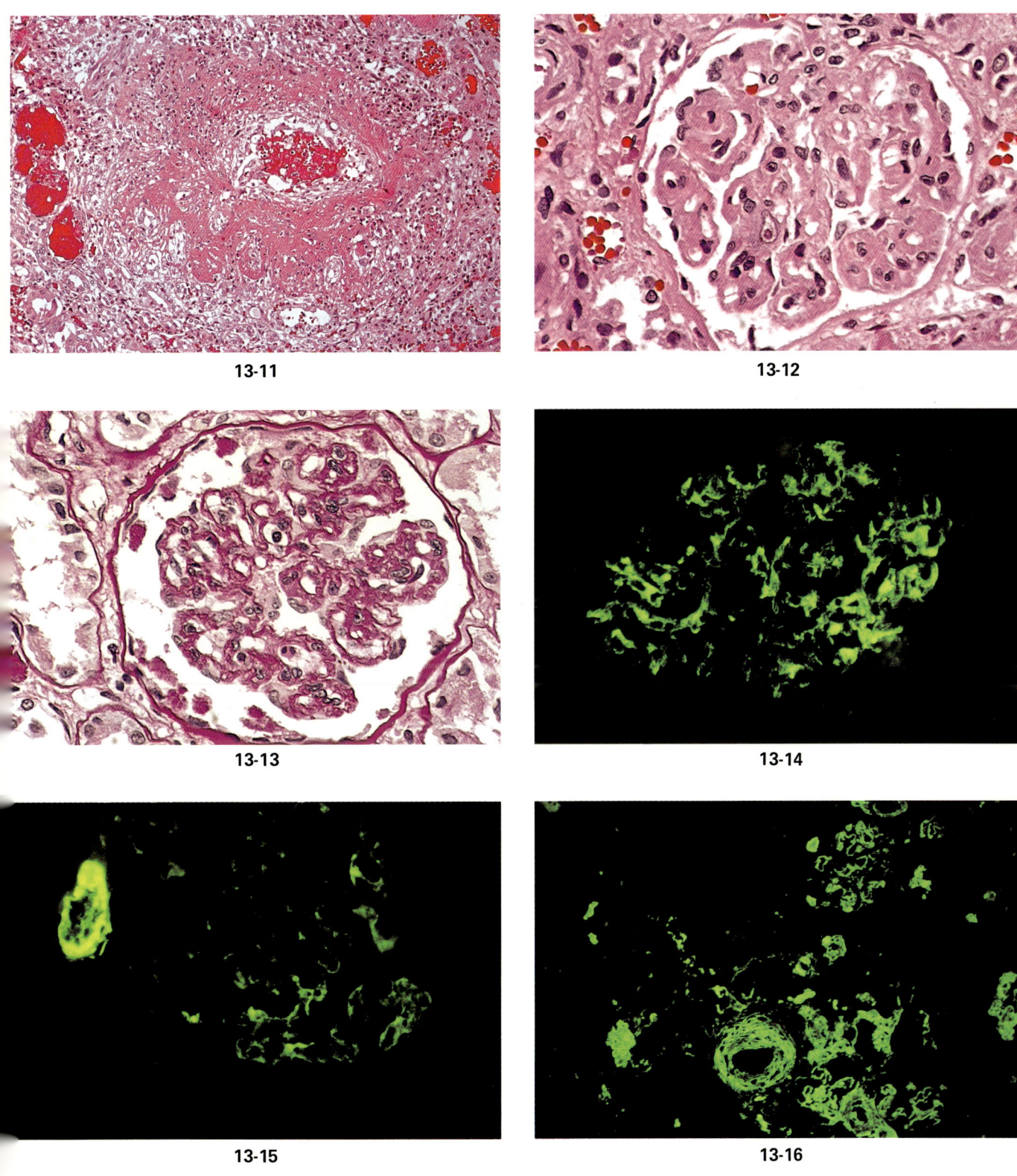

GLOMERULAR LESIONS IN VASCULAR DISEASES

BENIGN NEPHROSCLEROSIS

Fig. 13-17 Benign nephrosclerosis. Electron micrograph. Part of a glomerular tuft showing collapsed wrinkled capillaries and loose fibrous tissue filling most of the urinary space (U) and capillary lumina (L).   x 7,000.

MALIGNANT NEPHROSCLEROSIS

Fig. 13-18 Electron micrograph. Malignant nephrosclerosis. Part of a hyperplastic juxtaglomerular apparatus showing heavily granulated cells. x 6,600.

BM: basement membrane, JGC: juxtaglomerular cell, BC: Bowman's capsule, Cap: capillary.

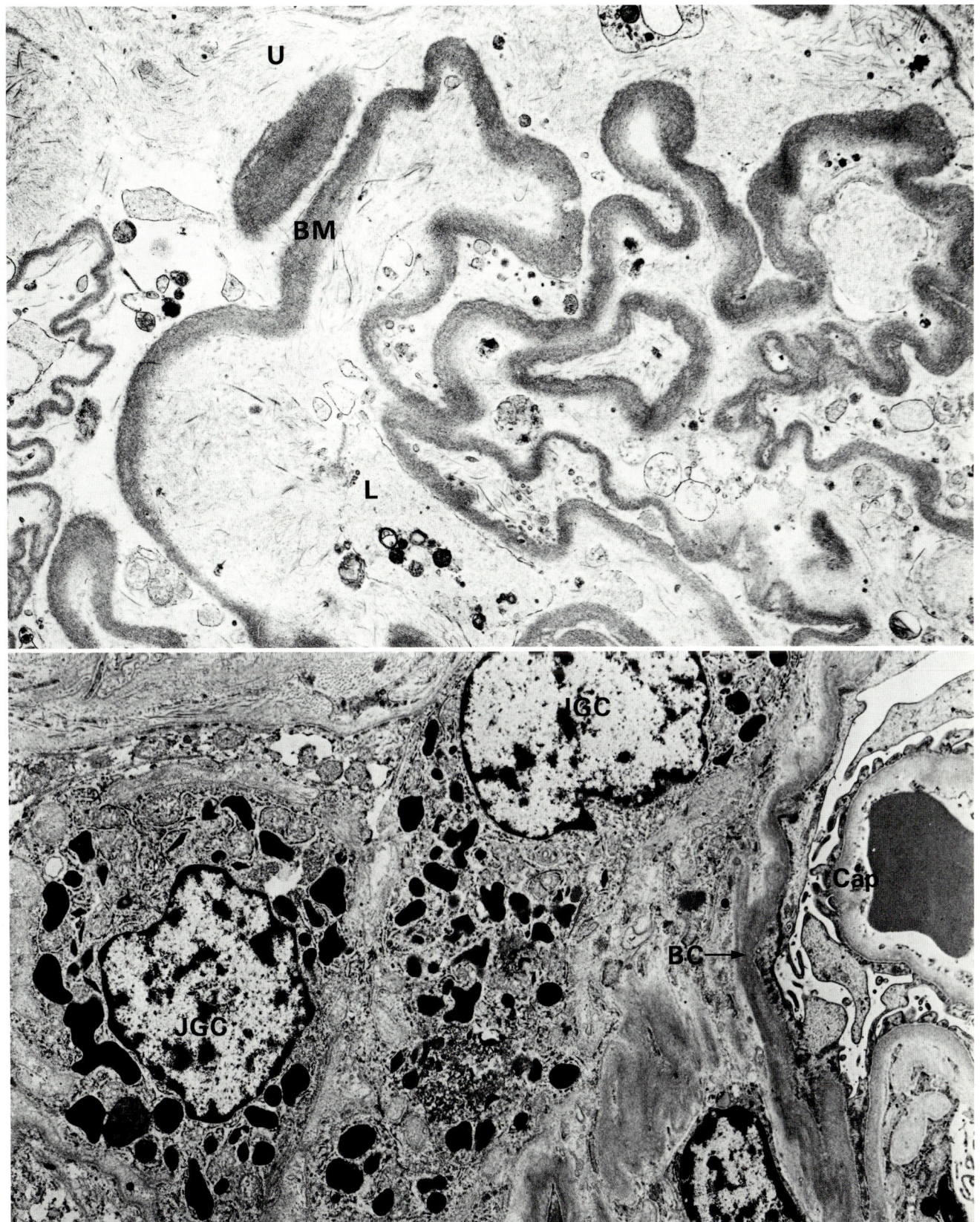

SCLERODERMA

Fig. 13-19 Electron micrograph. Same case as Fig. 13-12. Wall of a glomerular capillary showing subendothelial (paramesangial) electron dense deposits (D).
x 24,000.

Fig. 13-20 Electron micrograph. Walls of glomerular capillaries showing thickening and notching of the lamina densa of the basement membrane (BM). Note focal effacement of foot processes (FP) and microvilli (MV) in the urinary space.
x 16,000.

U: urinary space.

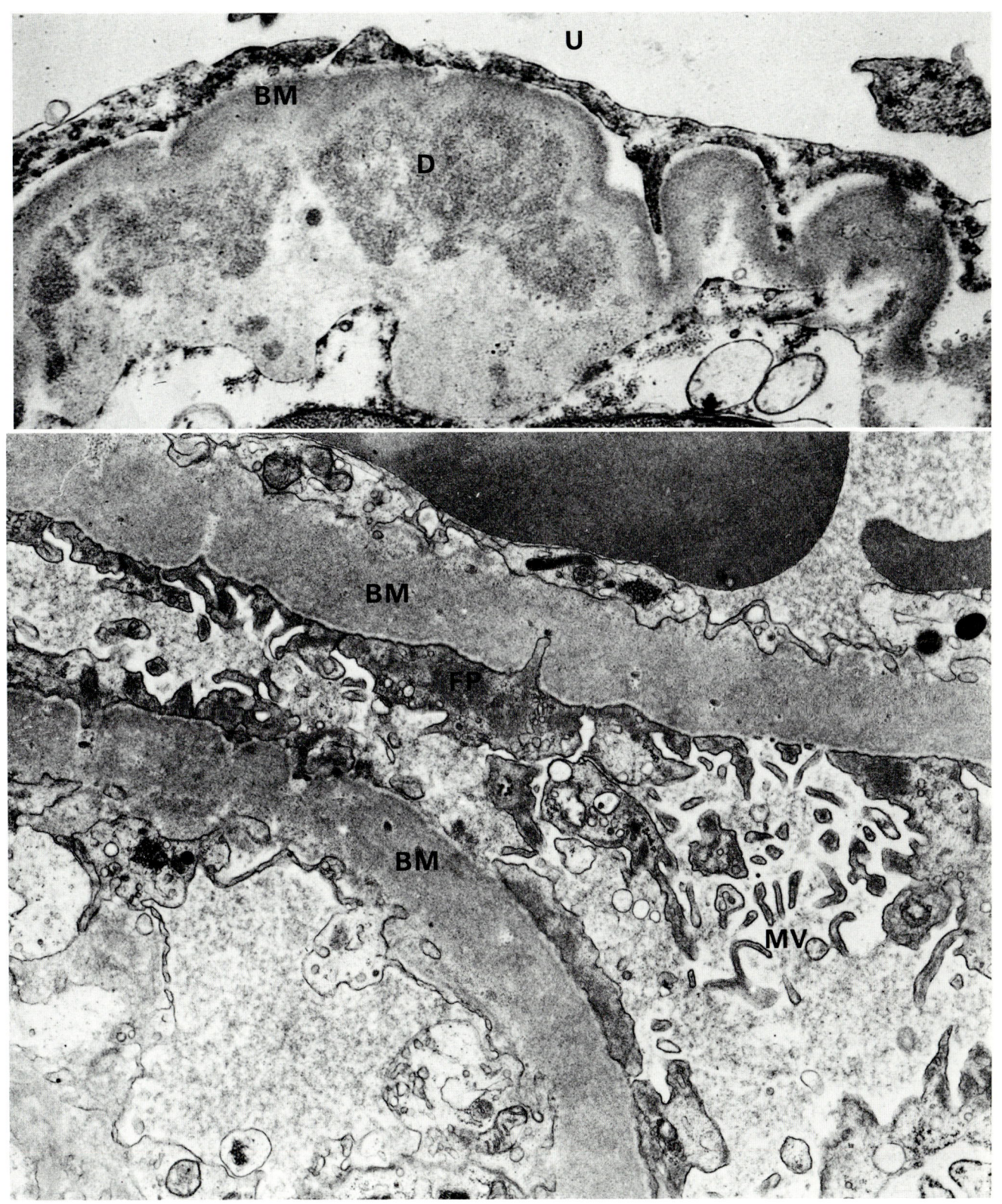

SCLERODERMA

Fig. 13-21 Electron micrograph. Part of a glomerular tuft showing collapse of the capillaries (Cap) and hyperplasia of cells in the urinary space, forming a small crescent (Cr). Note dark fat droplets in cell cytoplasm at right lower edge of the picture. × 3,000.

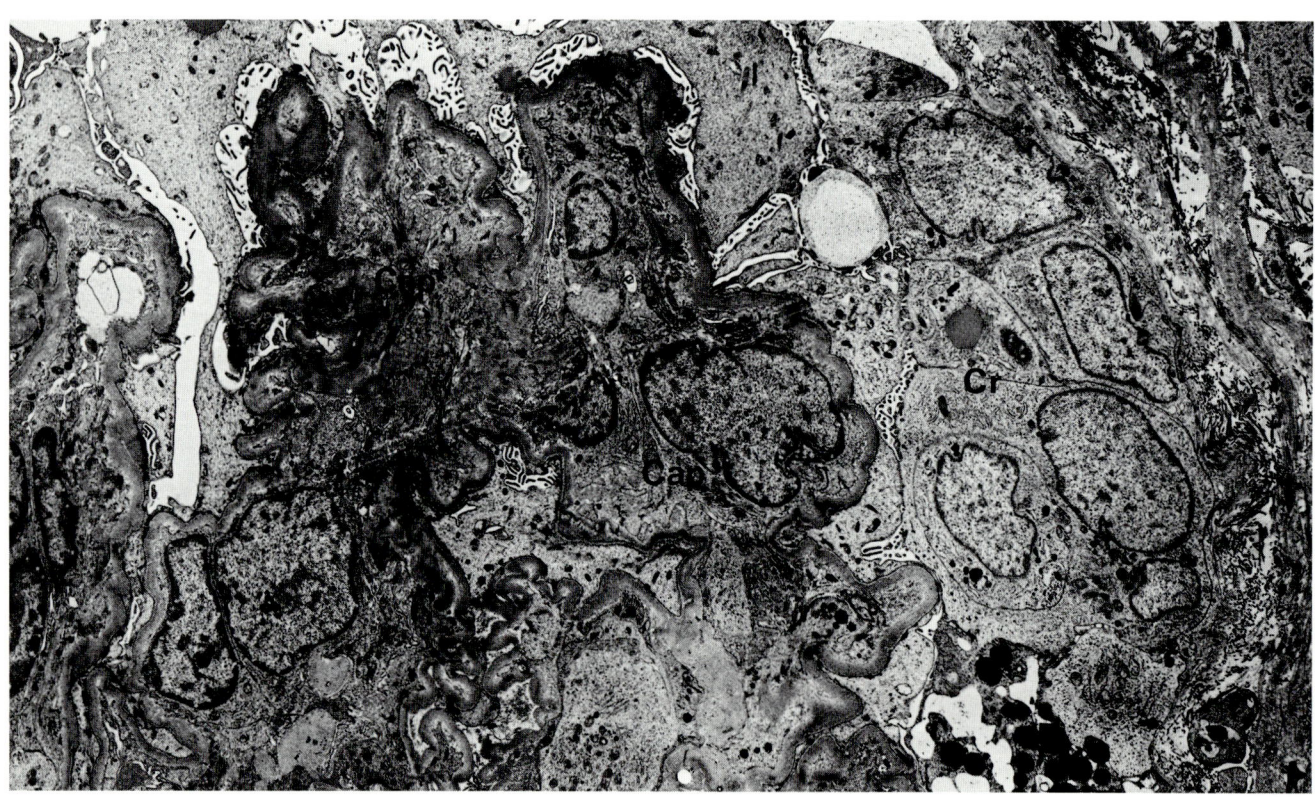

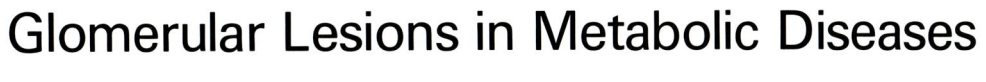

CHAPTER 14

Diabetic Glomerulosclerosis
(Figs. 14-1 to 14-18)

Diabetic Glomerulosclerosis

Definition: Glomerular disease associated with diabetes mellitus and probably related to it genetically or pathogenetically. This definition excludes intercurrent glomerular alterations such as diffuse proliferative or membranous glomerulonephritis, those secondary to vascular disease (diabetic or non-diabetic) or to pyelonephritis.

The most characteristic feature is probably the uniform thickening of glomerular capillary basement membrane. This is associated with an increase in mesangial matrix, which is much more marked than any increase in cellularity which may occur. The typical diabetic nodules arise from a localized exaggeration of this process. Hyaline deposits (so-called "exudative" or "insudative" lesions) may be present in capillary walls and Bowman's capsule. The presence of hyaline material in both afferent and efferent arterioles is also characteristic.

Clinical Manifestations: The main symptom of diabetic glomerulosclerosis is proteinuria. If sensitive methods are used, increase in protein excretion is found in many patients at the time diabetes is recognized, particularly after exercise. With time proteinuria becomes more pronounced and can be detected by standard laboratory methods. At first it is intermittent, but becomes fixed and more abundant, attaining nephrotic levels in some patients. Appreciable proteinuria and nephrotic syndrome are more common in juvenile diabetes, and generally are harbingers of progressive renal disease, ending in failure in a few years. Proteinuria is frequently accompanied by microscopic hematuria and by hypertension of moderate degree. The combination of severe proteinuria, hypertension and renal insufficiency has been called in the past the Kimmelstiel-Wilson *syndrome*.

Light Microscopy: Early in the disease the glomeruli enlarge, but retain normal architecture. The most constant change is widening of the glomerular mesangium and of Bowman's capsule. At first these are mild and similar to changes seen in hypertension and in senile arteriosclerosis. However in time they progress to a point where they can be recognized as so-called diffuse diabetic glomerulosclerosis. The widened mesangium contains increased amounts of matrix but relatively few cells. At the same time capillary basement membranes become thickened, though this change is more easily recognized on electron microscopy. Aneurysmal dilatation of capillaries is quite common.

In perhaps one-quarter of cases, mesangial thickening in the lobular center progresses to nodular formations. This form, nodular glomerulosclerosis, is considerably more specific for diabetes. The nodules consist of compacted matrix with perhaps a scattering of cells along the periphery. The matrix often shows a layered arrangement with silver stains such as periodic acid silver methenamine. This layering, as well as the tendency to peripheral location in the tuft and uneven distribution in the glomeruli, distinguishes nodular diabetic glomerulosclerosis from a similar lesion in advanced lobular glomerulonephritis. The only other conditions that show glomerular nodules are multiple myeloma or other plasma cell dyscrasias with light chain excretion.

Thickening of Bowman's capsule often leads to formation of fibrous crescents. On occasion true cellular crescents occur. Tubular basement membranes are also thickened, often out of proportion to the degree of cell atrophy, and may be accompanied by interstitial fibrosis.

A second very common change is the formation of hyaline (exudative or insudative) lesions. These are not specific for diabetes, but are more frequent and more prominent in this disease and occur earlier in the evolution of glomerular obsolescence. Hyaline deposits may be seen in the Bowman's capsule ("capsular drop") and in the expanded mesangium, but the most characteristic location is the lumen of a dilated capillary along the periphery of the tuft. An analogous lesion, known as capillary aneurysm, occurs in the retina of the eye. Hyalin is strongly acidophilic, stains red with trichrome dyes (in contradistinction to the mesangial nodules which stain blue or green) and contains a variety of serum proteins and lipids.

Arterioles are also affected by deposition of hyalin in their intima and media. This hyaline arteriolosclerosis often involves both the afferent and the efferent arterioles.

Progression of glomerular changes ends in complete sclerosis, often combined with prominent hyaline deposits.

Electron Microscopy: Thickineing of the glomerular basement membranes is a very early sign of diabetes, concomittant with the increase of the mesangial matrix. At first this thickening is segmental and mild, but later it becomes striking, with basement membranes attaining the width 5–10 times that of normal. Electron microscopy also demonstrates development of thick strands of mesangial matrix and their aggregation into nodules. Early hyaline deposits can be seen under the endothelium of the capillaries and in the expanded mesangium as granular electrondense accumulations.

In some cases of diabetes accompanied by nephrotic syndrome, lesions other than diabetic glomerulosclerosis are found, such as Minimal Change, or Membranous Glomerulonephiritis. The thickened tubular basement membranes often show a layered structure. Hyaline deposits in the arterioles lie primarily in the subendothelial space, but may extend into the media.

Immunofluorescence Microscopy: Interrupted linear deposits of immunoglobulins, especially of IgG, are fairly common in the earlier stages of diabetic glomerulosclerosis. They are usually accompanied by other plasma proteins such as albumin and fibrinogen. The immunoglobulins cannot be eluted by procedures that elute them from immune complexes, and are believed to represent non-specific trapping rather than immune binding. Occasionally small deposits of IgM and C3 are found in the mesangium. Deposits of immunoglobulin can also occur along the tubular basement membranes.

GLOMERULAR LESIONS IN METABOLIC DISEASES

DIABETIC GLOMERULOSCLEROSIS

Fig. 14-1 Diabetic glomerulosclerosis. Early diffuse sclerosis showing mild mesangial thickening and thickening of the Bowman's capsule.
PAS stain. x 390.

Fig. 14-2 Slightly more advanced diffuse diabetic glomerulosclerosis. Mesangium is somewhat more prominent. The capillary basement membranes appear thickened.
PAS Stain. x 390.

Fig. 14-3 Immunofluorescence microscopy. Early diffuse glomerulosclerosis. Weak deposits of IgG along capillary basement membranes and along tubular basement membranes. x 260.

Fig. 14-4 Diffuse and nodular diabetic glomerulosclerosis. A well formed nodule is seen towards one o'clock and a less compact nodule towards eight o'clock.
PAS stain. x 260.

Fig. 14-5 Nodular diabetic glomerulosclerosis. Compact nodules staining blue.
Trichrome stain. x 260.

Fig. 14-6 Nodule of diabetic glomerulosclerosis showing a layered structure.
PASM stain. x 1,000.

DIABETIC GLOMERULOSCLEROSIS

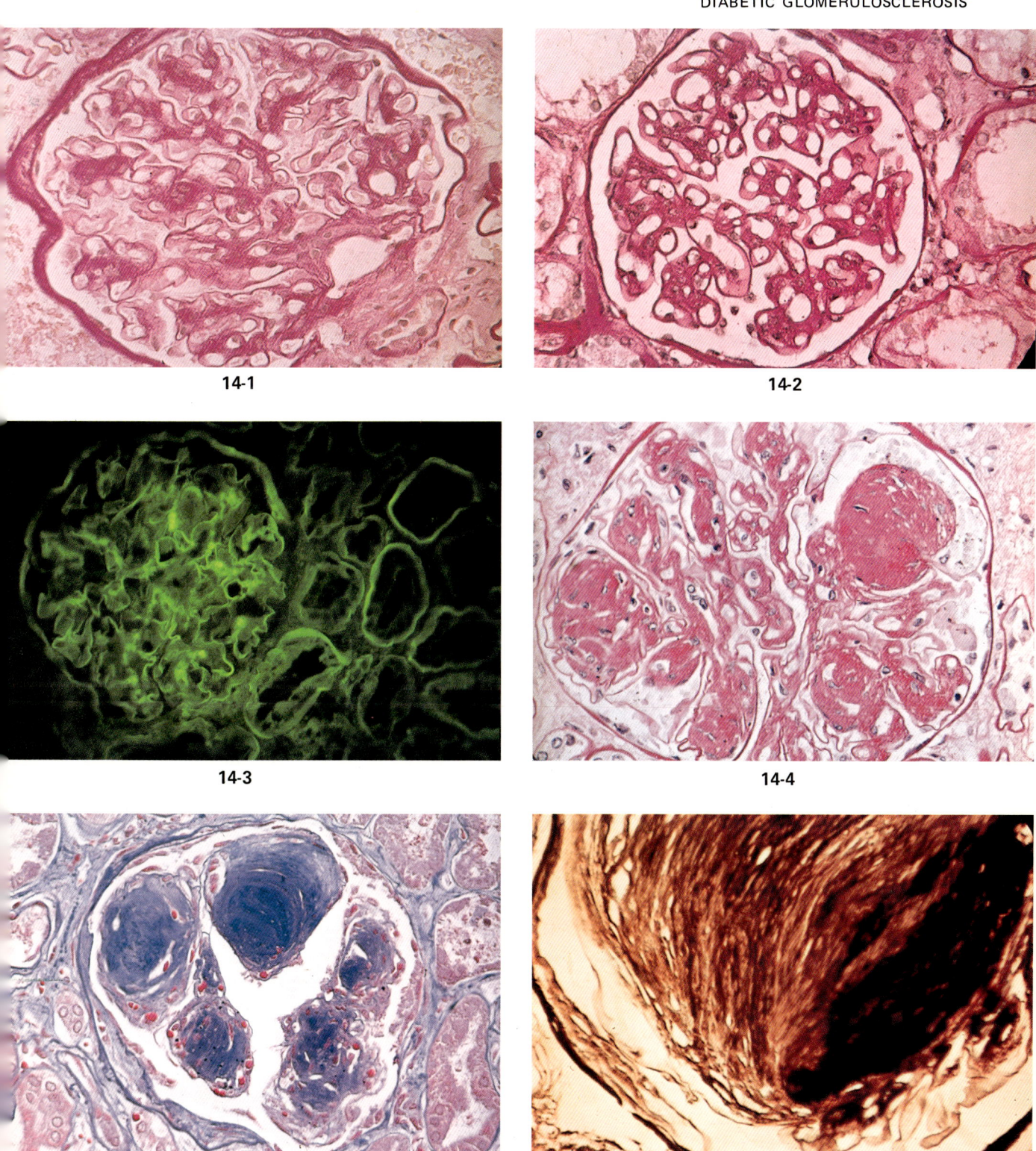

14-1

14-2

14-3

14-4

14-5

14-6

GLOMERULAR LESIONS IN METABOLIC DISEASES

DIABETIC GLOMERULOSCLEROSIS

Fig. 14-7 Exudative or hyaline lesions in diabetic glomerulosclerosis. Hyalin stains red and is sometimes vacuolated. Mesangium, basement membranes and Bowman's capsule stain blue.
Trichrome stain.   x 410.

Fig. 14-8 Retinal preparation showing a capillary aneurysm.
PAS stain.

Fig. 14-9 Diabetic glomerulosclerosis. Thickening of tubular basement membranes.
PAS stain.   x 260.

Fig. 14-10 Immunofluorescence microscopy. IgG deposits along tubular basement membranes.   x 260.

DIABETIC GLOMERULOSCLEROSIS

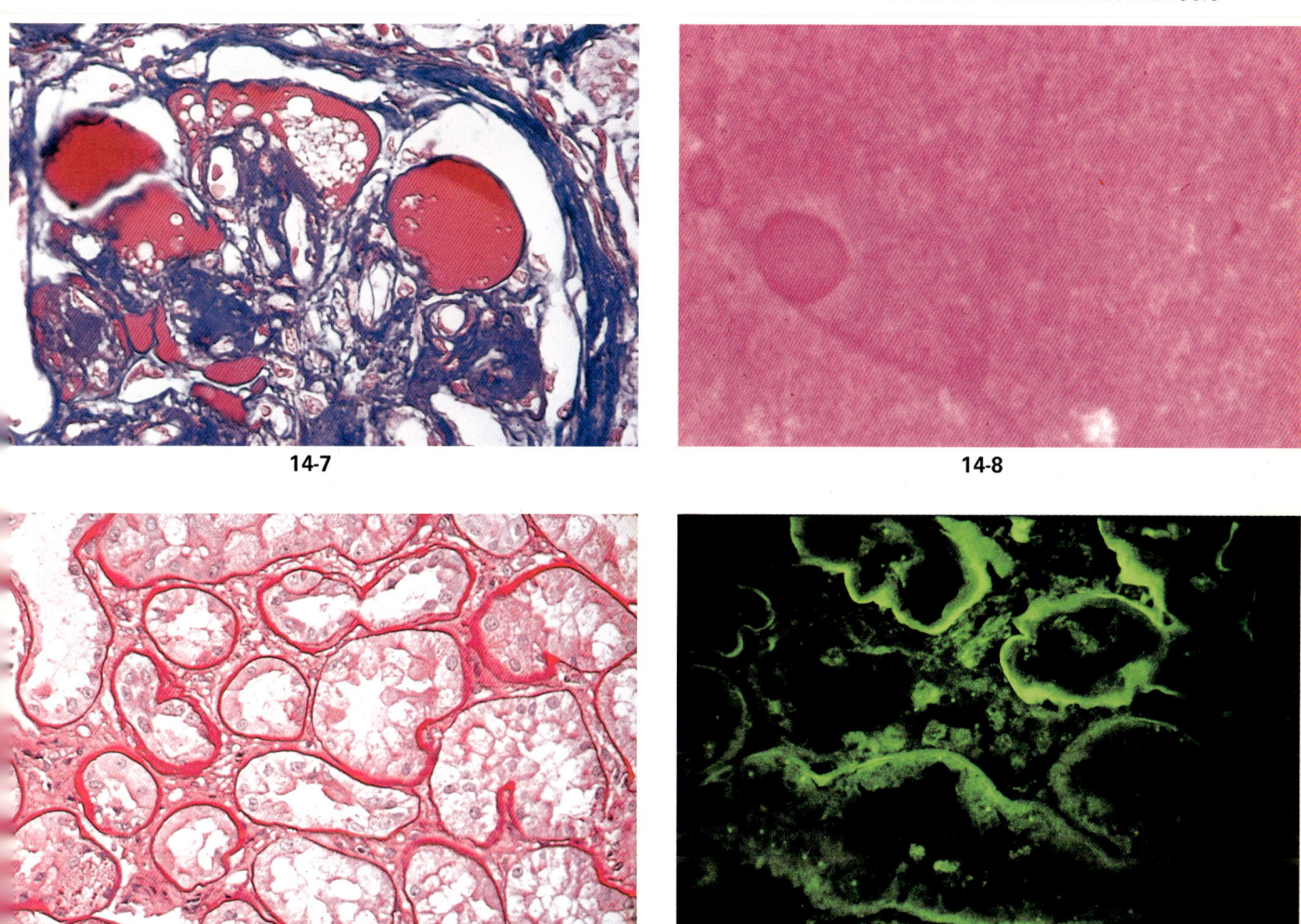

14-7

14-8

14-9

14-10

DIABETIC GLOMERULOSCLEROSIS

Fig. 14-11 Electron micrograph. Early diffuse diabetic glomerulosclerosis. Part of a glomerulus showing widening of the mesangium with two mesangial cells (MC) and increased amount of matrix (MM). Some of the capillary basement membranes (BM) are thickened and some are quite thin.   x 4,600.

Fig. 14-12 Electron micrograph. Moderately advanced diffuse diabetic glomerulosclerosis. The mesangium contains a slightly increased number of cells (MC) and a large amount of matrix (MM). The capillary basement membranes (BM) are focally thickened with small scattered electron dense deposits (D) in the lamina densa.   x 4,600.

U: urinary space.

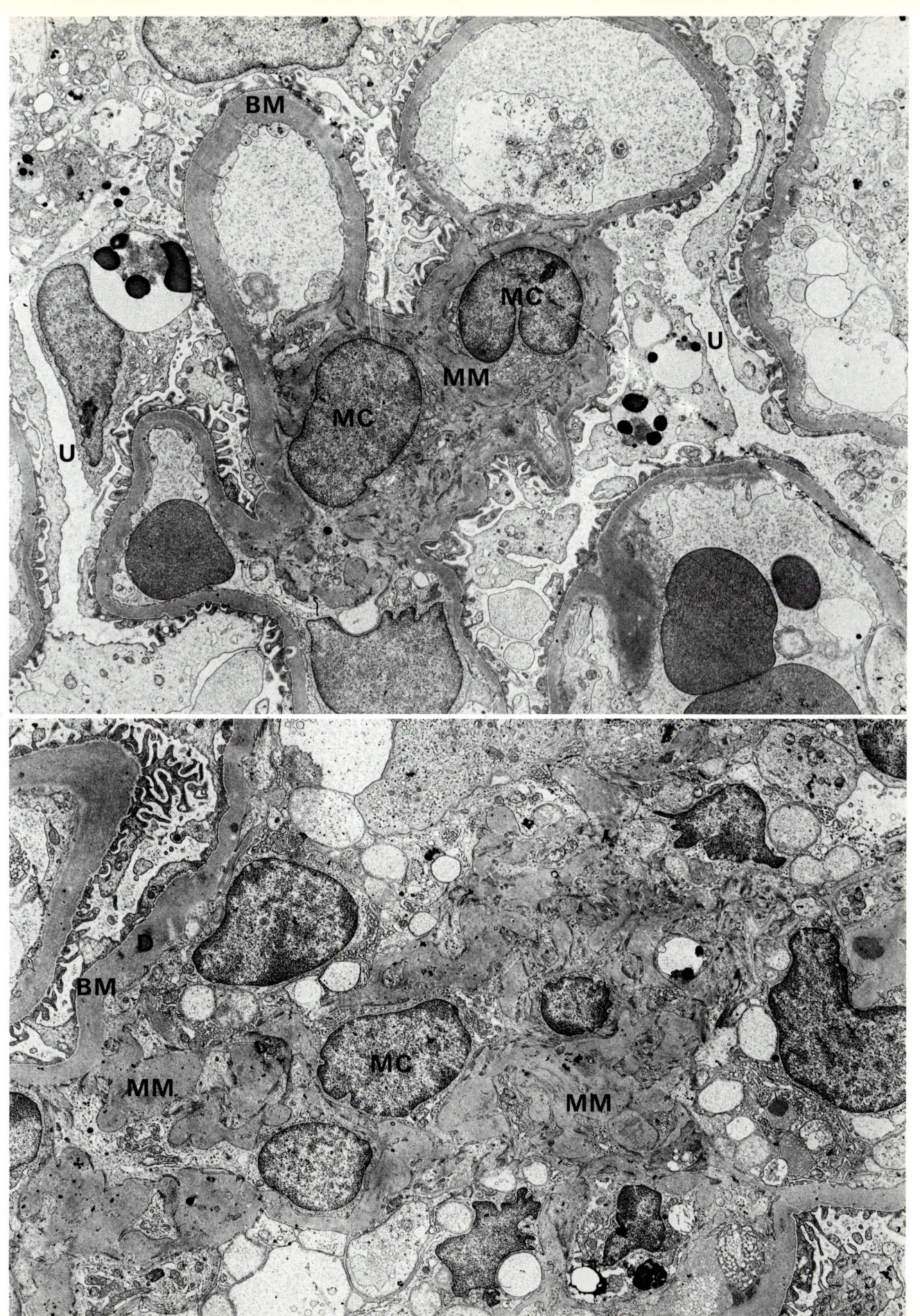

DIABETIC GLOMERULOSCLEROSIS

Fig. 14-13 Electron micrograph. Markedly thickened basement membrane (BM) in a case of diabetic glomerulosclerosis. Most of the thickening appears to be on the epithelial side of the original basement membrane (arrows). x 20,000.

Fig. 14-14 Electron micrograph. Glomerular capillary basement membrane (BM) in a patient with diabetes and nephrotic syndrome. The changes are those of membranous nephropathy, stage 3.   x 18,000.

L: capillary lumen,   U: urinary space,   D: deposit,   En: endothelial cell, P: podocyte.

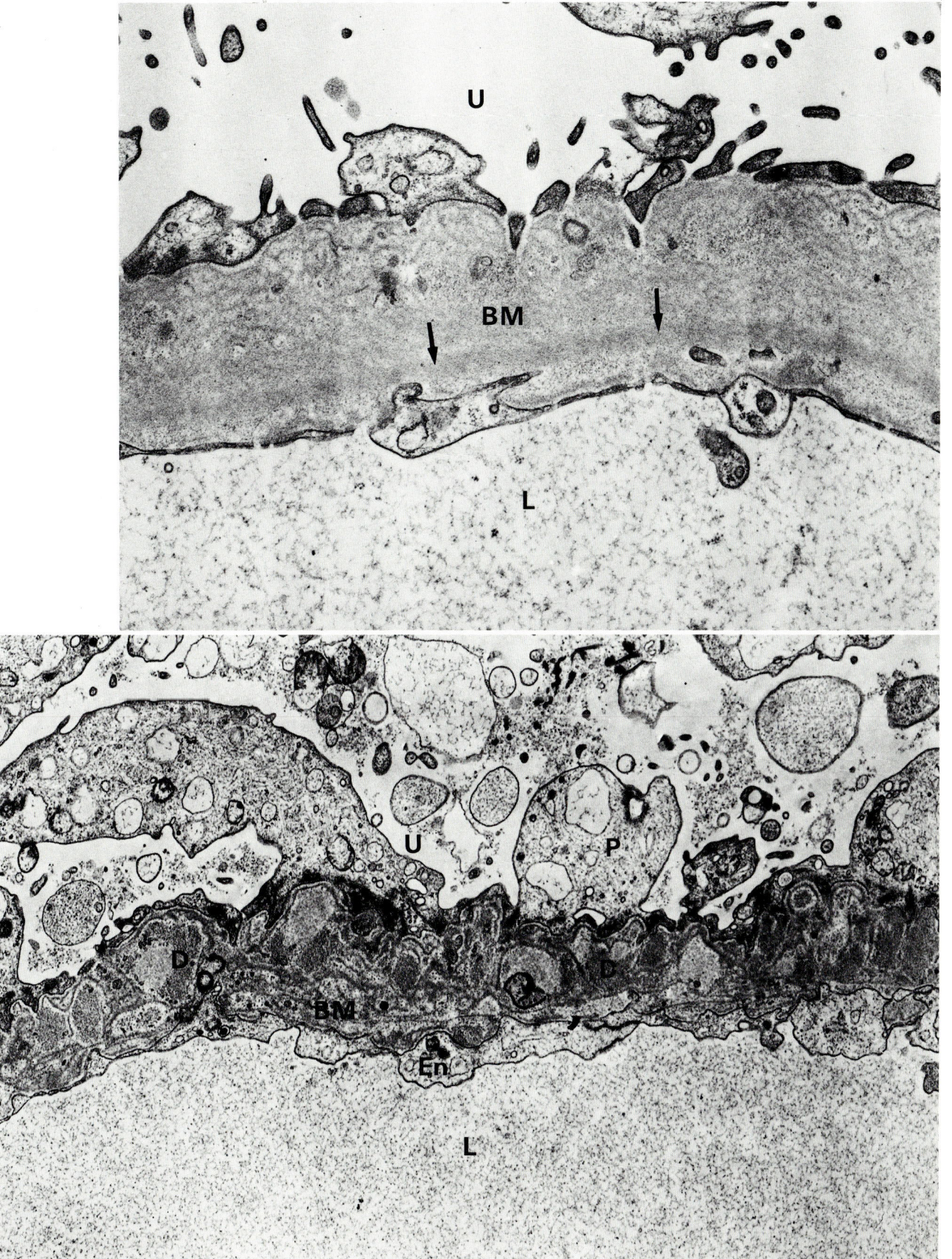

DIABETIC GLOMERULOSCLEROSIS

Fig. 14-15 Electron micrograph. Mesangial expansion, thickening of capillary basement membrane (BM) and hyaline (H) lesion filling the capillary lumen.
× 11,000.

Fig. 14-16 Electron micrograph. Typical nodule (MN) of diabetic glomerulosclerosis showing a finely layered structure. The nodule is surrounded by a less compacted mesangial matrix (MM).   × 6,400.

P: podocyte, BMM: basement membrane material.

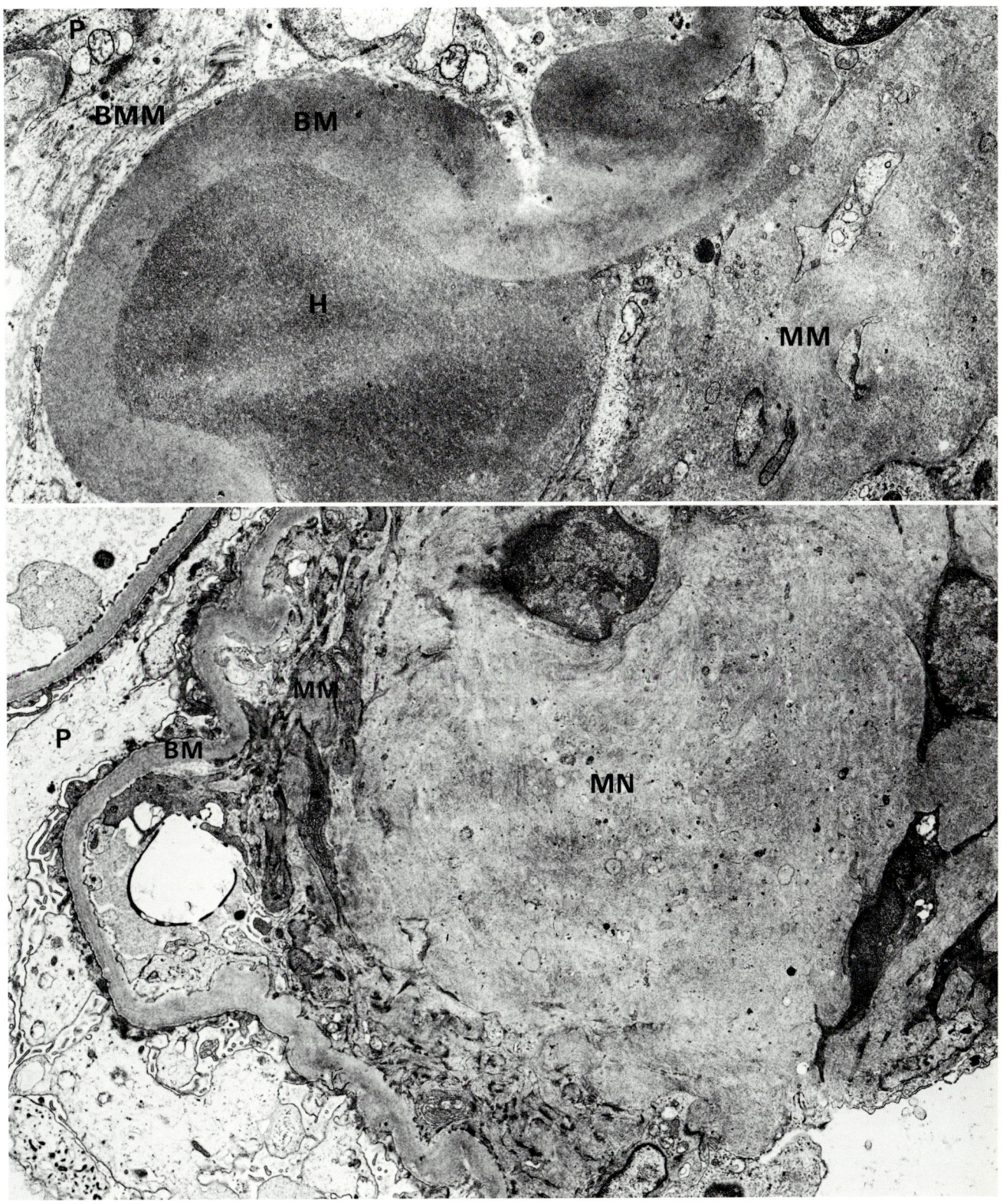

GLOMERULAR LESIONS IN METABOLIC DISEASES

DIABETIC GLOMERULOSCLEROSIS

Fig. 14-17 Electron micrograph. Diabetic glomerulosclerosis. Markedly thickened and layered tubular basement membrane (TBM).   x 16,000.

Fig. 14-18 Electron micrograph. Hyalinization of a renal arteriole in a diabetic patient. Hyaline (H) deposits lie under the endothelium (En) extending into the media.   x 6,700.

TC: tubular cell.

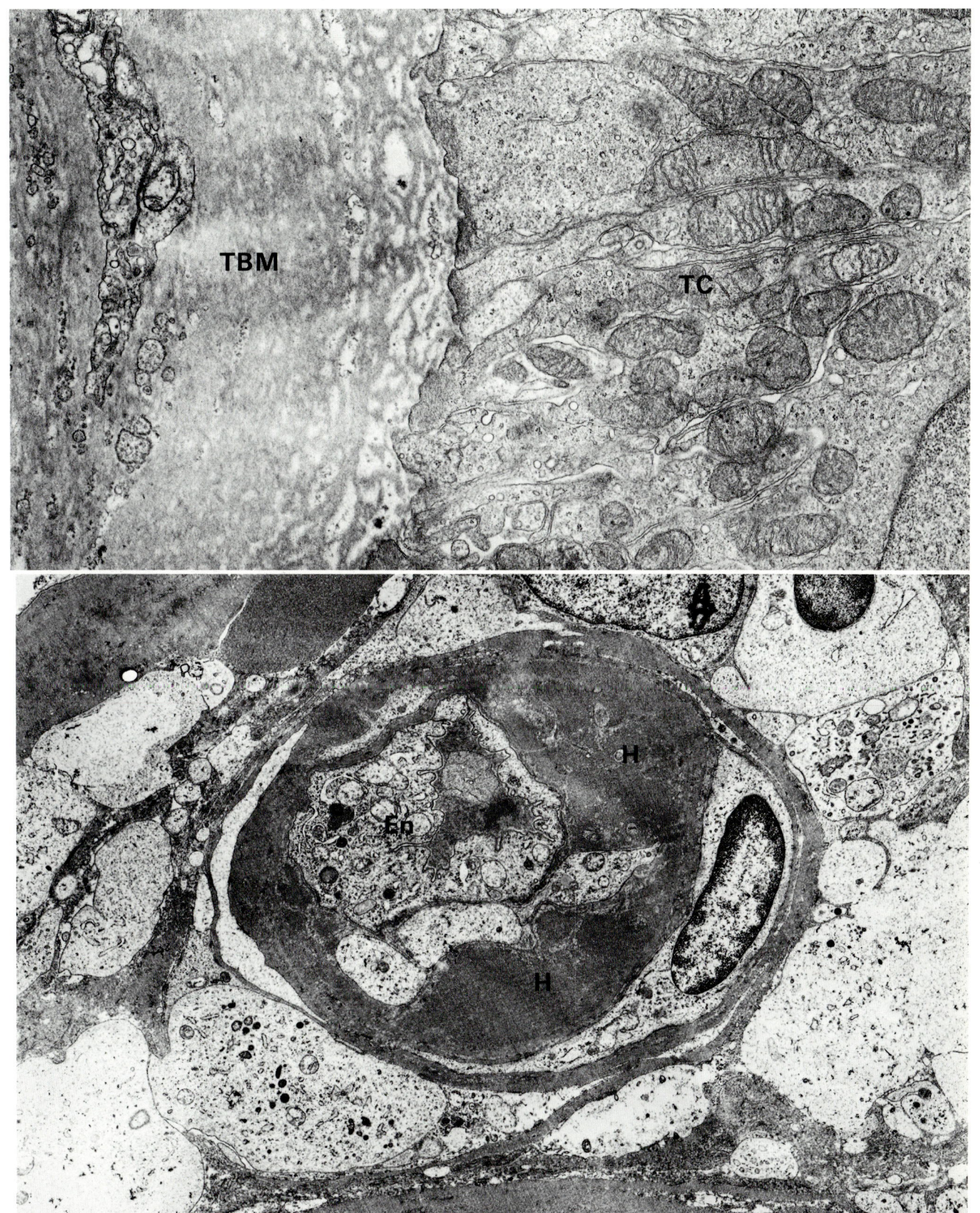

CHAPTER 15

Amyloidosis
    (Figs. 15-1 to 15-10 and Figs. 15-25 to 15-26)
Multiple Myeloma
    (Figs. 15-11 to 15-14 and Figs. 15-27 to 15-30)
Waldenstrom's Macroglobulinemia
    (Figs. 15-15 to 15-16 and Fig. 15-31)
Cryoglobulinemia
    (Figs. 15-17 to 15-24 and Figs. 15-32 to 15-36)

Renal Amyloidosis

Definition: Glomerular disease resulting from deposition of amyloid in the mesangium and the capillary walls. Identification is best achieved using Congo red staining, viewed with polarized light to give the typical apple green color. Amyloid may also be identified using its metachromatic reaction or by electron microscopy. Deposits of amyloid also occur in the walls of blood vessels and in the interstitial tissue.

Clinical Manifestations: Glomerular involvement is most constant in secondary amyloidosis due to chronic infections (tuberculosis, syphilis, osteomyelitis), degenerative diseases (rheumatoid arthritis) or malignancies (carcinoma, Hodgkin's disease), but occurs also in primary amyloidosis, amyloidosis of multiple myeloma and that of familial Mediterranean fever. The main clinical sign is proteinuria often associated with nephrotic syndrome. Renal failure develops at a variable rate, sometimes quite rapidly, indicating rapid increase of amyloid deposits, or renal vein thrombosis, but occasionally for unexplained reasons. Hypertension when it occurs is most frequently associated with azotemia and is seen mainly in secondary amyloidosis. Patients with primary amyloidosis have a tendency to develop hypotension. A few patients show defects in urinary concentrating ability, or salt wasting, probably related to interstitial rather than to glomerular amyloid deposits.

Light Microscopy: Amyloid is found both in the glomerular mesangium and in the capillary walls. In the mesangium it forms nodules of various sizes, or more diffuse infiltrates which expand the intercapillary space and compress the lumina. Capillary wall deposits occupy subendothelial space, infiltrate the basement membrane and appear in a pattern of perpendicular projections ("spicules") on the epithelial side. These spicules are like other amyloid deposits, metachromatic with crystal violet and toluidine blue, reddish with Congo red (with dichroic-red and green-coloration under partly polarized light), and yellowish-green with Thioflavin-T in a fluorescence microscope. In addition, spicules often stain with silver (PASM), while most amyloid deposits are silver-negative. Patients with many spicules appear to have a more rapidly progressive course. There are occasional reports of resolution of amyloid deposits after eradication of chronic infection.

Amyloid also involves arterioles, arteries and peritubular interstitial tissue. Such deposits do not necessarily correlate with glomerular involvement.

Electron Microscopy: Amyloid is composed of fine non-branching fibrils, 7–10 nm in diameter, arranged in criss-crossing bundles. Amyloid fibrils in the spicules tend to lie perpendicularly to the basement membrane, and are sometimes covered by a layer of apparently newly formed basement membrane, perhaps an indication of healing or scarring. Areas of epithelial denudation are quite common.

Immunofluorescence Microscopy: Occasionally irregular staining deposits of IgG and C3 are associated with amyloid. Albumin and fibrinogen may also be present. Amyloid frequently exhibits autofluorescence. L amyloid (light chain) reacts with antisera to light chains, and A amyloid with AA antisera.

Nephropathy in Dysproteinemias

The term dysproteinemia applies to quantitative or qualitative changes of gamma globulins, essentially immunoglobulins and their fragments. These changes are most often associated with neoplastic proliferation of specific hemopoietic cells of the lymphocyte-plasma cell species. However, dysproteinemia may occur in non-neoplastic conditions. Some immunoglobulins have the property of precipitating at low temperature and redissolving upon warming. This is most frequently seen in mixed cryoglobulinemia which most likely represents immune complexes. Cryoglobulinemia may be due to neoplastic cell proliferation, may be idiopathic, or may accompany renal diseases, particularly various forms of glomerulonephritis.

Multiple Myeloma

Definition: Renal manifestations are common in multiple myeloma but are mainly due to tubular damage. Glomerular lesions are quite rare and may vary from capillary wall thickening to mesangial nodules and exceptionally, to proliferative glomerulonephritis.

Clinical Manifestations: Proteinuria is a frequent finding. Its main component is light chain fragments of immunoglobulins which are not always detectable by the routine laboratory procedures, and are best demonstrated by immunoelectrophoresis. The amounts of albumin vary from trace to those in the nephrotic range. Acute or progressive chronic renal failure in multiple myeloma is due mainly to tubular damage by light chains, especially those of the lambda type, and also to dehydration, hypercalcemia or hyperuricemia. Acute failure may be precipitated by intravenous pyelography. Kappa chain proteinuria is sometimes associated with Fanconi's syndrome, due to damage of tubular cells.

Light Microscopy: In a small percentage of patients (5–15%) amyloid deposits are found in the glomeruli. Amyloid is responsible for most of the cases with nephrotic syndrome and for some cases of chronic renal failure. On occasion, mesangial nodules occur similar to Kimmelstiel-Wilson nodules of diabetes. Capillary walls may be thickened. Very rarely true proliferative glomerulonephritis is seen.

Tubular changes in multiple myeloma consist of dense, sometimes multi-layered intraluminal casts, often surrounded by multinucleated giant cells; tubular calcification, atrophy and peritubular interstitial fibrosis. On occasion nodules composed of plasma cells are seen in the interstitium.

Electron Microscopy: The mesangial nodules, when present, contain finely granular material, scattered collagen and non-periodic fibrils. They may be associated with ribbon-like granular deposits under the endothelium and around the tubular basement membranes. These deposits contain mainly kappa light chains. Occasionally the more usual electron dense deposits are found under the capillary endothelium or epithelium. Amyloid deposits show the typical fibrillar structure. Tubular cells may contain electron dense protein crystals.

Immunofluorescence Microscopy: Subendothelial and peritubular deposits give positive reaction for kappa chain. Deposits of immunoglobulins may occasionally be found in the glomeruli. The tubular casts contain a variety of proteins, including immunoglobulins, light chains of both types (lambda and Kappa), albumin and fibrinogen.

Waldenstrom's Macroglobulinemia

Definition: In Waldenstrom's macroglobulinemia there is neoplastic proliferation of lymphocyte-like cells and a monoclonal elevation of IgM. The glomerular lesions are similar to those of multiple myeloma, but in addition "plugging" of glomerular capillaries can occur caused by hyaline thrombi rich in IgM.

Clinical Manifestations: In contrast to multiple myeloma, tubular damage and chronic renal failure are rare. However, acute renal failure may occur in association with capillary hyaline thrombi. Proteinuria may reach the nephrotic range particularly when the patient has amyloidosis.

Light Microscopy: Amyloid deposits, mesangial nodules, thickening of basement membrane and on occasion proliferative glomerulonephritis are similar to those encountered in multiple myeloma. A more characteristic finding is the presence of hyaline thrombi in the glomerular capillaries. These are eosinophilic and stain strongly with PAS procedure; they often attain a large size. On occasion hyaline thrombi coexist with cellular proliferation. Interstitial infiltrates of lymphocytes and plasma cells are quite common.

Electron microscopy essentially confirms the light microscopic changes which are similar to those seen in multiple myeloma. The hyaline thrombi are dense and homogeneous. In their early stages they may appear as dense subendothelial or intra-endothelial globules.

Immunofluorescence microscopy typically shows IgM in the hyaline thrombi. The IgM is identical in its composition with that in the serum.

Cryoglobulinemia

Definition: Glomerular disease is much more frequent in patients with primary mixed cryoglobulinemia than with the monoclonal type. The glomerular disease must be distinguished from cases with proliferative glomerulonephritis with secondary cryoglobulinemia. The latter is usually minor or moderate in degree.

Clinical Manifestations: Acute nephritic syndrome is seen but rarely; it may be accompanied by severe oliguria or anuria. The presence of cutaneous vasculitis, purpura, arthralgias or splenomegaly may suggest the correct diagnosis. Spontaneous recovery is not uncommon, but some patients progress to chronic renal failure. About one-third of patients with cryoglobulinemia develop chronic progressive renal disease, manifested by proteinuria, nephrotic syndrome, microhematuria, hypertension and renal failure.

Light Microscopy: In the acute form, the changes in the glomeruli resemble those of diffuse lupus nephritis and also those of Waldenstrom's macroglobulinemia. There is diffuse cellular proliferation, tendency to lobulation, polymorphonuclear exudation and subendothelial and intraluminal deposits which stain strongly with eosin and PAS. In the chronic form the picture is less specific, varying from focal to diffuse mesangiocapillary or to membranous glomerulonephritis, but may be similar to that of the acute form. Crescents are occasionally present.

Electron Microscopy: The deposits are found

under the endothelium, in the lumen and under the epithelium. They often show a characteristic "organized" arrangement composed of parallel arrays of fibrils or tubules. The diameter of these structures varies from case to case but is constant in each individual case. In some instances protein crystals, visible by light microscopy are found in the epithelial or endothelial cells.

Immunofluorescence microscopy shows granular or "lumpy" deposits of either individual immunoglobulins or of mixed immunoglobulins, most commonly IgM and IgG but on occasion of other combinations. Complement components are usually present.

GLOMERULAR LESIONS IN METABOLIC DISEASES

AMYLOIDOSIS

Fig. 15-1　Renal amyloidosis. Glomerulus showing mild involvement by amyloid deposits, occupying mainly the slightly expanded mesangial areas. Amyloid has the appearance of pale structureless material.
H&E stain.　　　　　　　　　　　　　　　　　　　x 260.

Fig. 15-2　Advanced amyloid changes. Amyloid deposits in a sclerosed glomerulus.
Crystal violet stain.　　　　　　　　　　　　　　　x 260.

Fig. 15-3　Extensive involvement of glomerular mesangium by amyloid deposits. Amyloid stains pinkish red against purplish background.
Congo Red stain.　　　　　　　　　　　　　　　　x 260.

Fig. 15-4　Same glomerulus as in Fig. 15-3 under polarized light. The polarizer and the analyzer are incompletely crossed. Most amyloid deposits now stain strongly red but small bundles are pale green and some are yellow. These colors are due to orientation of the amyloid bundles in relation to the polarized light.
Congo Red stain. Polarized light.　　　　　　　　x 260.

Fig. 15-5　Same glomerulus as in Fig. 15-3 under polarized light. The polarizer and analyzer are slightly over-crossed. Many bundles previously stained red are now pale green while other bundles have become red.
Congo Red stain. Polarized light.　　　　　　　　x 260.

Fig. 15-6　Immunofluorescence microscopy. Large irregularly distributed deposits of IgG.
　　　　　　　　　　　　　　　　　　　　　　　　x 260.

AMYLOIDOSIS

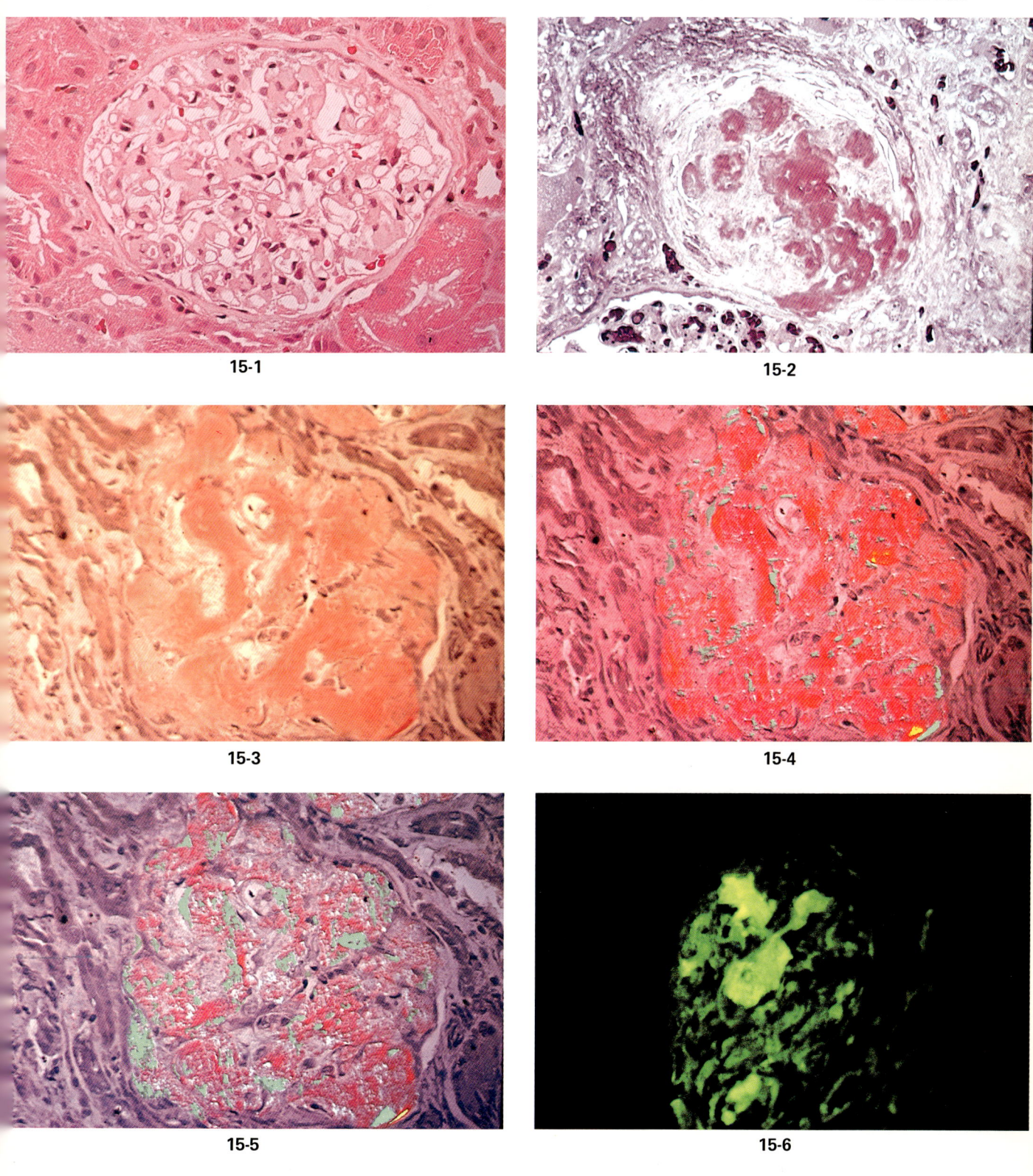

15-1

15-2

15-3

15-4

15-5

15-6

245

GLOMERULAR LESIONS IN METABOLIC DISEASES

AMYLOIDOSIS

Fig. 15-7 Amyloid involvement of capillary walls. Capillary walls are thickened and show variable staining with silver. At three o'clock a bunch of "spicules" can be seen.
Chromotrope Silver-Methenamine stain.   x 1,000.

Fig. 15-8 Same case as Fig. 15-7. There is involvement of the mesangium and of capillary walls. Spicules are seen along the capillary at nine o'clock.
Thioflavin T stain.   x 410.

Fig. 15-9 Slight glomerular involvement by amyloid and massive involvement of a small artery.
PAS stain.   x 260.

Fig. 15-10 Minimal amyloid deposits in the glomerular mesangium.
Thioflavin T stain.   x 410.

MULTIPLE MYELOMA

Fig. 15-11 Multiple myeloma. Case of light chain disease. Glomerulus showing homogeneous mesangial nodules with a few cell nuclei along the periphery. These nodules strongly resemble nodular diabetic glomerulosclerosis.
PAS stain.   x 260.

Fig. 15-12 Multiple myeloma. Light chain disease. Proliferative glomerulonephritis with a fibroepithelial crescent.
H&E stain.   x 260.

MULTIPLE MYELOMA

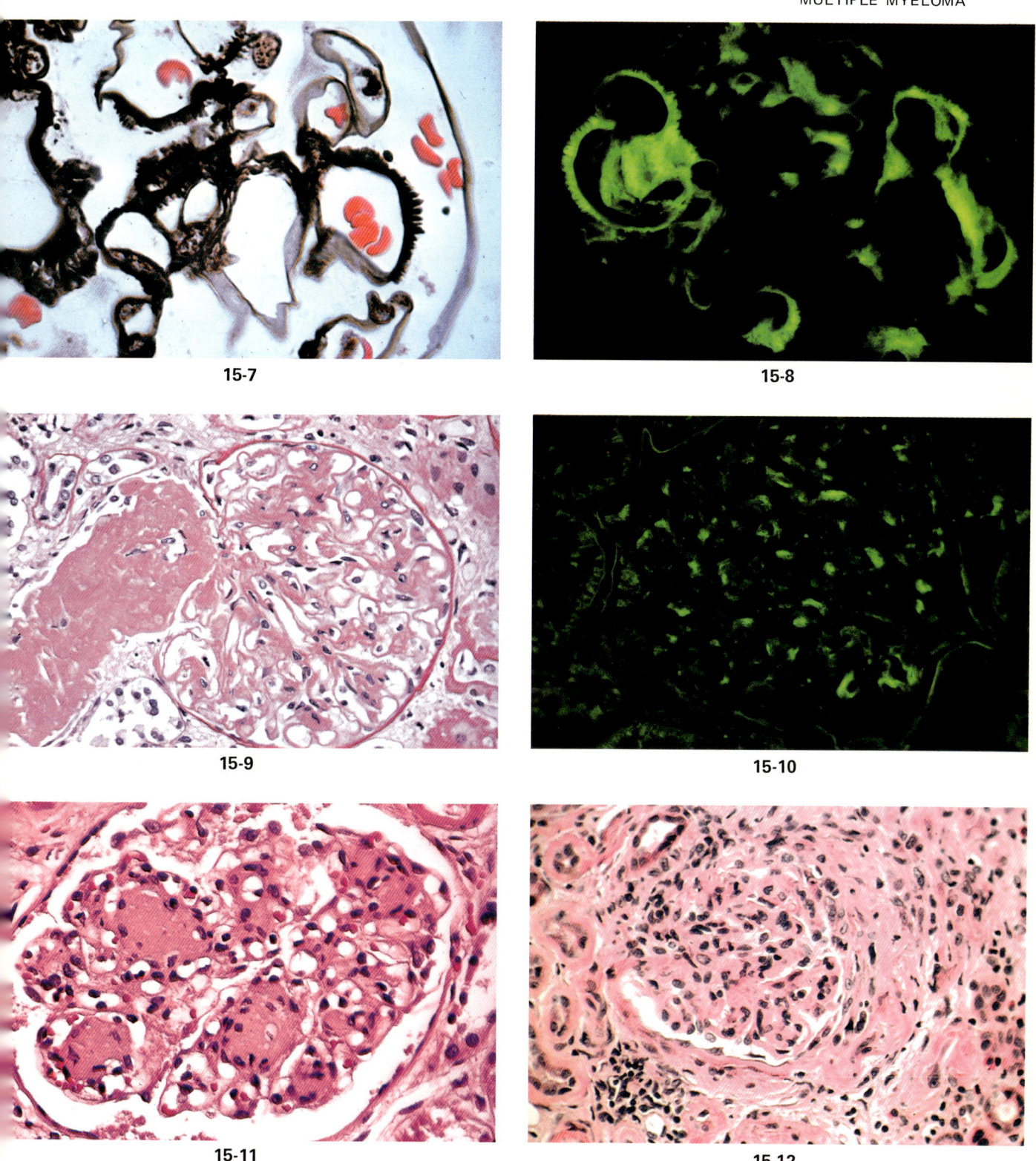

15-7

15-8

15-9

15-10

15-11

15-12

247

GLOMERULAR LESIONS IN METABOLIC DISEASES

MULTIPLE MYELOMA

Fig. 15-13 Immunofluorescence microscopy. Same case as Fig. 15-12. Peritubular deposits of kappa light chain. × 150.

Fig. 15-14 Same case as Fig. 15-12 after recovery. There is persistence of mild hypercellularity.
H&E stain. × 260.

WALDENSTROM'S MACROGLOBULINEMIA

Fig. 15-15 Waldenstrom's macroglobulinemia. Part of a glomerulus showing large dense hyaline thrombi in the glomerular capillaries.
PAS stain. × 410.

Fig. 15-16 Same case as Fig. 15-15. Glomerulus showing enlargement and moderate cellular proliferation. A hyaline thrombus is seen in the peripheral capillary towards seven o'clock.
H&E stain. × 410.

CRYOGLOBULINEMIA

Fig. 15-17 Cryoglobulinemia in a patient with a malignant lymphoma (chronic lymphatic leukemia? Waldenstrom's macroglobulinemia?). Extensive deposits of material stainable with PAS in the glomerular capillaries and mesangium. Some cellular proliferation is also present.
PAS stain. × 410.

Fig. 15-18 Immunofluorescence microscopy. Same case as Fig. 15-17. Extensive granular deposits of IgM, mainly along the capillary walls. Stains for IgG and IgA were negative. × 260.

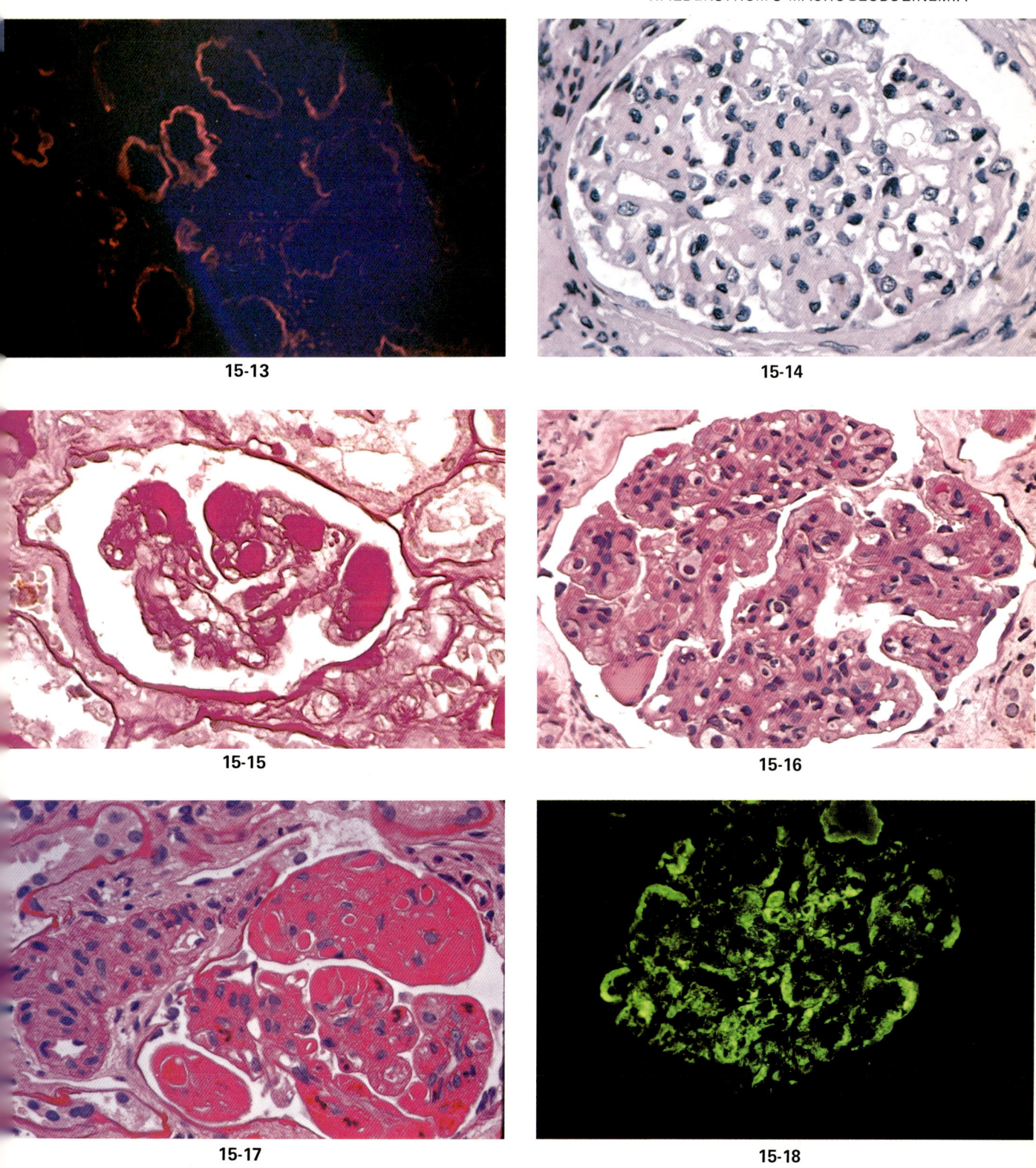

CRYOGLOBULINEMIA

Fig. 15-19 Immunofluorescence microscopy. Same case as Fig. 15-17. Kappa chain antigen distributed in the same manner as IgM. No lambda chain demonstrated. x 260.

Fig. 15-20 Immunofluorescence microscopy. Same case as Fig. 15-17. Complement (C3) also shows distribution similar to that of IgM. x 260.

Fig. 15-21 Mixed cryoglobulinemia. The patient, a 36 year old woman, had a high cryoglobulin level in the serum (634 mg/100 ml.) consisting of IgM and IgG. The picture shows a glomerulus with mesangial proliferation, and deposits of PAS positive material in the capillary lumina, along the capillary walls and in the mesangium.
PAS stain. x 260.

Fig. 15-22 Same case as Fig. 15-21. Slight cellular proliferation is noted. The capillaries along the top of the illustration contain finely crystalline material.
H&E stain. x 410.

Fig. 15-23 Same case as Fig. 15-21. Second biopsy one year later. Crystalline deposits are still visible (left side of the picture). There is also appreciable cellular proliferation.
H&E stain. x 260.

Fig. 15-24 Same case as Fig. 15-21. Skin biopsy taken shortly after the second renal biopsy. The patient had a cutaneous purpurice rash. Vascular lesions in the dermis show subendothelial deposits of pinkish material which narrow the lumen. There is also inflammatory perivascular infiltrate containing many polymorphonuclear leukocytes.
H&E stain. x 260.

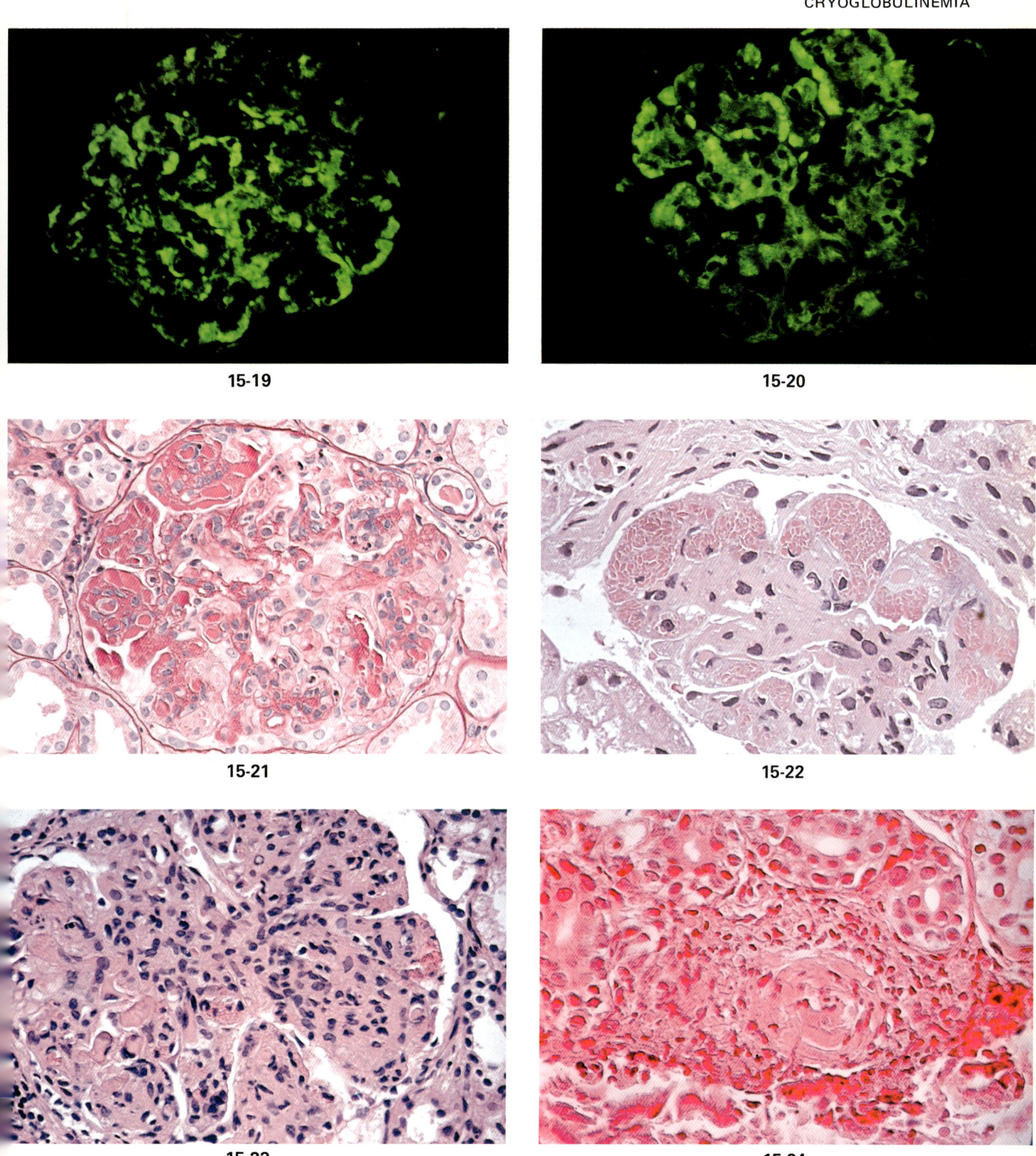

AMYLOIDOSIS

Fig. 15-25 Electron micrograph. Typical fibrillar structure of amyloid (Am) deposits. Many fibrils that are cut across are seen as black dots. x 81,000.

Fig. 15-26 Electron micrograph. Amyloid (Am) involvement of glomerular basement membrane showing deposits under the endothelium (En), in the basement membrane (BM) and under the epithelium. The lamina densa is attenuated. The subepithelial deposits from spicules consisting of parallel bundles of amyloid fibrils. x 17,000.

MC: mesangial cell, FP: foot process, U: urinary space.

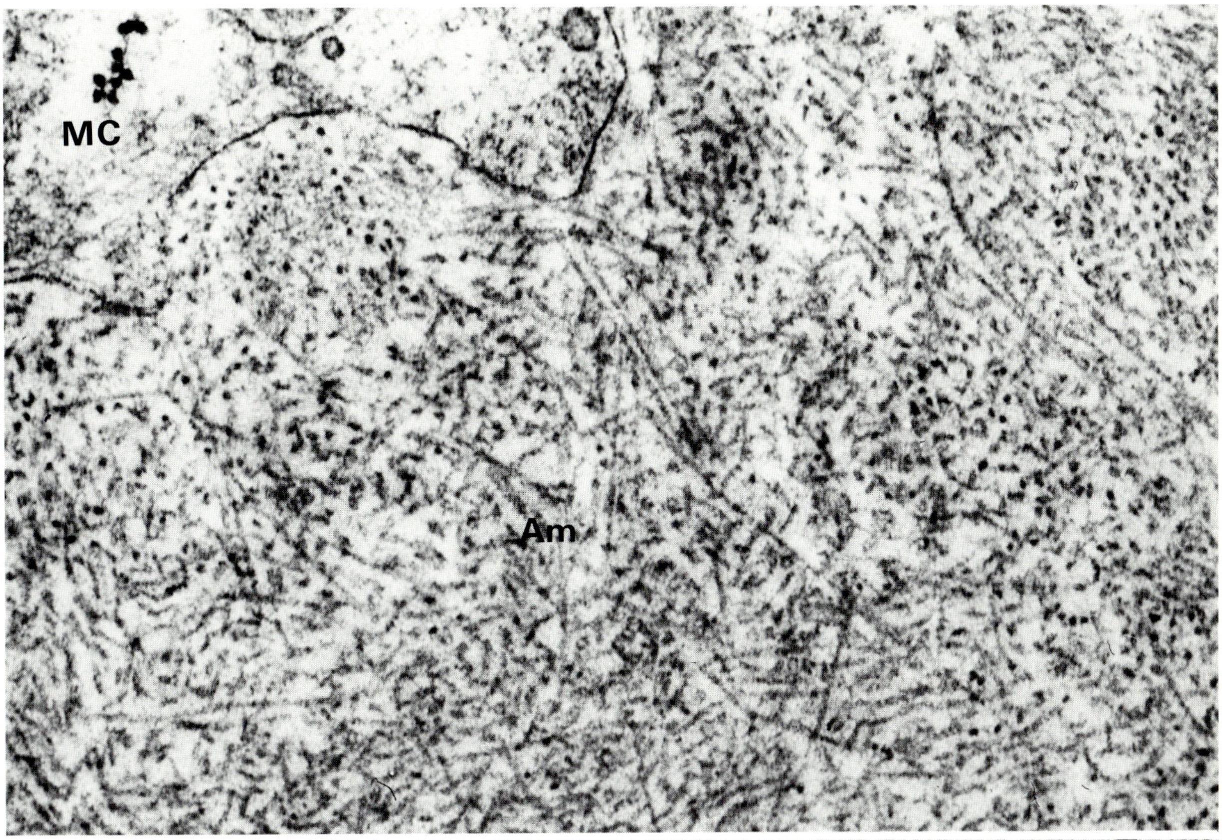

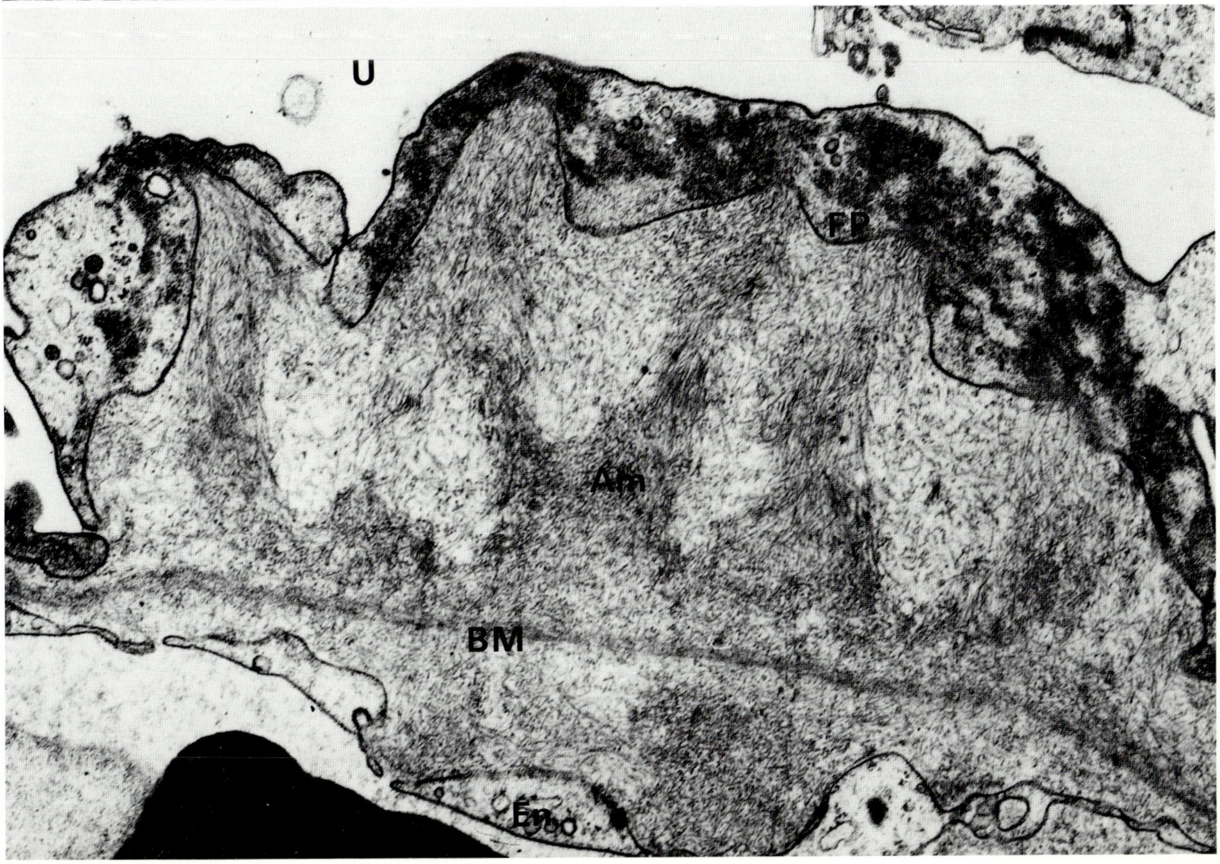

GLOMERULAR LESIONS IN METABOLIC DISEASES

MULTIPLE MYELOMA

Fig. 15-27 Electron micrograph. Multiple myeloma. Kappa light chain disease. Mesangial nodule consisting of masses of matrix (MM) enclosing scattered cells. The capillary lumina are almost completely compressed. × 4,000.

Fig. 15-28 Electron micrograph. Multiple myeloma. Kappa light chain disease. A thin layer of dense granular deposit (D) lies under the endothelium (En) extending into the inner part of the basement membrane (BM). Similar deposits (D) are seen in the thickened mesangial matrix (MM) (right side of picture).
× 16,000.

U: urinary space, MC: mesanginal cell.

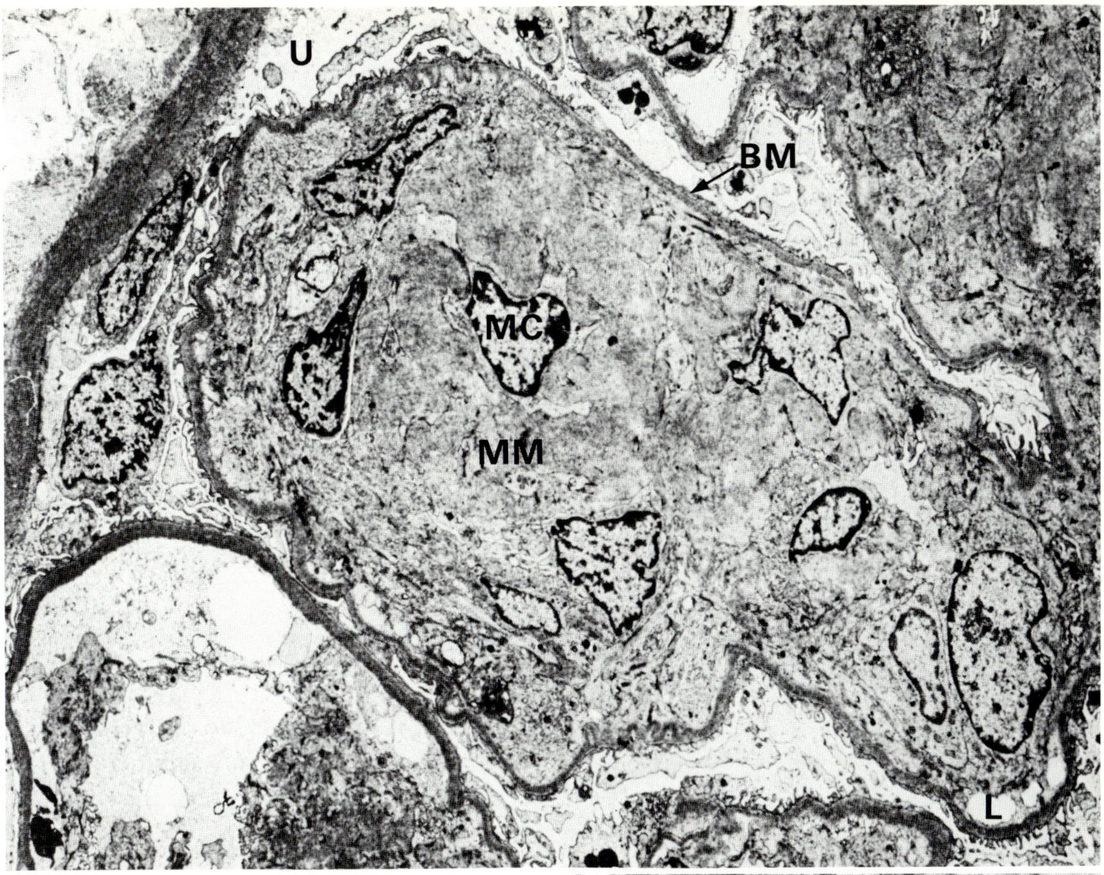

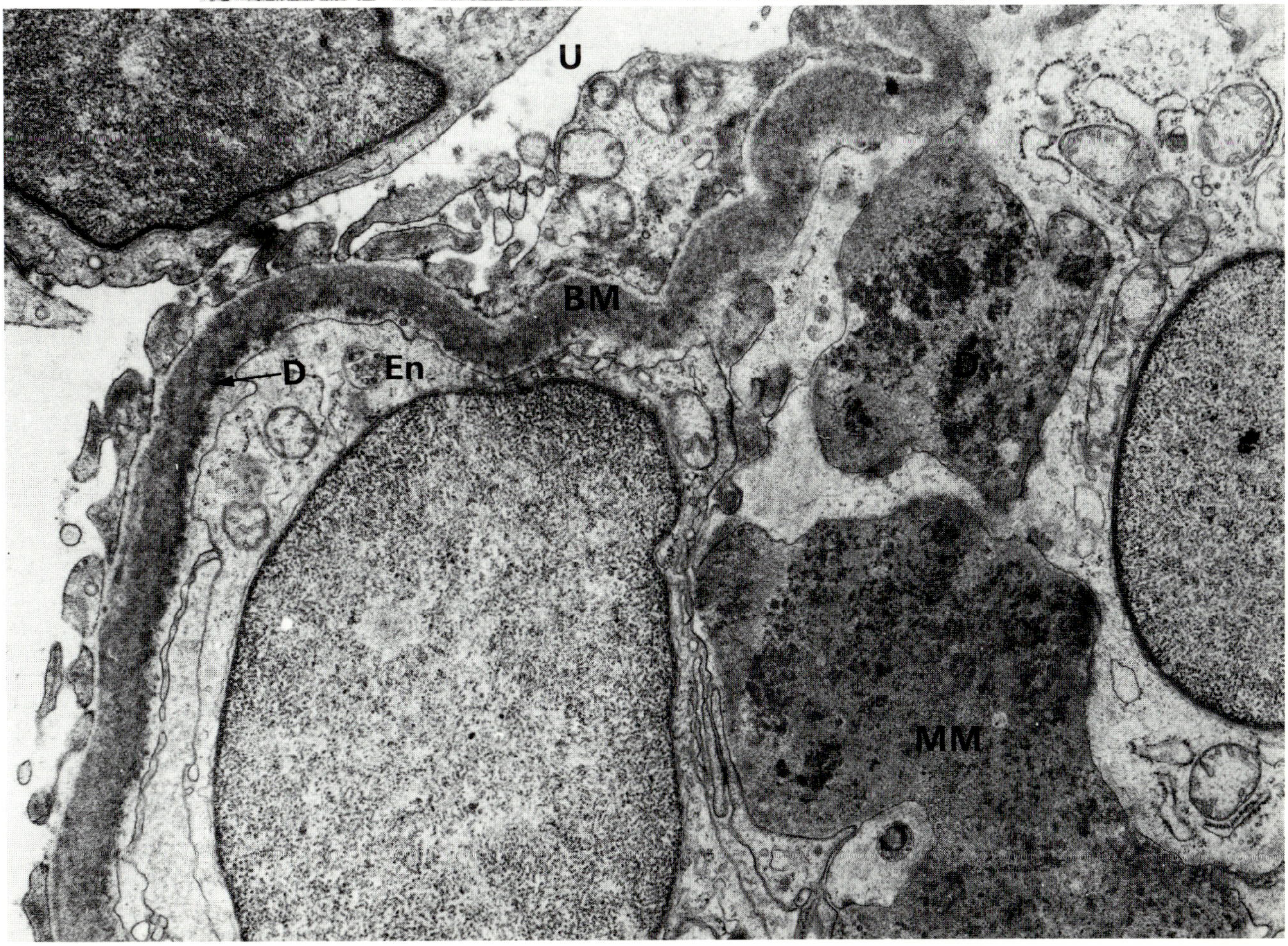

MULTIPLE MYELOMA

Fig. 15-29 Electron micrograph. Another case of kappa light chain disease. Part of a capillary wall showing a layer of dense granular deposit (D) under the endothelium (En) extending into the basement membrane (BM).
x 30,000.

Fig. 15-30 Electron micrograph. Kappa light chain disease. Layers of dense granular deposit (D) along the tubular basement membrane (TBM).
x 11,000.

U: urinary space, TC: tubular cell.

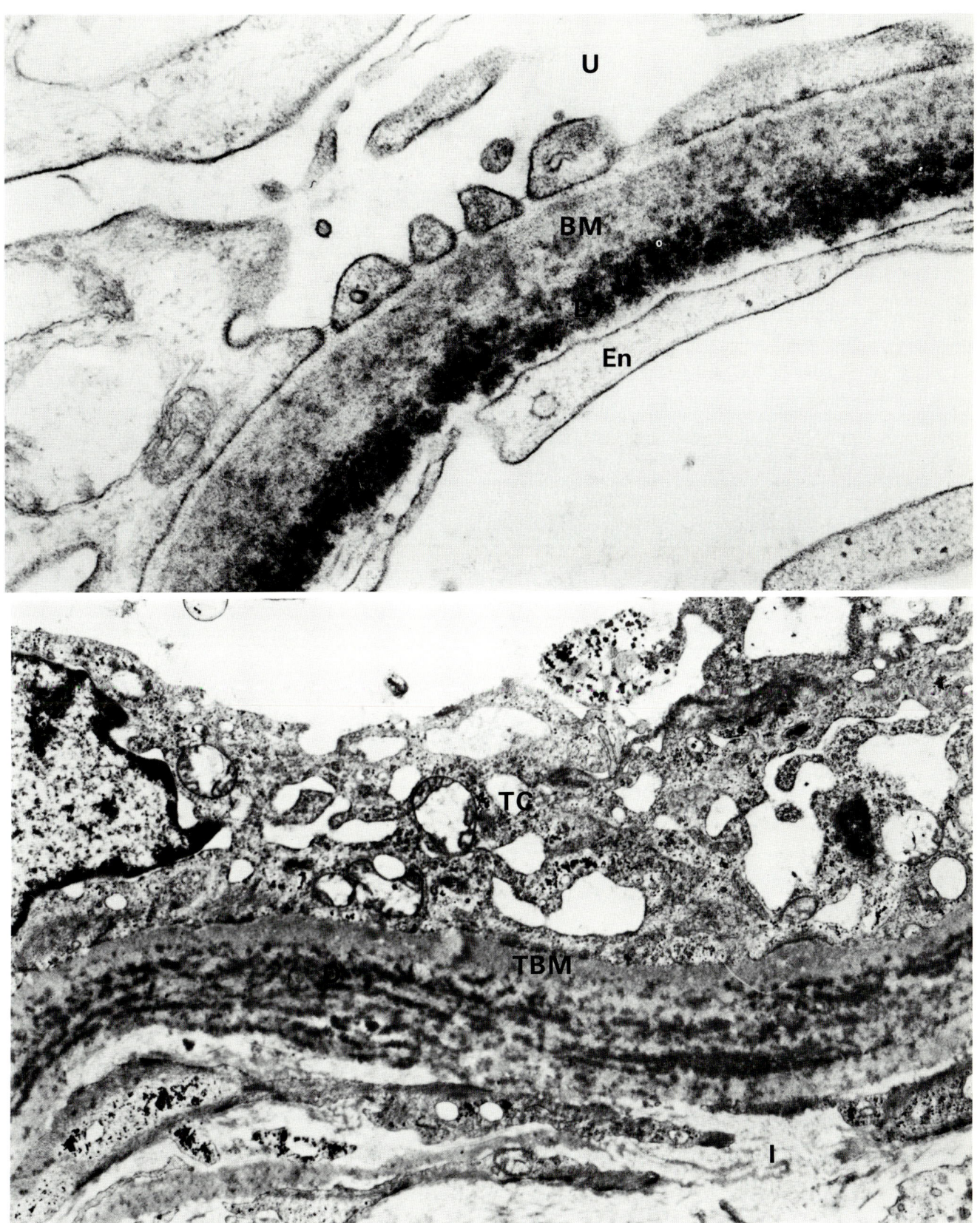

WALDENSTROM'S MACROGLOBULINEMIA

Fig. 15-31 Electron micrograph. Same case as Fig. 15-16. Part of a glomerular tuft showing mesangial proliferation and numerous globular deposits (D) of varying size and density along the endothelium of the capillary. Note the mesangial interposition (MI). × 4,000.

CRYOGLOBULINEMIA

Fig. 15-32 Electron micrograph. Same case as Fig. 15-17. IgM cryoglobulinemia showing "tubular" deposits in the glomerulus (arrows). Though in this case "tubular" pattern is associated with monoclonal cryoglobulinemia, it is more often seen in mixed cryoglobulinemia, such as IgM-IgG. × 48,000.

Fig. 15-33 Case of IgG cryoglobulinemia. Electron micrograph showing fibrillar subendothelial deposits (D). Vague periodicity is noted in the longitudinal sections of the fibrils. In cross sections, the fibrils appear to have hollow centers. × 54,000.

L: capillary lumen, P: podocyte, BM: basement membrane, MM: mesangial matrix, MC: mesangial cell, En: endothelial cell.

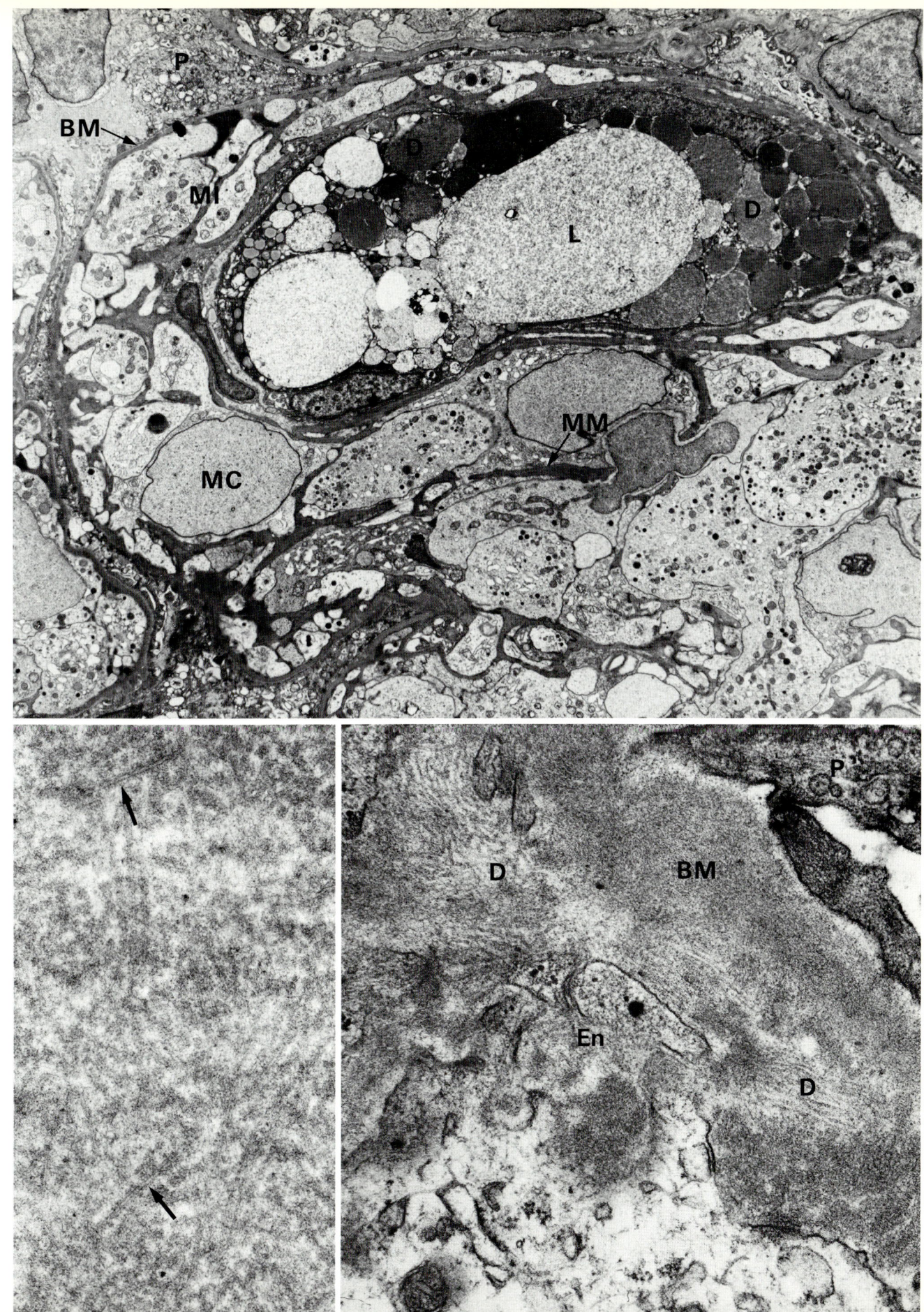

CRYOGLOBULINEMIA

Fig. 15-34 A case of pure monoclonal IgG kappa cryoglobulinemia in an elderly male. Electron micrograph showing subendothelial and mesangial electron dense deposits (D) consisting of aggregates of rounded or elongated structures.
× 10,000.

Fig. 15-35 Electron micrograph. Inset. Same case as Fig. 15-34. High magnification of a deposit showing curved tubular structures in longitudinal section and in cross section. There is a resemblance to "fingerprints" × 90,000.

Fig. 15-36 Electron micrograph. Mixed cryoglobulinemia IgM-IgG. Same case as Fig. 15-21. Rhomboid and rounded crystals in the cytoplasm of the glomerular endothelium (En). × 14,000.

BM: basement membrane, U: urinary space, P: podocyte.

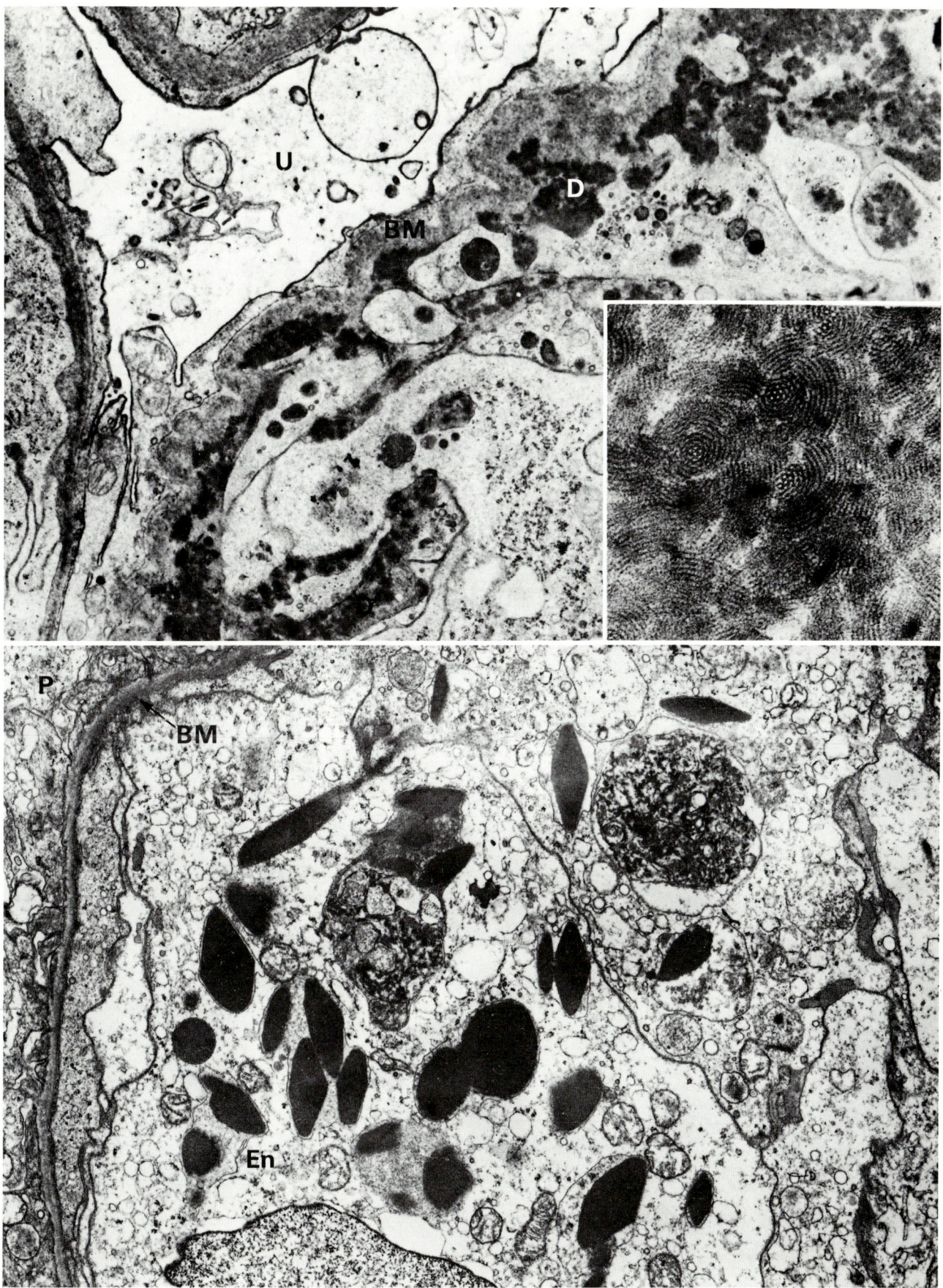

CHAPTER 16

Nephropathy of Liver Disease
    (Figs. 16-1 to 16-8 and Figs. 16-17 to 16-21)
Nephropathy of Sickle Cell Disease
    (Figs. 16-9 to 16-14 and Figs. 16-22 to 16-23)
Nephropathy of Cyanotic Congenital Heart Disease
    (Figs. 16-15 to 16-16 and Fig. 16-24)

Nephropathy of Liver Disease

Definition: Structural abnormalities of glomeruli found in patients with hepatitis and with liver cirrhosis. They consist of mesangial proliferation and sclerosis or in more severe cases, mesangiocapillary or membranous glomerulonephritis or a combination of the two.

Clinical Manifestations: Many patients have no renal manifestations. Those with a more severe glomerular disease may have mild proteinuria and hematuria, microscopic or macroscopic. Renal failure is usually the result of hemodynamic disturbances rather than glomerular damage. Elevation of serum IgA and depression of C3 is not uncommon. Mixed cryoglobulinemia is also quite common.

Light Microscopy: The changes vary from mild mesangial widening to those resembling mesangial or mesangiocapillary glomerulonephritis with mesangial and lobular sclerosis. In some cases there is a picture of membranous glomerulonephritis. It has been noted that poststreptococcal glomerulonephritis with a typical histological picture is more common in patients with cirrhosis.

Electron Microscopy: Mesangial cell proliferation and matrix deposition vary with the severity of the lesion. Dark irregular particles may be seen in the mesangium and in the subendothelial space. They lie in the centers of clear zones which impart a "moth-eaten" appearance to the affected areas*. In some cases the more common type of electron dense deposits are also present in the mesangium, under the endothelium and under the epithelium.

Immunofluorescence Microscopy: Scattered deposits of IgG, IgM, IgA and C3 are often found. In patients with cirrhosis IgA is particularly prominent. In those with hepatitis B, Hbs antigen and Hbs antibodies may be present, probably in the form of immune complexes. Hb_e antigen has been demonstrated in some cases.

---

* These particles are similar to those seen in lecithin cholesterol acyltransferase deficiency (see there) and may have the same basis, that is, a disturbance in the composition of serum lipids.

Nephropathy of Sickle Cell Disease

Definition: Renal disease in patients with hemoglobin S (homozygous) or S and A (heterozygous). This disease is usually manifested by hematuria, concentrating defect and sometimes progressive renal insufficiency, due to tubulo-interstitial disease, especially papillary necrosis, and to "sludging" of erythrocytes in the medullary capillaries. In some cases there is glomerular involvement accompanied by proteinuria and nephrotic syndrome.

Clinical Manifestations of Glomerular Disease include massive proteinuria, hypoalbuminemia, hypercholesteremia and edema. It is not known whether glomerular disease per se leads to renal failure.

Light Microscopy: In many cases only minor changes are seen. Other patients have focal segmental glomerulosclerosis, and still others show a lesion resembling mesangiocapillary glomerulonephritis, with cellular proliferation, increase of mesangial matrix and thickening of capillary walls. Occasionally granules of iron (hemosiderin) are found in the glomerular and also in the tubular cells.

Electron Microscopy: In addition to cellular proliferation and deposition of matrix in the mesangial areas, mesangial interposition occurs in the capillary wall. Electron dense deposits may be found in the mesangium, under the endothelium and in the basement membrane, but this occurs infrequently.

Immunofluorescence Microscopy: Granular deposits of IgG and C3 have been noted along the capillary walls and in the mesangium. It is of interest that C3 level in the serum is usually normal.

Nephropathy of Cyanotic Congenital Heart Disease and in Pulmonary Hypertension

Definition: Glomerular enlargement and mesangial widening with mild cellular proliferation and increase in matrix observed in patients with cardiac and pulmonary disease that is accompanied by hypoxia, cyanosis and polycythemia.

Clinical Manifestations: There are few if any clinical manifestations, seldom more than mild proteinuria. On rare occasion hematuria, hypertension and azotemia have been reported.

Light Microscopy: The glomeruli are enlarged and congested, the capillaries often dilated. The mesangium is widened, sometimes considerably so, with increase in cells and intercellular material (mesangial matrix). On occasion true mesangial nodules are formed. These changes may bear considerable resemblance to those of mesangial glomerulonephritis and even to diabetic glomerulosclerosis.

Electron Microscopy shows mesangial cell proliferation and increase in matrix often accompanied by fine collagen fibrils. The basement membrane is often focally thickened and sometimes altered in density. Foot processes are variably effaced.

Immunofluorescence Microscopy: Inconstant deposits, mainly of IgM, may be found in the mesangium or along the capillary walls.

NEPHROPATHY OF LIVER DISEASE

Fig. 16-1 Hepatic glomerulosclerosis in a case of liver cirrhosis. Glomerular enlargement with mesangial widening and increase of matrix and cells.
PAS stain. × 260.

Fig. 16-2 Advanced stage of hepatic glomerulosclerosis. Mesangial expansion and sclerosis with mild cellularity.
PAS stain. × 260.

Fig. 16-3 Hepatic glomerulosclerosis. Glomerulus showing moderate cellular proliferation and fine lipid deposits (stained red).
Oil Red O stain. × 410.

Fig. 16-4 Immunofluorescence microscopy. Hepatic glomerulosclerosis. Deposits of IgA mainly in the mesangium. × 260.

Fig. 16-5 Hepatitis B and nephrotic syndrome in an 11-year-old girl from Cameroon, Africa. This glomerulus shows mild mesangial expansion and slight capillary wall thickening.
PAS stain of an Epon section. × 260.

Fig. 16-6 Immunofluorescence microscopy. Same case as Fig. 16-5. Numerous granular deposits of IgA mainly along capillary walls. × 260.

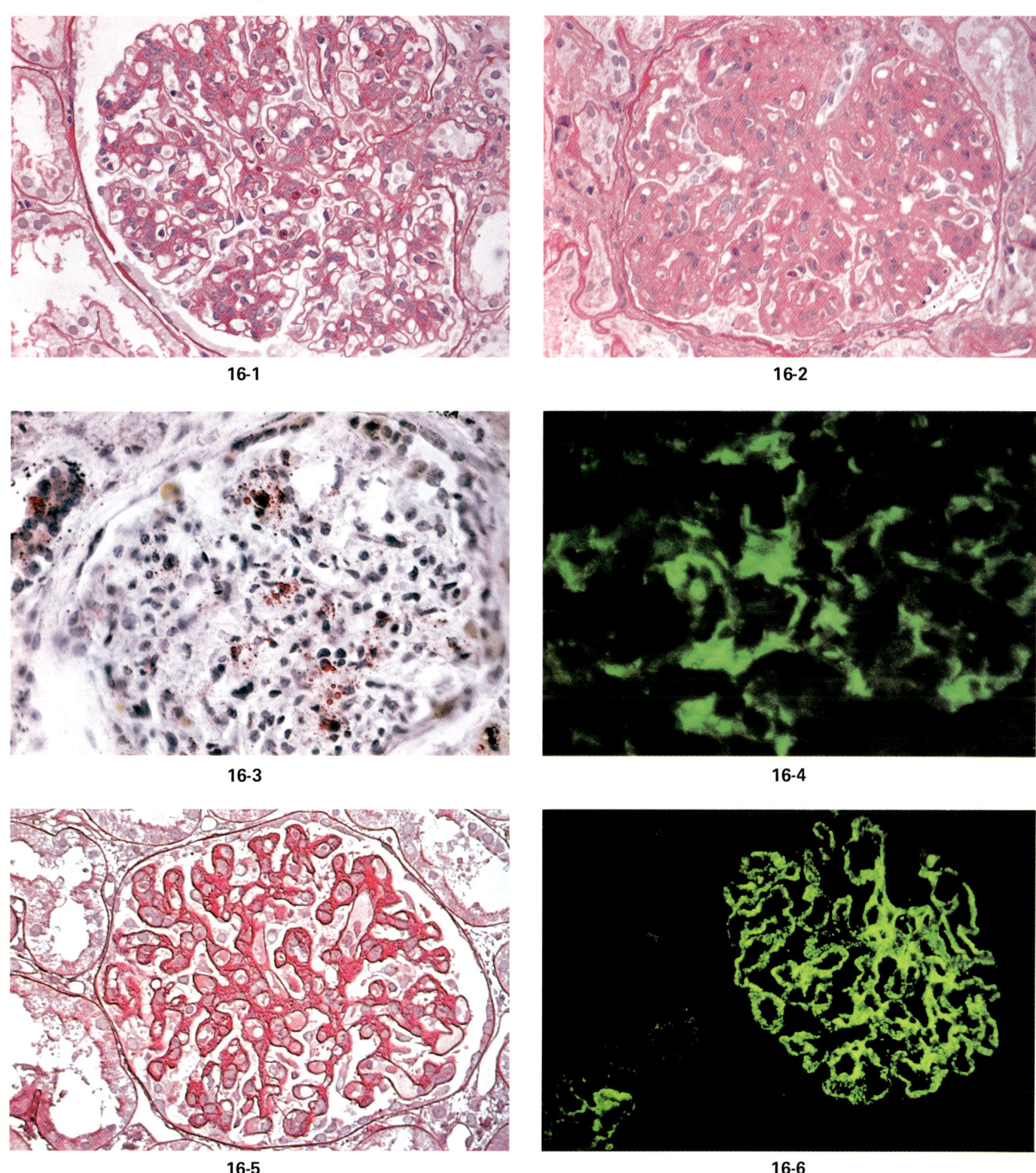

GLOMERULAR LESIONS IN METABOLIC DISEASES

NEPHROPATHY OF LIVER DISEASE

Fig. 16-7 Immunofluorescence microscopy. Same case as Fig. 16-5. Finely granular deposits of C3 along capillary walls. × 260.

Fig. 16-8 Immunofluorescence microscopy. Same case as Fig. 16-5. Small granular deposits of HB_s antigen along the glomerular capillary walls. × 410.

NEPHROPATHY OF SICKLE CELL DISEASE

Fig. 16-9 Sickle cell disease (SS hemoglobin). Sudden death during exercise. Massive sickling of red blood cells in the glomerular capillaries.
H&E stain. × 410.

Fig. 16-10 Sickle cell disease. Glomerulus showing segmental cellular proliferation (right side of picture). There is a suggestion of a thrombus in the lobule towards four o'clock.
PAS stain. × 410.

Fig. 16-11 Sickle cell disease and nephrotic syndrome. Large glomerulus showing mesangial expansion and sclerosis, and segmental thickening of capillary walls.
PAS stain. × 260.

Fig. 16-12 Sickle cell disease. Renal biopsy showing sclerosis of many glomeruli, focal tubular atrophy and tubular dilatation with many casts.
PAS stain. × 41.

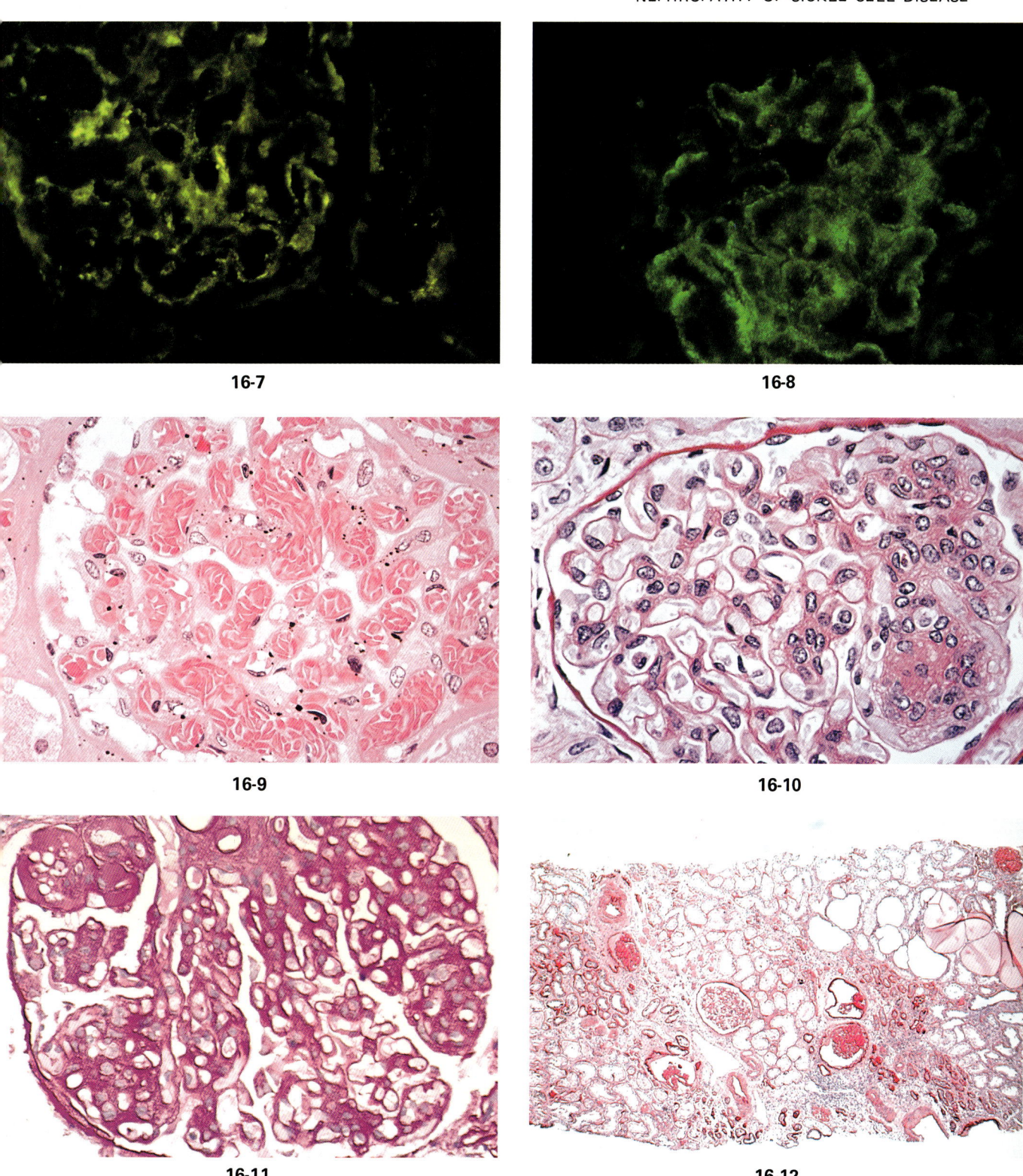

NEPHROPATHY OF SICKLE CELL DISEASE

Fig. 16-13 Same case as Fig. 16-12. Glomerular collapse and sclerosis.
PAS stain. × 260.

Fig. 16-14 Sickle cell disease. Deposits of iron in the tubular cells.
Gomori stain. × 260.

NEPHROPATHY OF CYANOTIC CONGENITAL HEART DISEASE

Fig. 16-15 Cyanotic congenital heart disease in a child. Glomerular enlargement and slight mesangial widening with increase of cells.
H&E stain. × 260.

Fig. 16-16 Cyanotic congenital heart disease in a child. A more advanced change with considerable cellularity, mesangial expansion and partial obliteration of capillaries. This appearance may be mistaken for proliferative glomerulonephritis.
H&E stain. × 260.

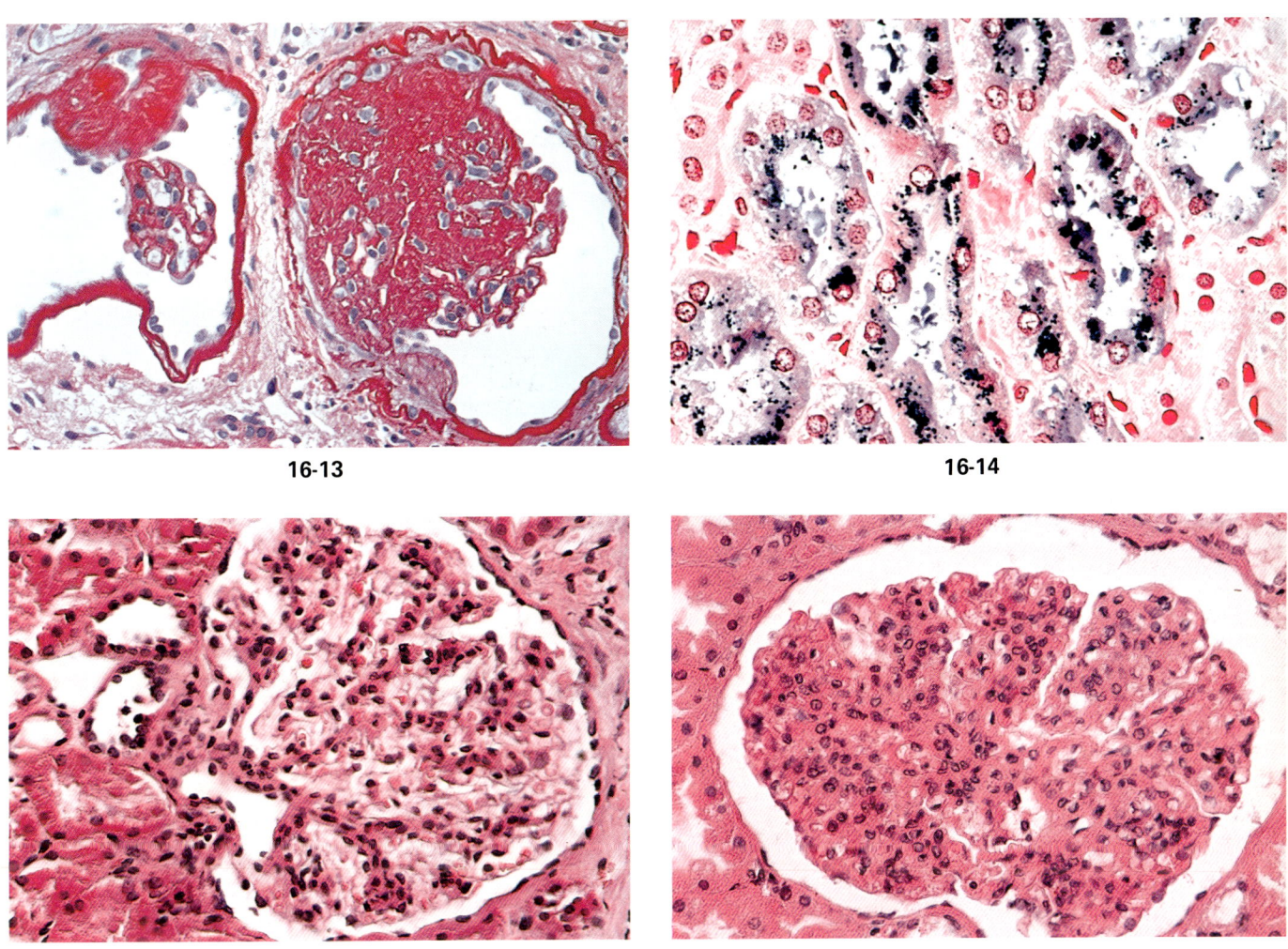

NEPHROPATHY OF LIVER DISEASE

Fig. 16-17 Electron micrograph. Same case as Fig. 16-2. Part of a glomerular tuft showing numerous small white lacunae (l) in the mesangial matrix (MM) containing dark irregular granules.   x 6,400.

Fig. 16-18 Electron micrograph. Inset. Part of the glomerular tuft showing a large clear space in paramesangial area filled with aggregates of dark irregular granules.   x 25,000.

U: urinary space, BM, bm: basement membrane, FP: foot process, MC: mesangial cell, L: capillary lumina.

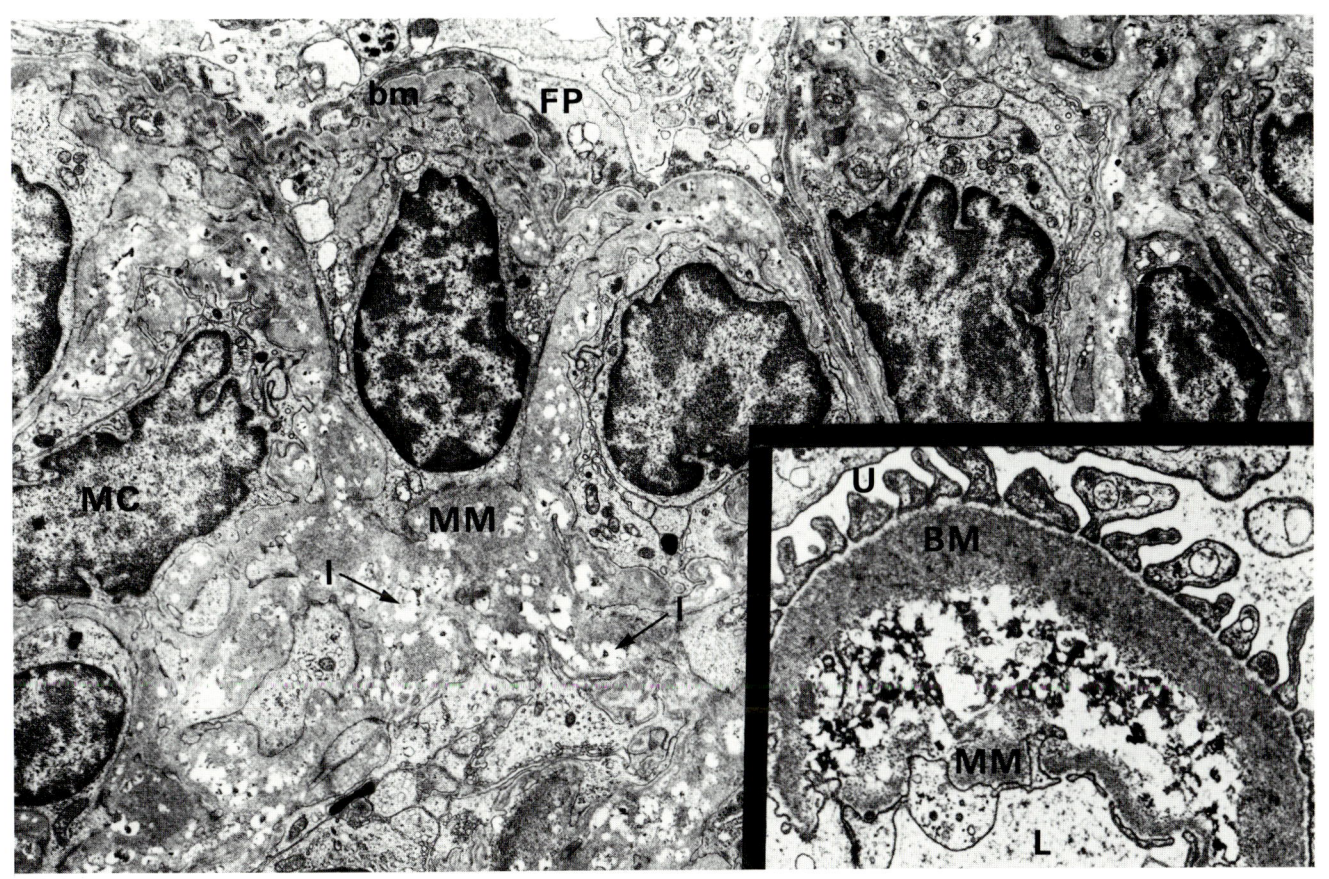

GLOMERULAR LESIONS IN METABOLIC DISEASES

NEPHROPATHY OF LIVER DISEASE

Fig. 16-19 Electron micrograph. Same case as Fig. 16-5. Irregular electron dense subendothelial deposits (D) infiltrating the basement membrane (BM).
x 18,000.

Fig. 16-20 Electron micrograph. Same case as Fig. 16-5. Another area in the same glomerulus showing subepithelial deposits (D). The foot processes (FP) are extensively effaced.
x 15,000.

U: urinary space, En: endothelial cell, P: podocyte.

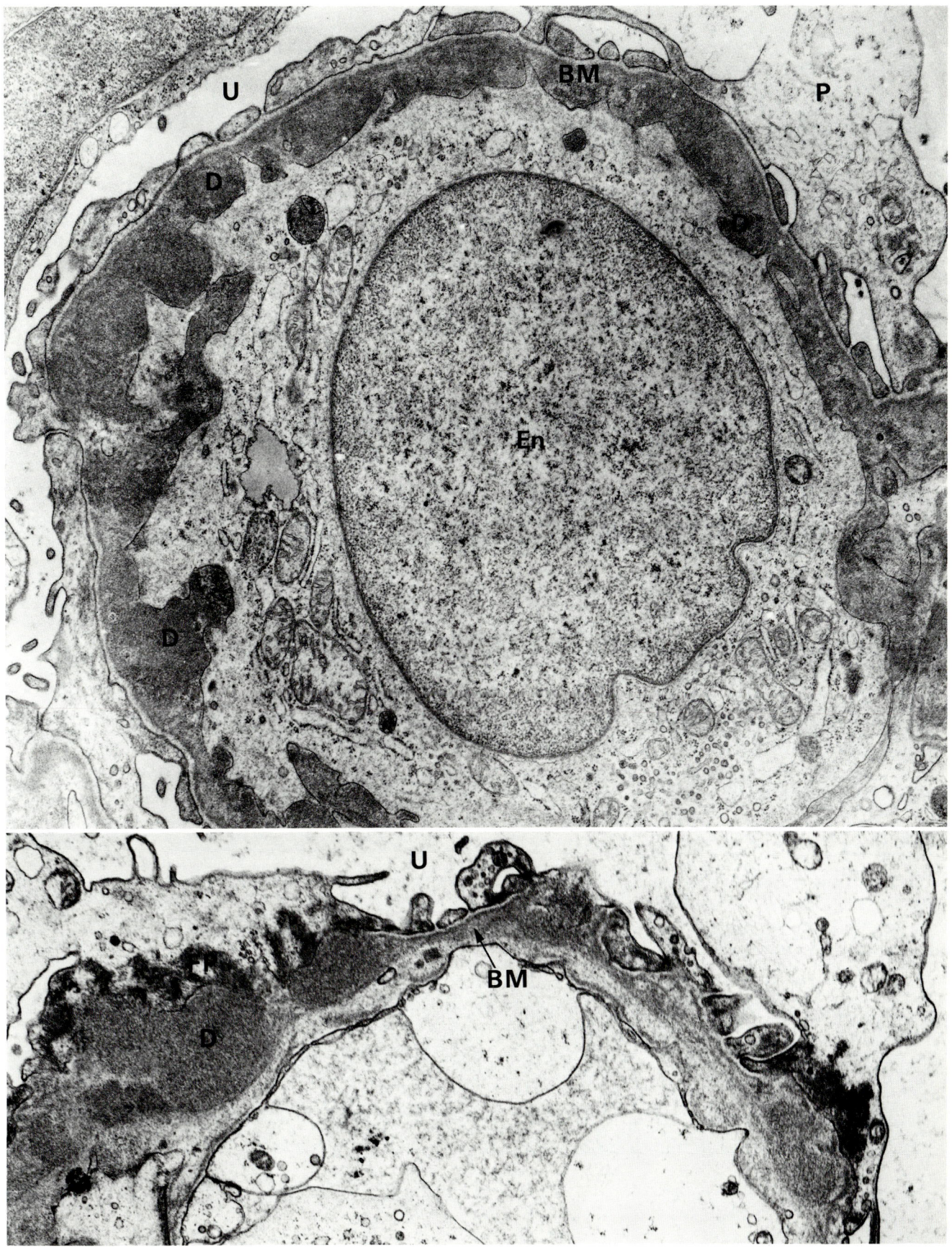

NEPHROPATHY OF LIVER DISEASE

Fig. 16-21 Electron micrograph. Same case as Fig. 16-5. Another area in the same glomerulus showing mesangial proliferation and mesangial interposition. There are electron dense deposits (D) in the interposed mesangium (right side and top of the picture). In many areas the deposits have apparently disappeared and the thickened capillary wall has a "plexiform" appearance.
x 9,000.

NEPHROPATHY OF SICKLE CELL DISEASE

Fig. 16-22 Electron micrograph. Sickle cell disease. Red blood cells showing thin crystals of hemoglobin S.   x 21,000.

BM: basement membrane, U: urinary space.

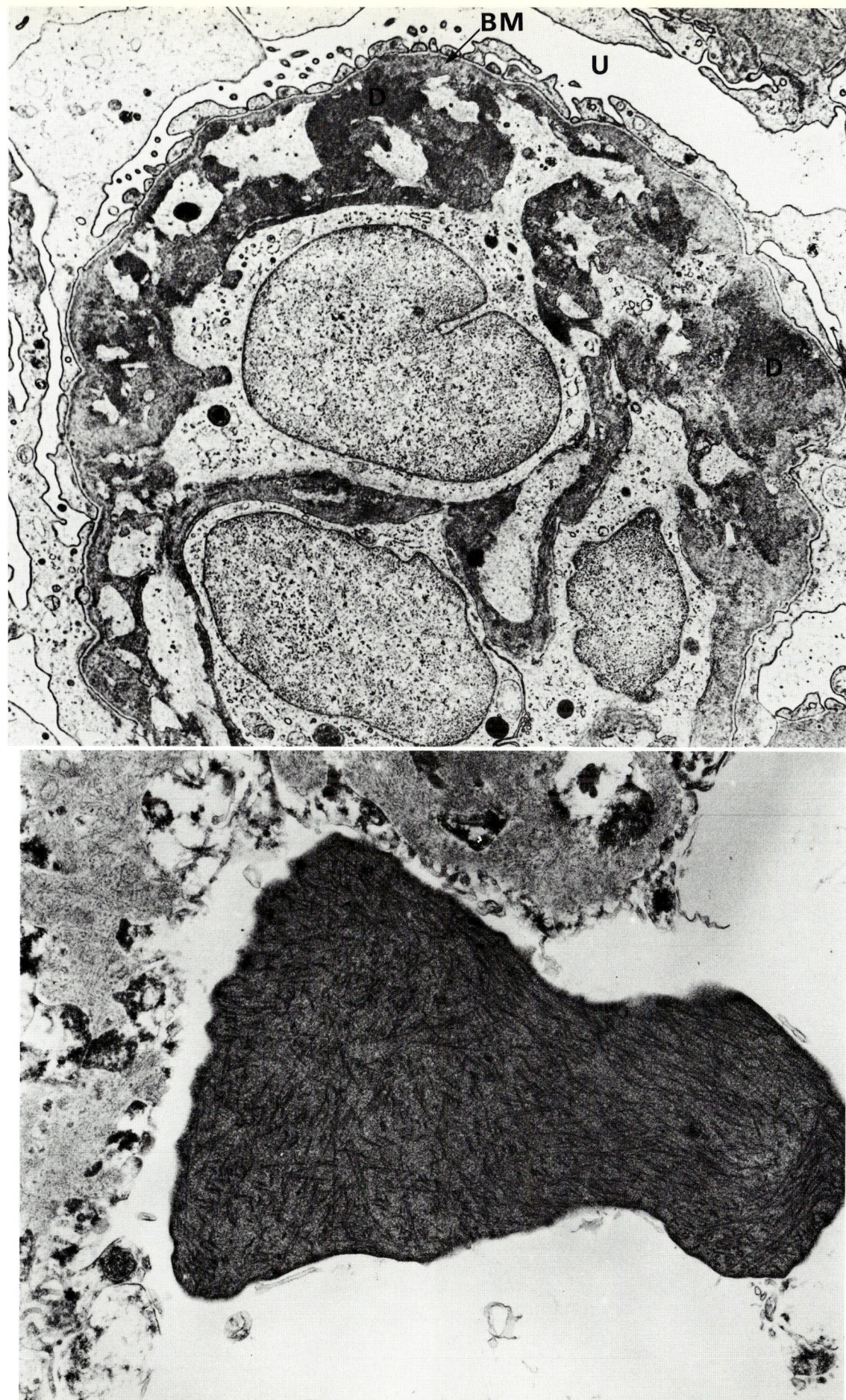

GLOMERULAR LESIONS IN METABOLIC DISEASES

NEPHROPATHY OF SICKLE CELL DISEASE

Fig. 16-23 Electron micrograph. Part of a glomerular tuft in a case of sickle cell disease and nephrotic syndrome. The capillary lumina (L) contain distorted red blood cells (RBC). There is mesangial interposition (MI) circling the capillary. The basement membrane (BM) is thin. The foot processes are extensively effaced. x 6,400.

NEPHROPATHY OF CYANOTIC CONGENTIAL HEART DISEASE

Fig. 16-24 Electron micrograph. Part of a glomerular capillary wall showing mesangial interposition, thickening of the basement membrane (BM) and focal loss of foot processes. x 25,000.

U: urinary space, MC: mesangial cell, MM: mesangial matrix, P: podocyte.

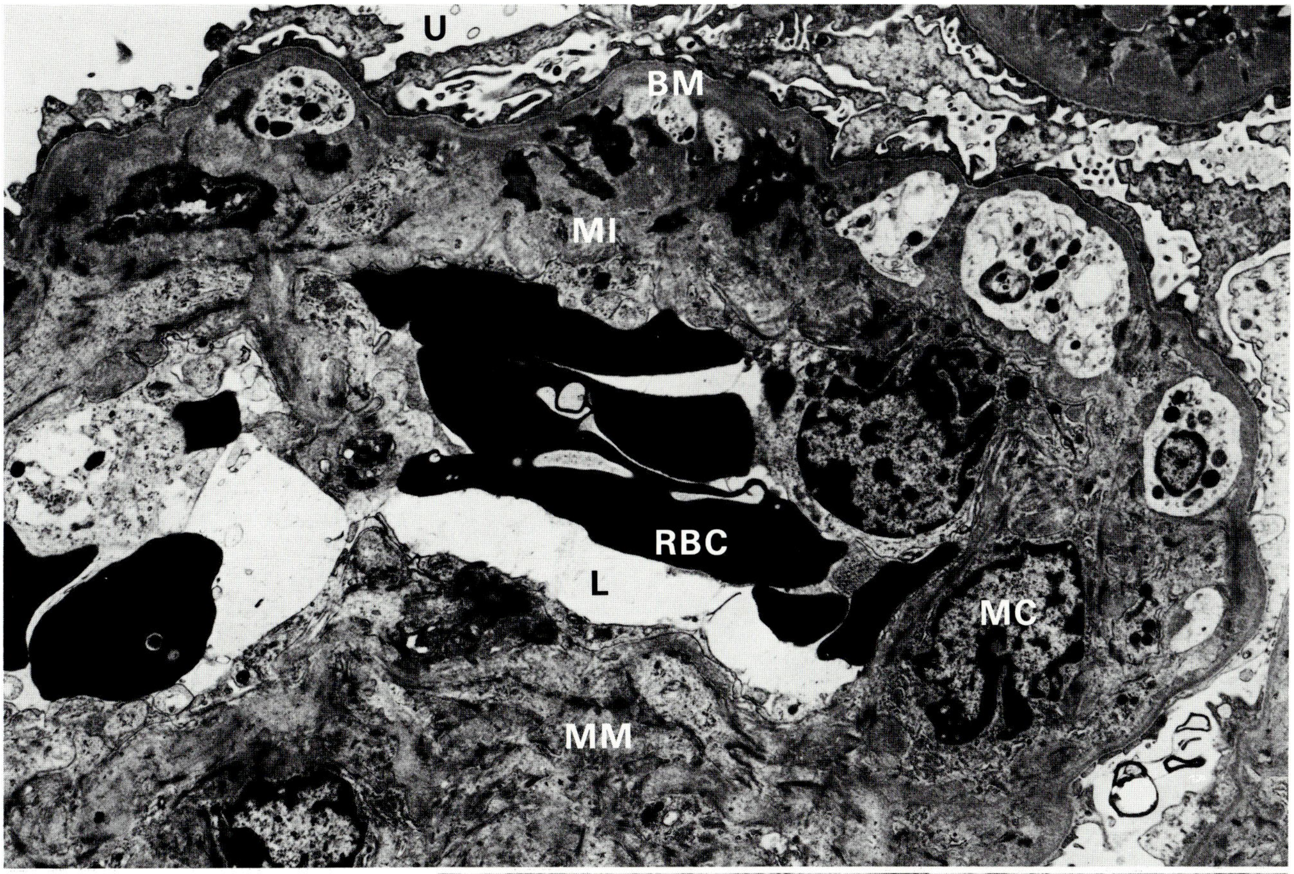

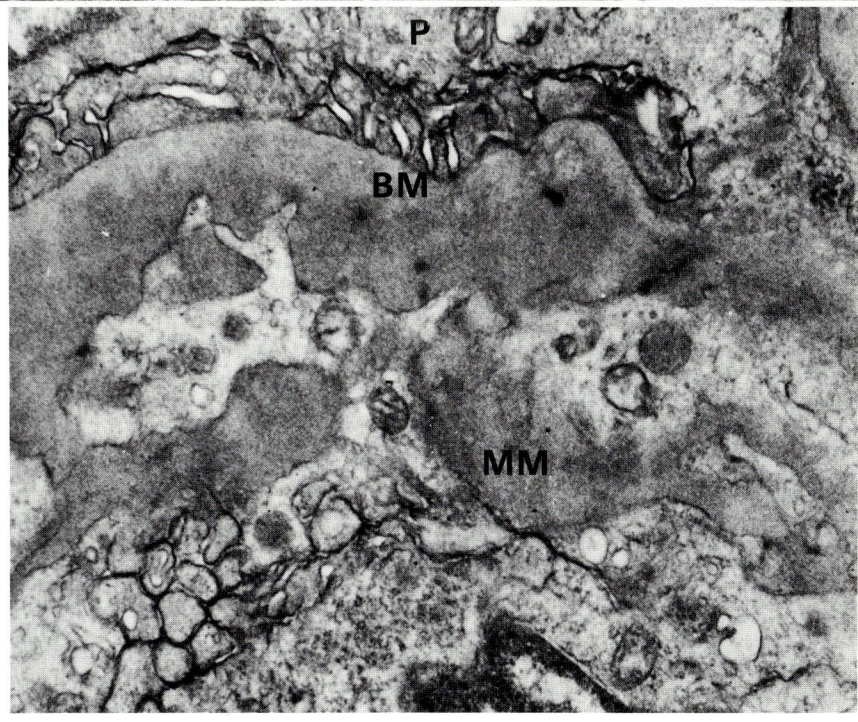

Hereditary Nephropathies

CHAPTER 17

Alport's Syndrome
(Figs. 17-1 to 17-4 and Figs. 17-15 to 17-16)
Thin Basement Membrane Syndrome
(Fig. 17-5 and Fig. 17-17)
Nail-Patella Syndrome
(Figs. 17-6 to 17-8 and Figs. 17-18 to 17-19)
Congenital Nephrotic Syndrome (Finnish Type)
(Figs. 17-9 to 17-11 and Figs. 17-20 to 17-21)
Infantile Nephrotic Syndrome (French Type)
(Figs. 17-12 to 17-14)

Alport's Syndrome

Definition: Hereditary renal disease, probably an autosomal dominant (modulated usually by the presence of Y chromosome) involving glomeruli, tubules and interstitial tissue. In some cases it probably represents a new mutation. When associated with neurosensory deafness and sometimes also with ocular abnormalities, it is known as Alport's syndrome.

Clinical Manifestations: The disease affects both sexes but runs a more severe course in the male. Hearing deficit is most noticeable in the high frequency range. It occurs in over half the patients, and is occasionally the sole manifestation, but is usually associated with progressive renal disease. Various types of eye changes are present in about 10% of patients.

Renal symptoms begin very early in life although may not be discovered until years later. Microscopic or gross hematuria is seen most frequently, but proteinuria is a common accompaniment, occasionally leading to nephrotic syndrome. Renal insufficiency develops gradually, first manifesting in males in the second decade of life and progressing to failure in the majority over a period of 10–20 years. The onset of renal insufficiency in females usually occurs later and is considerably less frequent. Many women live to old age despite bouts of hematuria.

Hereditary glomerulopathy is probably not a single entity, but rather a group of syndromes. Some cases of Alport's syndrome are accompanied by mental retardation and hyperprolinemia, and others by thrombocytopenia and giant platelets. Whether they are the same as Alport's syndrome is not known. There are also families with similar renal symptomatology but without hearing or ocular defects, and families in whom renal disease is more severe in females.

Light Microscopy: In the early stages glomerular changes are minor or entirely absent. With progression, focal mesangial proliferation and focal segmental areas of sclerosis and hyalinization appear, eventually leading to the picture of diffuse sclerosing glomerulonephritis. Occasionally capillary wall thickening may be recognized. In some cases "foam cells" are seen in the glomeruli.

Tubular changes consist of vacuolation of cell cytoplasm and thickening of basement membranes. Interstitial infiltration by inflammatory cells and fibrosis may suggest the diagnosis of pyelonephritis. A characteristic change is accumulation of vacuolated "foam cells". This is non-specific but in the presence of normal blood lipid levels, and absence of interstitial inflammation, is strongly suggestive of Alport's syndrome.

Abnormalities of structure have been also observed in the eye and in the inner ear.

Electron Microscopy: The most characteristic change is segmental thickening and splitting of the glomerular basement membrane into many parallel layers, with clear spaces and small dense particles between the layers. Alternating with, and perhaps in some cases, preceding the above change, is segmental *thinning* of the lamina densa to 1/3–1/4 that of normal. These basement membrane abnormalities are not present in every case; actually they are found in the minority of patients, perhaps because of insufficient sampling, or because the lesions have not yet developed, or because the case represents a different syndrome. Severe thickening and splitting of basement membranes in the absence of other glomerular changes is almost diagnostic of Alport's syndrome. Minor degrees of splitting may accompany a variety of glomerular diseases. Thickening and splitting of tubular basement membranes is frequent but less specific than the glomerular changes; it is often seen in nephrotic syndrome. The same is true of the interstitial foam cells.

Immunofluorescence Microscopy: As a rule no immunoglobulins are found in the glomeruli. Occasional and minor deposits of C3 have been reported.

Benign Recurrent Hematuria

Definition: A non-progressive renal disease manifested by repeated attacks of hematuria. This is probably a heterogeneous group, which includes focal and segmental glomerulonephritis, perhaps early stages of Alport's syndrome, exertional hematuria, as well as familial glomerular disease characterized by marked thinning of the basement membranes.

Thin Basement Membrane Syndrome

Clinical Manifestations: Attacks of hematuria, gross or microscopic, are brought about by intercurrent infection, by exertion, or occur spontaneously. Mild proteinuria may be also noted. Children and adults are affected. Long-term follow-ups are scanty and it is possible that some cases do progress to renal failure.

Light Microscopy: In a considerable proportion of patients, in whom lower urinary tract disease has been excluded by careful study, glomeruli show no abnormalities by light microscopy or by electron and immunofluorescence microscopy, or perhaps only an increased number of totally sclerosed glomeruli. In some of these cases the renal origin of hematuria is confirmed by the presence of red cell casts in the tubular lumina. The absence of glomerular lesions may be the result of insufficient sampling, particularly if such lesions are focal and involve only a small percentage of glomeruli. In other cases the characteristic change cannot be recognized by light microscopy and require electron microscopy.

Electron Microscopy may demonstrate segmental thinning of the basement membranes as a sole lesion. The lamina densa is usually reduced, in at least some capillaries, to half its normal thickness or less, and may measure as little as 60–80 nm. In children it is important to exclude the early stage of Alport's syndrome, before the development of basement membrane thickening and splitting. However, there are indications that some patients who only show thinning of the basement membrane, may also progress to renal failure.

Immunofluorescence Microscopy: Deposits of immunoglobulins and complement are generally absent.

Nail-Patella Syndrome (Osteo-onychodysplasia)

Definition: Glomerular disease associated with the syndrome of bony abnormalities and dysplasia of nails.

Clinical Manifestations: The disease is inherited as autosomal dominant. Bony changes consist of absence of patellae, iliac protrusions (horns) and subluxation of radial heads. Nails may be atrophic, or soft or longitudinally ridged. Ocular anomalies have been noted on occasion.

Renal symptoms occur in about half the patients and consist mainly of proteinuria, generally mild, but on occasion in the nephrotic range. Microscopic hematuria may be present. Some of the patients progress to renal failure.

Light Microscopy: In patients with urinary abnormalities, at first only minor changes are seen, although focal thickening of capillary basement membranes may be noted. With more advanced disease, mesangial widening, focal cellularity and sclerosis develop, followed by focal segmental sclerotic lesions and eventually by diffuse glomerular sclerosis. Tubular atrophy and interstitial fibrosis accompany the glomerular lesions.

Electron Microscopy: The characteristic finding, which is seen also in the absence of other glomerular changes, is the occurrence of short bundles of collagen in the thickened lamina densa of the glomerular basement membranes. The collagen lies in the centers of pale areas (lacunae) and is also pale and sometimes difficult to identify. It is best demonstrated after staining with phosphotungstic acid. The collagen shows typical periodicity, and is also found in the mesangial matrix.

Immunofluorescence Microscopy: Usually there is no evidence of immune deposits. Only in rare instances the presence of small amounts of IgM and C3 have been reported.

Congenital Nephrotic Syndrome (Finnish Type)

Definition: The syndrome of massive proteinuria and inanition which develops shortly after birth, predominantly in children of Finnish extraction. The syndrome is inherited as an autosomal recessive.

Clinical Manifestations: The infants are usually premature and of low birth weight, but the placenta is larger than normal. The nephrotic syndrome may be present at birth or develops during the first three months of life and does not respond to therapy. Most of the affected individuals die of metabolic disturbances or intercurrent infections. Very few survive beyond the first year of life.

Light Microscopy: Many glomeruli are immature. The mature glomeruli show mild to moderate mesangial proliferation and some sclerosis. Advanced sclerosis occurs only late in the disease. A very characteristic but not an invariable lesion is the presence of small cysts in the cortex, especially near the corticomedullary junction ("microcystic disease"), arising by dilatation of the proximal tubules. Arteriolar medial hypertrophy is commonly present and may also be a striking feature on histologic examination.

Electron Microscopy shows diffuse loss of foot processes and other changes in the podocytes, typical of nephrotic syndrome. The basement membranes are thin. Mesangial cellularity and sclerosis are usually present.

Immunofluorescence Microscopy: No specific changes have been registered.

Infantile Nephrotic Syndrome (French Type)
(Diffuse Mesangial Sclerosis)

Definition: Familial nephrotic syndrome which develops during the first year of life and is probably inherited as autosomal recessive.

Clinical Manifestations: The nephrotic syndrome may appear as early as the first week after birth, but usually after three months. There is a steady progression to renal insufficiency, terminating in uremia between the ages of one and three years.

Light Microscopy: The glomeruli show mesangial and later global sclerosis without significant cell proliferation. They become small and contract into rounded masses that are covered by a layer of epithelium. Bowman's spaces are often moderately dilated. The lesion is usually uniform, involving all glomeruli. There is corresponding tubular atrophy with interstitial fibrosis.

Electron Microscopy: Loss of foot processes and edema of podocytes are typical of nephrotic syndrome. Basement membrane may be severely altered and irregularly thickened. Sclerosis is due to progressive increase of mesangial matrix.

Immunofluorescence Microscopy: No deposits reported.

HEREDITARY NEPHROPATHIES

ALPORT'S SYNDROME

Fig. 17-1   Alport's syndrome in a young boy. Glomerulus showing no significant abnormalities on light microscopy.
PAS stain. × 410.

Fig. 17-2   Alport's syndrome in a 15-year-old girl. Numerous "foam cells" are seen in the interstitium.
H&E stain. × 260.

Fig. 17-3   Alport's syndrome in a teen-age boy. Numerous lipid droplets in the renal interstitium and in the tubular cells.
Oil Red O stain. × 410.

Fig. 17-4   Another case of Alport's syndrome in a teen-age boy. Glomerular sclerosis with slight cell proliferation and capsular adhesions. There is also tubular atrophy and dilatation. This picture resembles sclerosing glomerulonephritis.
H&E stain. × 260.

ALPORT'S SYNDROME

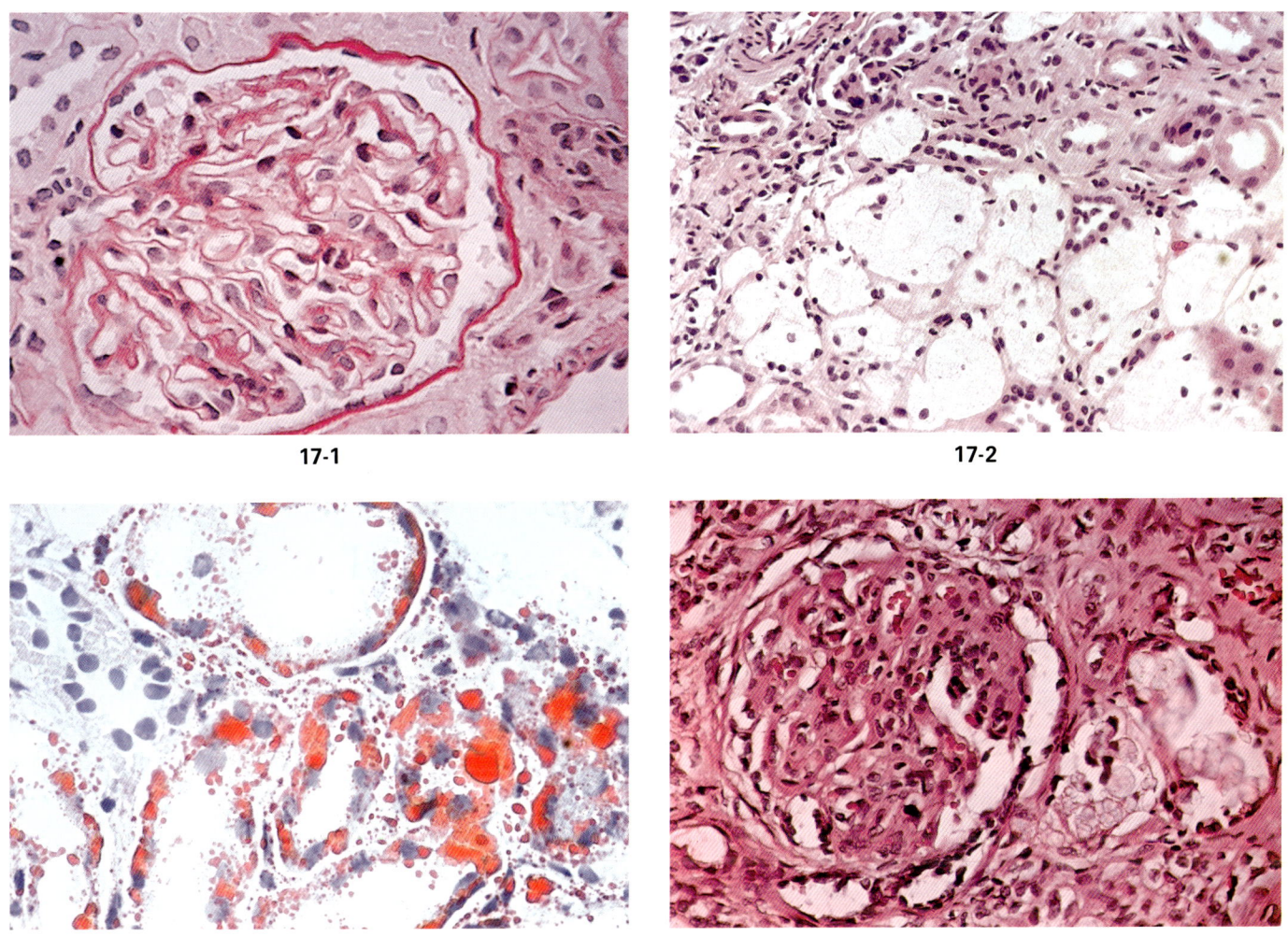

17-1

17-2

17-3

17-4

THIN BASEMENT MEMBRANE SYNDROME

Fig. 17-5 Thin basement membrane syndrome. Recurrent hematuria in a 20-year-old female. Neither glomeruli nor tubules show any significant changes on light microscopy.
PAS stain. × 260.

NAIL-PATELLA SYNDROME

Fig. 17-6 Nail-patella syndrome. Asymptomatic proteinuria in a young boy. Glomerulus showing slight and segmental capillary wall thickening.
PAS stain. × 410.

Fig. 17-7 Proteinuria and renal failure in an adult. Glomerulus shows segmental sclerosis and adhesions to the Bowman's capsule. There is beginning tubular atrophy.
PAS stain. × 260.

Fig. 17-8 Same case as in Fig. 17-7. Renal biopsy showing considerable glomerular sclerosis and tubular atrophy.
PAS stain. × 40.

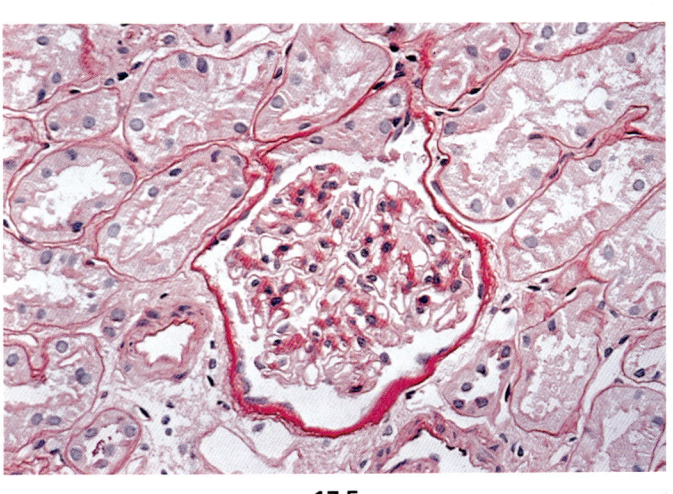

17-5

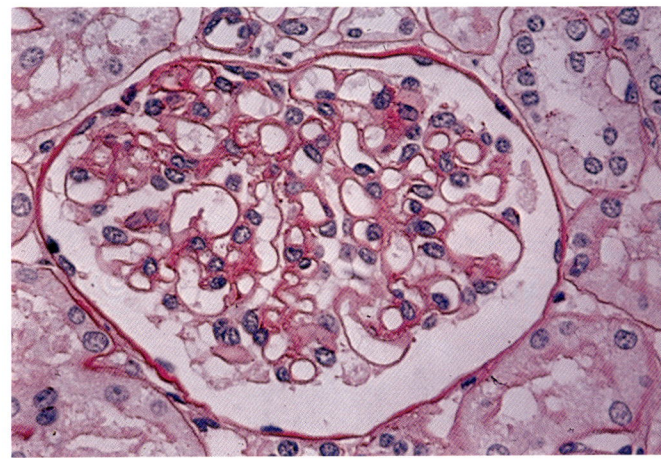

17-6

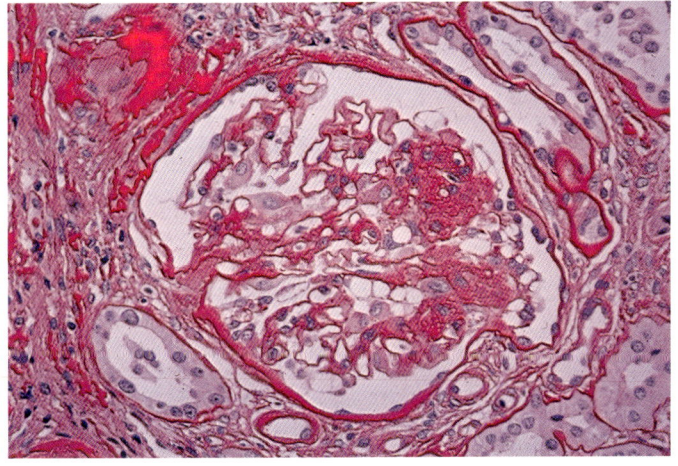

17-7

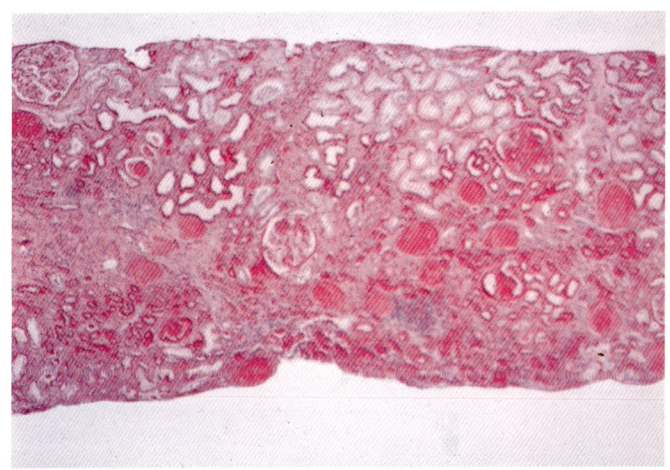

17-8

CONGENITAL NEPHROTIC SYNDROME (FINNISH TYPE)

Fig. 17-9 Congenital nephrotic syndrome in an infant. There is obvious mesangial hypercellularity.
H&E stain.   x 640.

Fig. 17-10 A more advanced stage of congenital nephrotic syndrome in a young child. There is mesangial and more diffuse sclerosis of the glomerulus with loss of capillary lumina.
PAS stain.   x 510.

Fig. 17-11 General appearance of renal cortex in a young child with congenital nephrotic syndrome. Numerous microcysts are present.
H&E stain.   x 150.

INFANTILE NEPHROTIC SYNDROME (FRENCH TYPE)

Fig. 17-12 Infantile nephrotic syndrome (French type). Renal biopsy in a child 18 months old. Nephrotic syndrome developed at the age of 16 months. At the time of biopsy there was also renal insufficiency. Some glomeruli show segmental sclerosis. The tubules are dilated.
PAS stain.   x 100.

Fig. 17-13 Same case as Fig. 17-12. Typical appearance of a glomerulus with slight mesangial proliferation and increase of matrix.
PAS stain.   x 410.

Fig. 17-14 Same case as Fig. 17-12. The child died five months after the biopsy. At autopsy some glomeruli were similar to those seen in the biopsy, but most of them showed considerable degree of sclerosis.
PAS stain.   x 100.

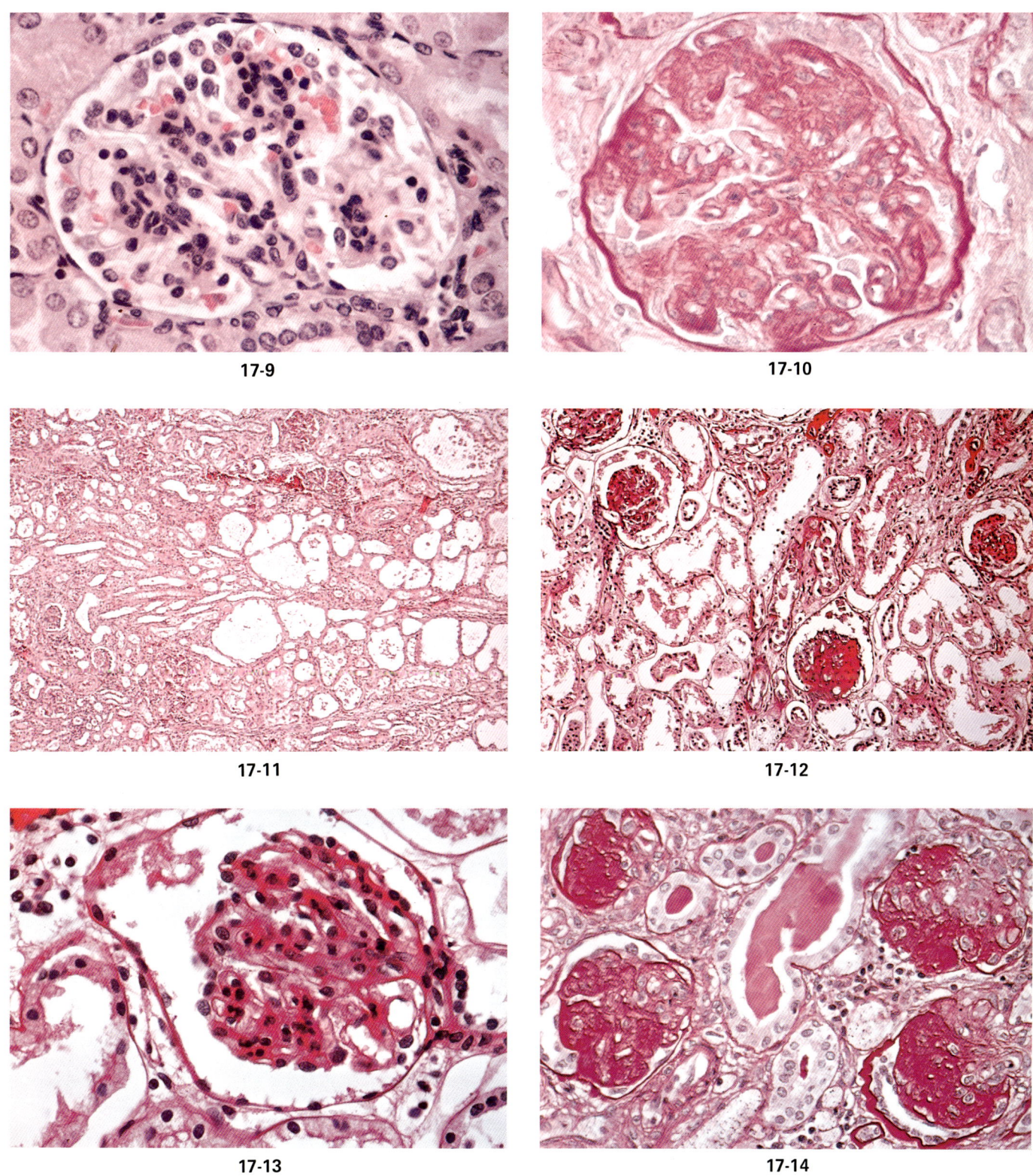

HEREDITARY NEPHROPATHIES

ALPORT'S SYNDROME

Fig. 17-15 Electron micrograph. Typical appearance of the glomerular basement membranes (BM) in Alport's syndrome. The upper capillary as well as part of the lower capillary shows thickening of the lamina densa with splitting into many layers and small dense particles between the layers. The left side of the basement membrane (BM) of the lower capillary is considerably thinned out.
× 13,000.

Fig. 17-16 Electron micrograph. Same case as Fig. 17-3. Thickening, splitting and focal thinning of the glomerular capillary basement membrane (BM) (arrows).
× 16,000.

L: capillary lumen, U: urinary space, P: podocyte.

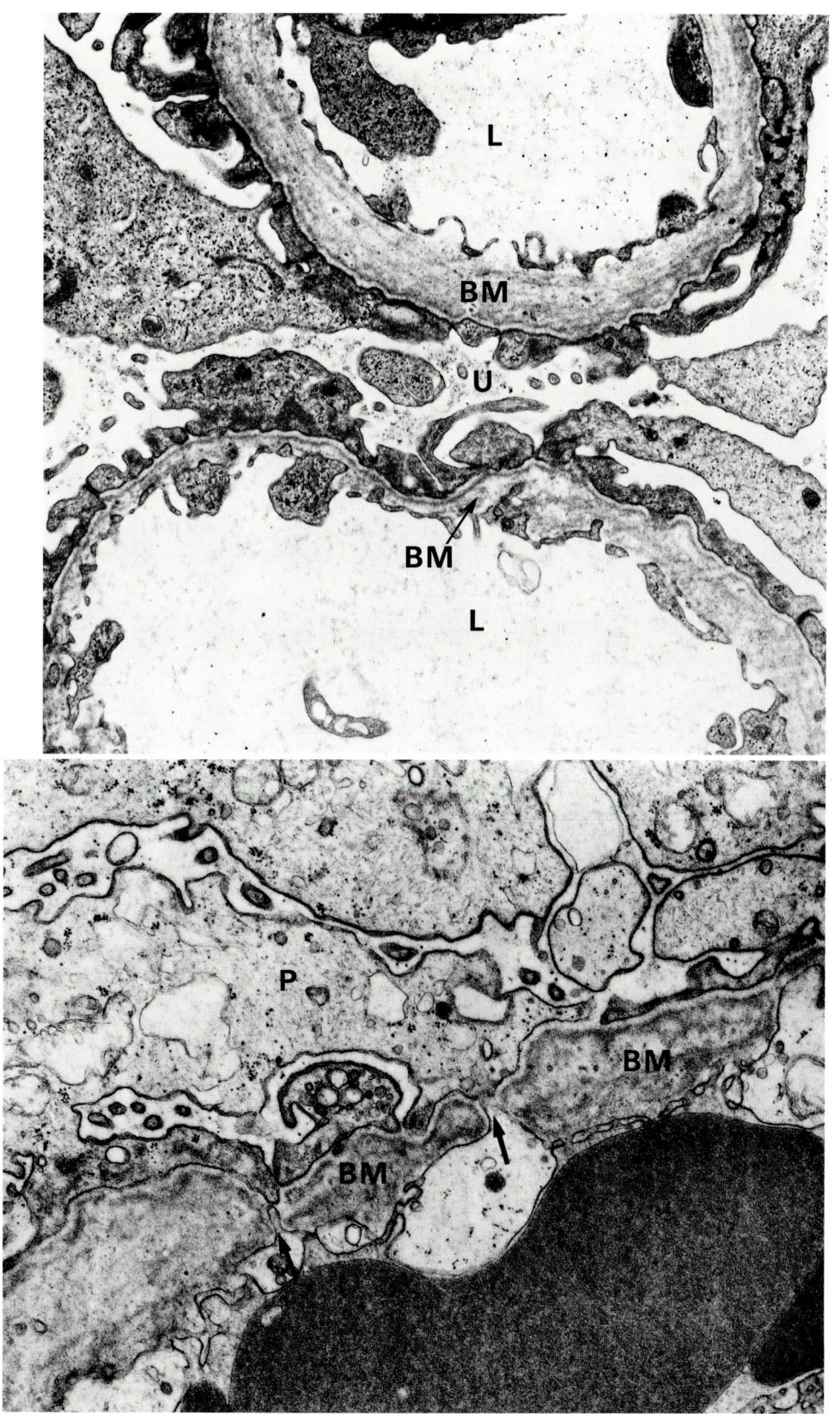

THIN BASEMENT MEMBRANE SYNDROME

Fig. 17-17 Electron micrograph. Thin basement membrane syndrome. The lamina densa of the peripheral glomerular basement membrane (bm) is strikingly thin. Lamina densa over the mesangium (left and right lower corners) is thickened.
x 9,900.

P: podocyte, L: capillary lumen.

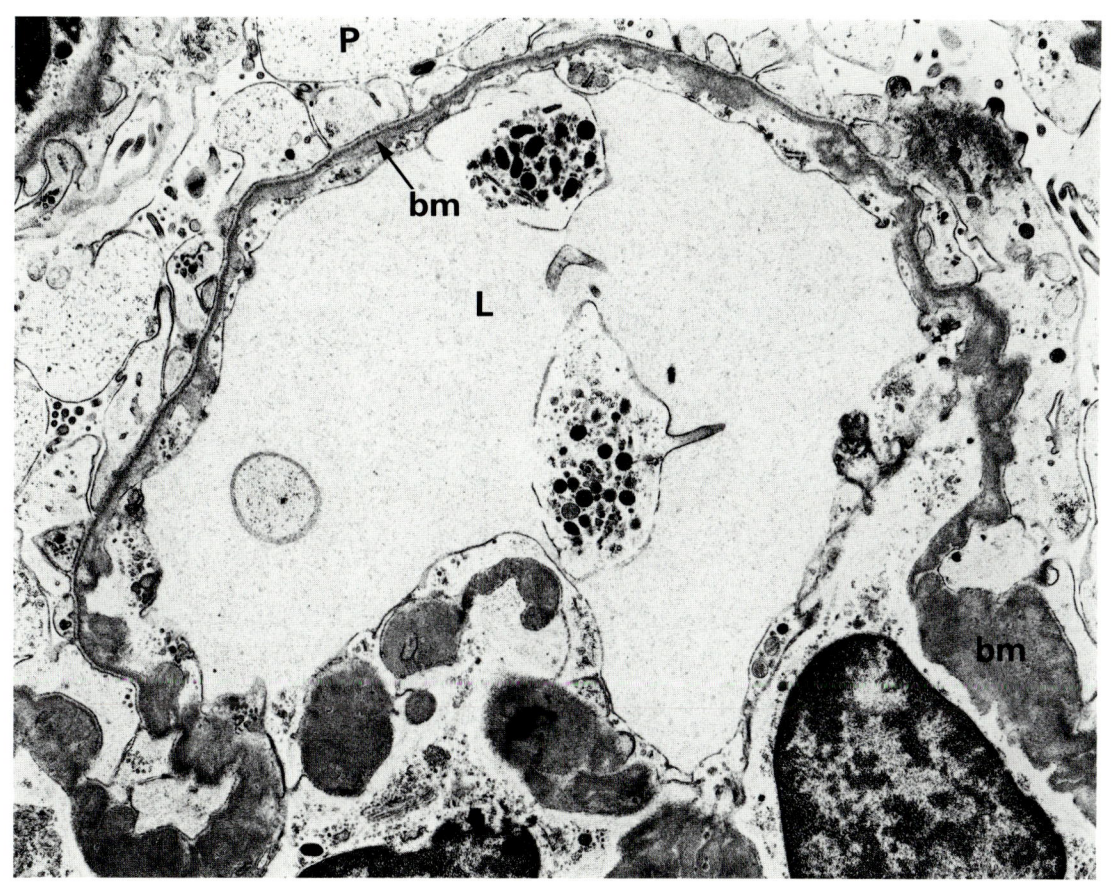

HEREDITARY NEPHROPATHIES

NAIL-PATELLA SYNDROME

Fig. 17-18 Electron micrograph. Same case as in Fig. 17-6. Part of a glomerular capillary showing thickening of the lamina densa with many irregular lucent areas (l).
x 13,000.

Fig. 17-19 Electron micrograph. Same case as in Fig. 17-6. The clear areas in the basement membranes (BM) contain thick bundles of collagen (Col), made visible by the special stain.
PTA stain.   x 40,000.

U: urinary space, BM: basement membrane, L: capillary lumen.

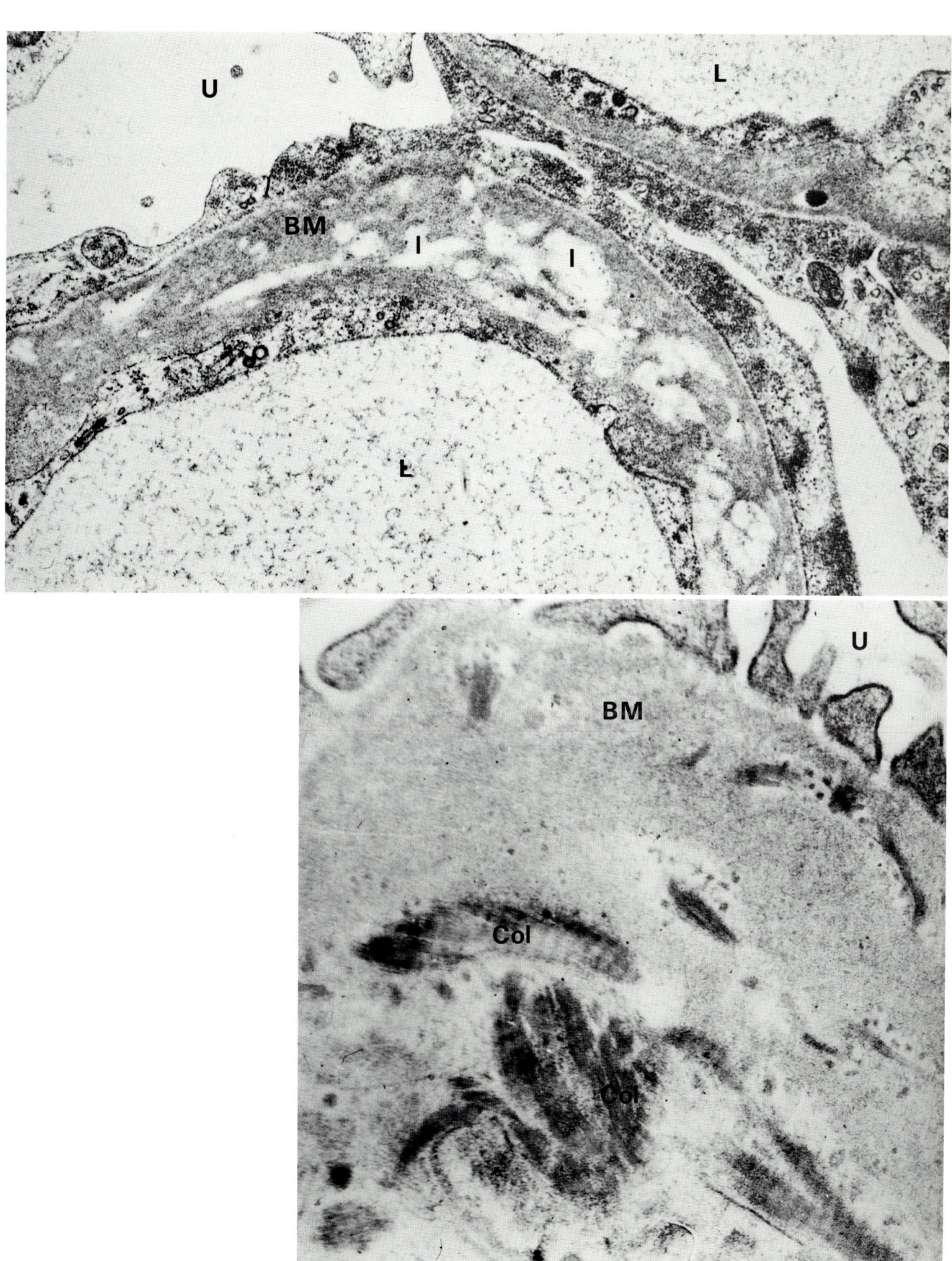

HEREDITARY NEPHROPATHIES

CONGENITAL NEPHROTIC SYNDROME (FINNISH TYPE)

Fig. 17-20 Electron micrograph. Congenital nephrotic syndrome. Glomerular capillary shows very thin basement membrane (arrows) and diffuse effacement of foot processes (FP). × 6,000.

Fig. 17-21 Electron micrograph. Congenital nephrotic syndrome in a young child. Glomerular lobule in the process of sclerosis. There is marked increase of mesangial matrix (MM), narrowing of the capillary lumina (L) and rather extensive loss of foot processes. × 2,000.

BC: Bowman's capsule, U: urinary space.

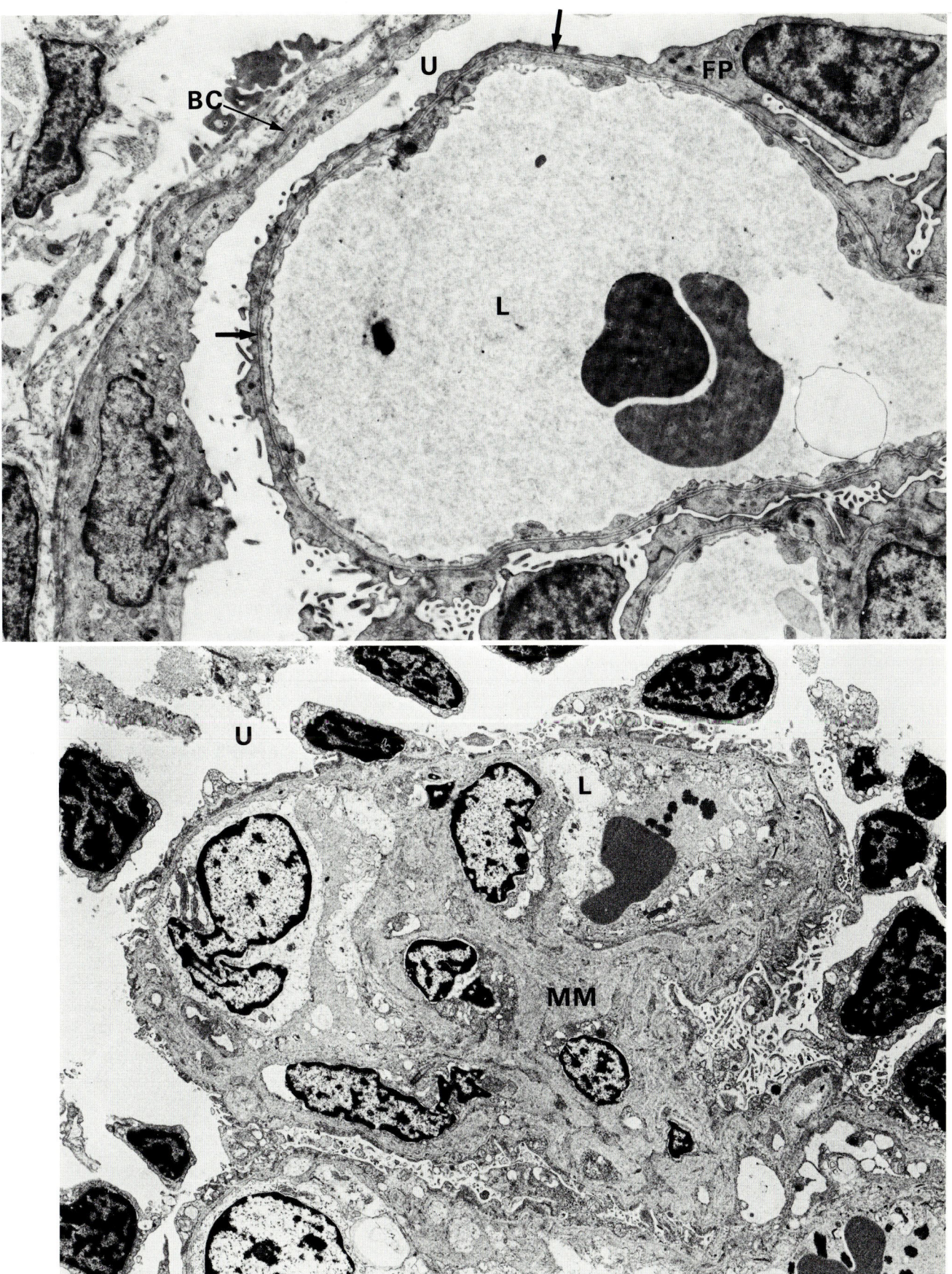

CHAPTER 18

Fabry's Disease
(Figs. 18-1 to 18-2 and Figs. 18-7 to 18-8)
Familial Lecithin-Cholesterol Acyl Transferase Deficiency
(Figs. 18-3 to 18-4 and Figs. 18-9 to 18-12)
I-Cell Disease
(Figs. 18-5 to 18-6)

Fabry's Disease

Definition: Renal disease due to deposition of glycosphingolipids, trihexosylceramide and to some extent dihexosylceramide, in the tissues. These substances accumulate in the cell lysosomes because of inherited deficiency of a specific enzyme, ceramide trioxidase (α-galactosyl hydrolase A). The mode of inheritance is x-linked recessive.

Clinical Manifestations: In hemizygous males the disease begins in childhood and runs a progressive course. Some of the heterozygous females are also affected, but usually later in life and less severely. Systemic manifestations include cutaneous and mucosal hemangiomata (angiokeratomas), attacks of inexplicable pain in the extremities, corneal dystrophy, coronary heart disease, and cerebral involvement, including strokes. Diagnosis is established by demonstrating deficiency of the enzyme, ceramide trioxidase, in leukocytes, cultured fibroblasts or hair follicles. Renal symptoms consist of proteinuria, microscopic hematuria and lipiduria, occasionally concentration defect and aminoaciduria. Renal failure develops in men in their 30's or 40's and sometimes earlier; it is uncommon in women, but may occur even in the absence of cutaneous lesions.

Light Microscopy: The typical finding is the presence of vacuolated epithelium in the glomerulus. The content of the vacuoles, the glycosphingolipid, is dissolved in formalin fixed tissues during processing and paraffin embedding, but can be demonstrated as fine granules in frozen sections, or better still after osmic acid fixation. This material is birefringent, stains with lipid stains and is strongly PAS positive. Similar material is also present in the mesangial and endothelial cells, in tubular cells, in the smooth muscle of the arterial walls and in the interstitial cells. With progression of disease, capillary wall thickening and mesangial sclerosis become evident in the glomeruli, and there is striking thickening of arterial walls with narrowing of the lumina.

(It must be noted that glomerular epithelial vacuolization of similar appearance is also a feature of other metabolic storage diseases, including mucopolysaccharidoses and mucolipidoses, and that specific diagnosis depends on supplemental clinical information; it should be noted also, however, that glomerular sclerosis and progression to renal failure are rarely found in these other conditions).

Electron Microscopy demonstrates dense whorled osmiophilic structures (myelin bodies) in cell cytoplasm, corresponding to the granules seen by light microscopy. These structures are particularly prominent in the epithelial cells.

Immunofluorescence Microscopy: Deposition of immunoglobulins or complement has not been reported.

Familial Lecithin-Cholesterol Acyl Transferase Deficiency

Definition: Glomerular lipidosis and progressive glomerular sclerosis occur in lecithin-cholesterol acyl transferase deficiency. This deficiency is inherited apparently as an autosomal recessive. The lack of the enzyme results in marked disturbances of lipid metabolism. Renal involvement is common.

Clinical Manifestations: This is a rare disease most often reported in the Scandinavian countries, particularly in Norway. It affects both sexes. The first manifestation is mild or moderate proteinuria which begins in the second decade of life or possibly earlier, and persists for the next 20–40 years. Mild microscopic hematuria may also be noted. Corneal opacities and moderately severe normochromic anemia are almost always found. The characteristic manifestation is change in the composition of serum lipids with increased levels of total cholesterol, triglycerides and phospholipids and almost complete lack of estrified cholesterol. Renal failure develops in the fourth or fifth decade of life and progresses rapidly often with nephrotic syndrome and hypertension.

Light Microscopy: Typically the glomeruli contain lipid-laden foam cells, lying in the capillary lumina and apparently representing altered endothelial cells. Foam cells are also present in the interstitium. Glomerular capillary basement membranes are thickened, and some glomeruli are sclerosed even in the early stages of the disease.

Electron Microscopy: The foam cells are filled with what appears to be neutral lipids. Thickening of the capillary basement membranes is caused by widening of the lamina rara interna and also lamina densa, with accumulation of partly membrane-bound dark particles lying in the centers of clear spaces. The overlying endothelium may become detached. Similar particles may be seen in the widened mesangium. In some cases serpiginous fibrillar deposits are seen in the subendothelial space. Deposits recur rapidly in the transplanted kidney.

I-Cell Disease (Mucolipidosis II)

Definition: This is an autosomal recessive disorder characterized by accumulation of various macromolecules, especially glycosaminoglycans and lipids in the lysosomes of connective tissue cells, histiocytes and renal epithelium. Cultured fibroblasts contain inclusions of accumulated glycosaminoglycans, hence the name "Inclusion Cell" or I-cell disease. The basic defect appears to be deficient retention of acid hydrolases by the lysosomes. The affected individuals show skeletal deformities, psychomotor retardation and cardiac insufficiency, and seldom survive childhood.

Clinical Manifestations: Renal manifestations are infrequent and if present are very mild. There may be slight proteinuria and hematuria as well as casts and leukocytes in the urinary sediment. Renal insufficiency is unusual.

Light Microscopy: Glomerular podocytes may be strikingly vacuolated and be accompanied by slight mesangial widening. The contents of the vacuolated cells stain strongly with colloidal iron and with Alcian blue indicating the presence of glycosaminoglycans.

HEREDITARY NEPHROPATHIES

FABRY'S DISEASE

Fig. 18-1 Fabry's disease. Glomerulus showing fine vacuolization of epithelial cells.
H&E stain. x 410.

Fig. 18-2 Fabry's disease. Advanced glomerular changes with mesangial sclerosis. The lipid laden cells are strikingly stained.
Formalin-osmium fixation, Sudan Black stain. x 260.

FAMILIAL LECITHIN-CHOLESTEROL ACYL TRANSFERASE DEFICIENCY

Fig. 18-3 Familial lecithin-cholesterol acyl transferase deficiency. Large glomerulus showing mesangial sclerosis with mild cellular proliferation.
PAS stain. x 390.

Fig. 18-4 Another case of familial lecithin-cholesterol acyl transferase deficiency. There is more advanced glomerular sclerosis and thickening and vacuolization of capillary walls.
Epon embedding, PASM stain. x 310.

I-CELL DISEASE

Fig. 18-5 I-cell disease in an 8-year-old girl who died of congestive heart failure. She had had 2—3+ albuminuria and hematuria as well as mild elevation of blood urea nitrogen. The glomerulus shows marked vacuolization of the epithelial cells (podocytes). Slight mesangial widening is present.
Trichrome stain x 260.

Fig. 18-6 Same case as Fig. 18-5. Intense blue staining of the content of the glomerular epithelial cells.
Colloidal iron stain. x 260.

I-CELL DISEASE

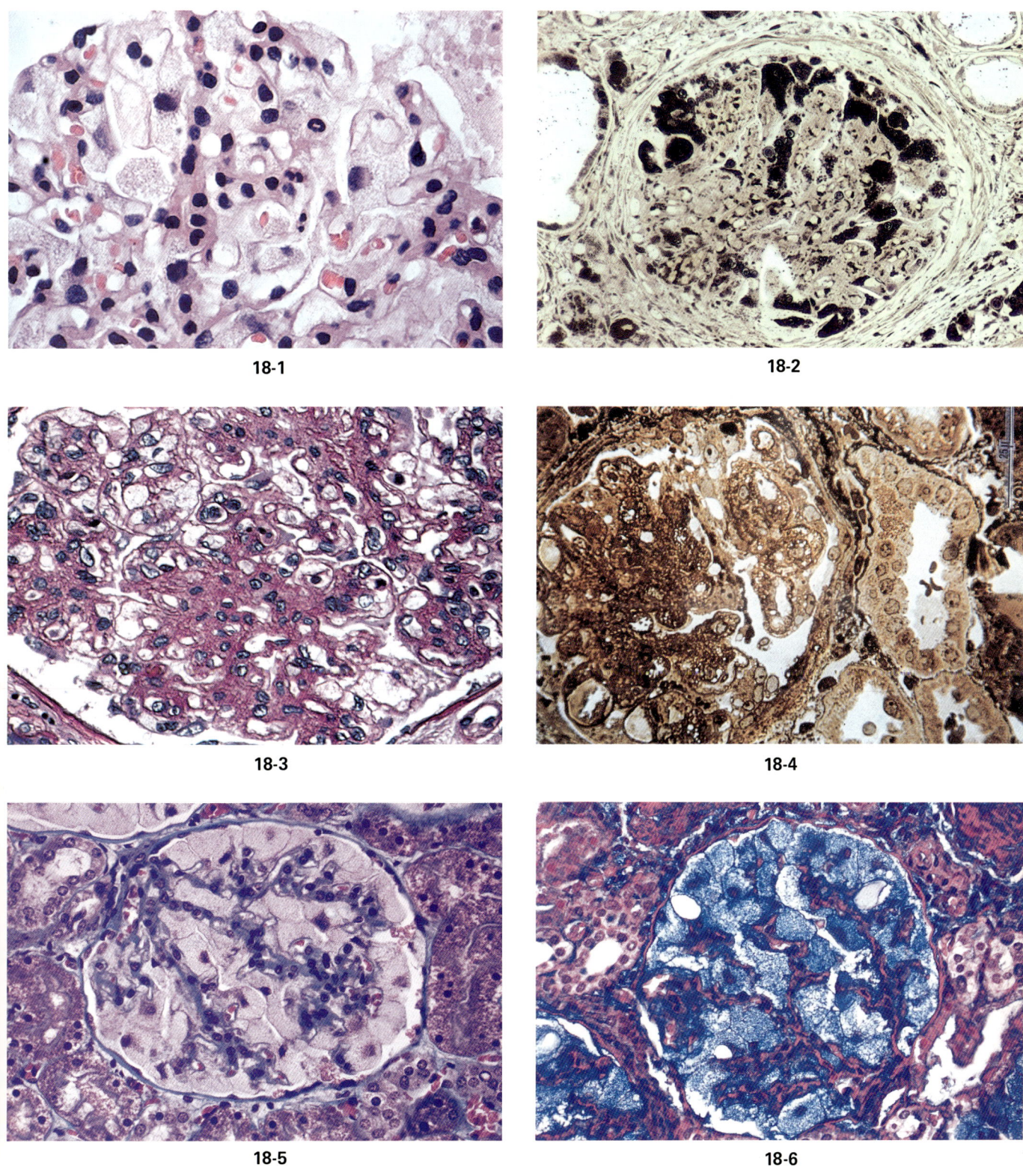

HEREDITARY NEPHROPATHIES

FABRY'S DISEASE

Fig. 18-7 Electron micrograph. Same case as Fig. 18-1. Part of a glomerular capillary. The epithelial cells (podocytes) (P) are markedly enlarged and are filled with dark lamellated structures.　　　　　　　　　　　　　　　×9,100.

Fig. 18-8 Electron micrograph. Same case as Fig. 18-2. Glomerular mesangium showing accumulation of matrix (MM) and numerous lamellated bodies in the cytoplasm of the mesangial cells (MC).　　　　　　　×4,600.

L: capillary lumen, BM: basement membrane, En: endothelial cell.

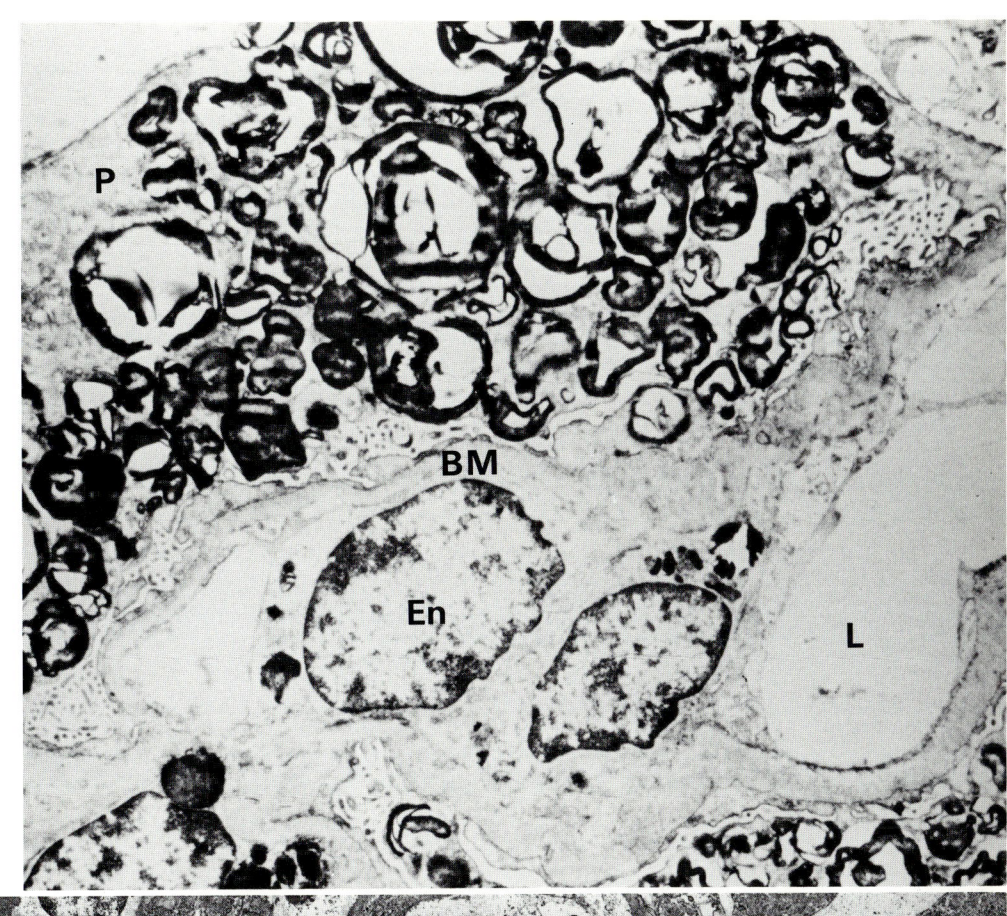

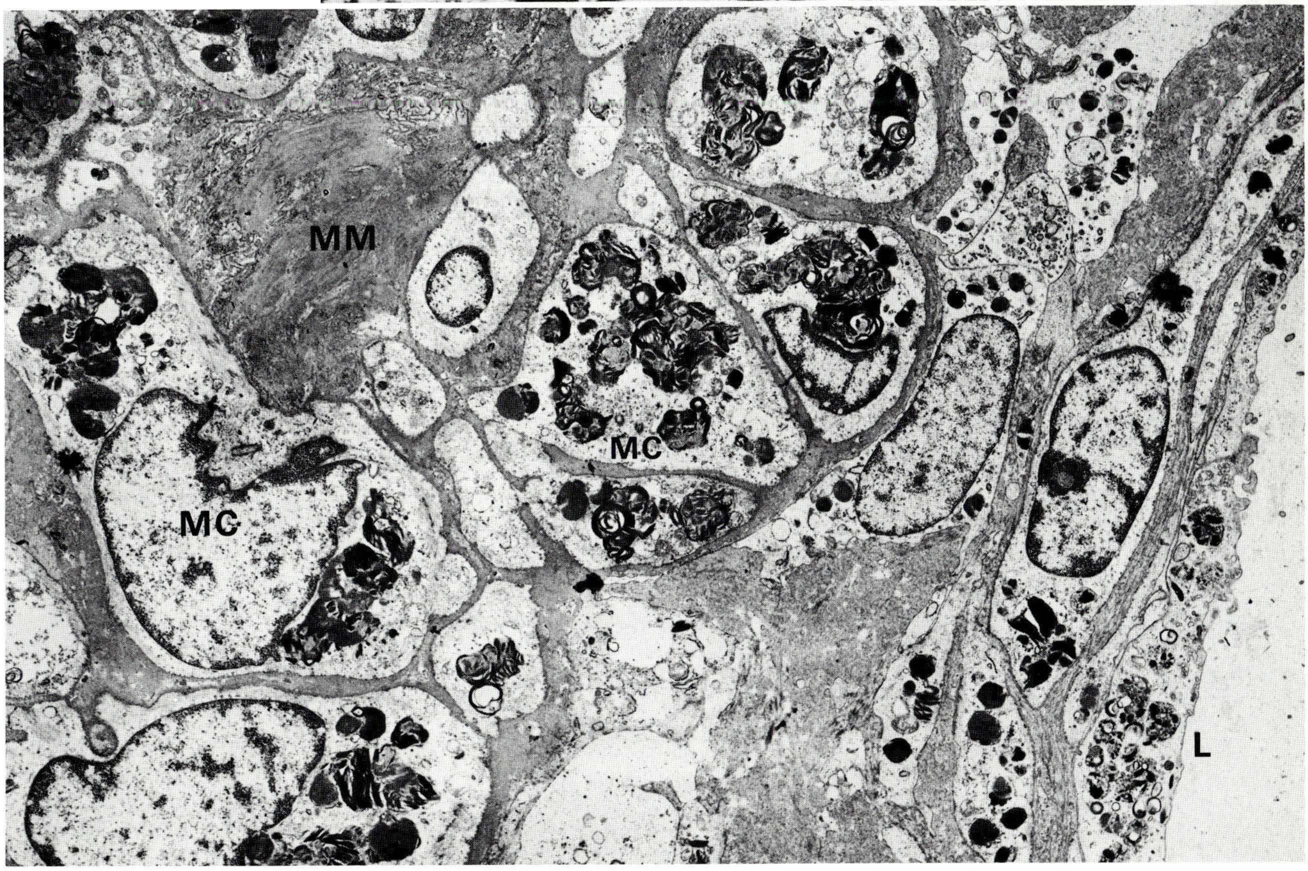

HEREDITARY NEPHROPATHIES

FAMILIAL LECITHIN-CHOLESTEROL ACYL TRANSFERASE DEFICIENCY

Fig. 18-9 Electron micrograph. Same case as Fig. 18-4. Part of a glomerular tuft showing enlargement and vacuolization of the mesangium (M) and numerous fine subendothelial vacuoles in some of the capillary loops. One cell is strikingly vacuolated ("foam cell") (FC). × 2,000.

Fig. 18-10 Electron micrograph. Same case as Fig. 18-4. Part of a glomerular capillary showing separation of the endothelium (En) from the basement membrane (BM) and accumulation of clusters of dark particles (compare with Nephropathy of Liver Disease, Fig. 16-18). × 28,000.

L: capillary lumen, U: urinary space.

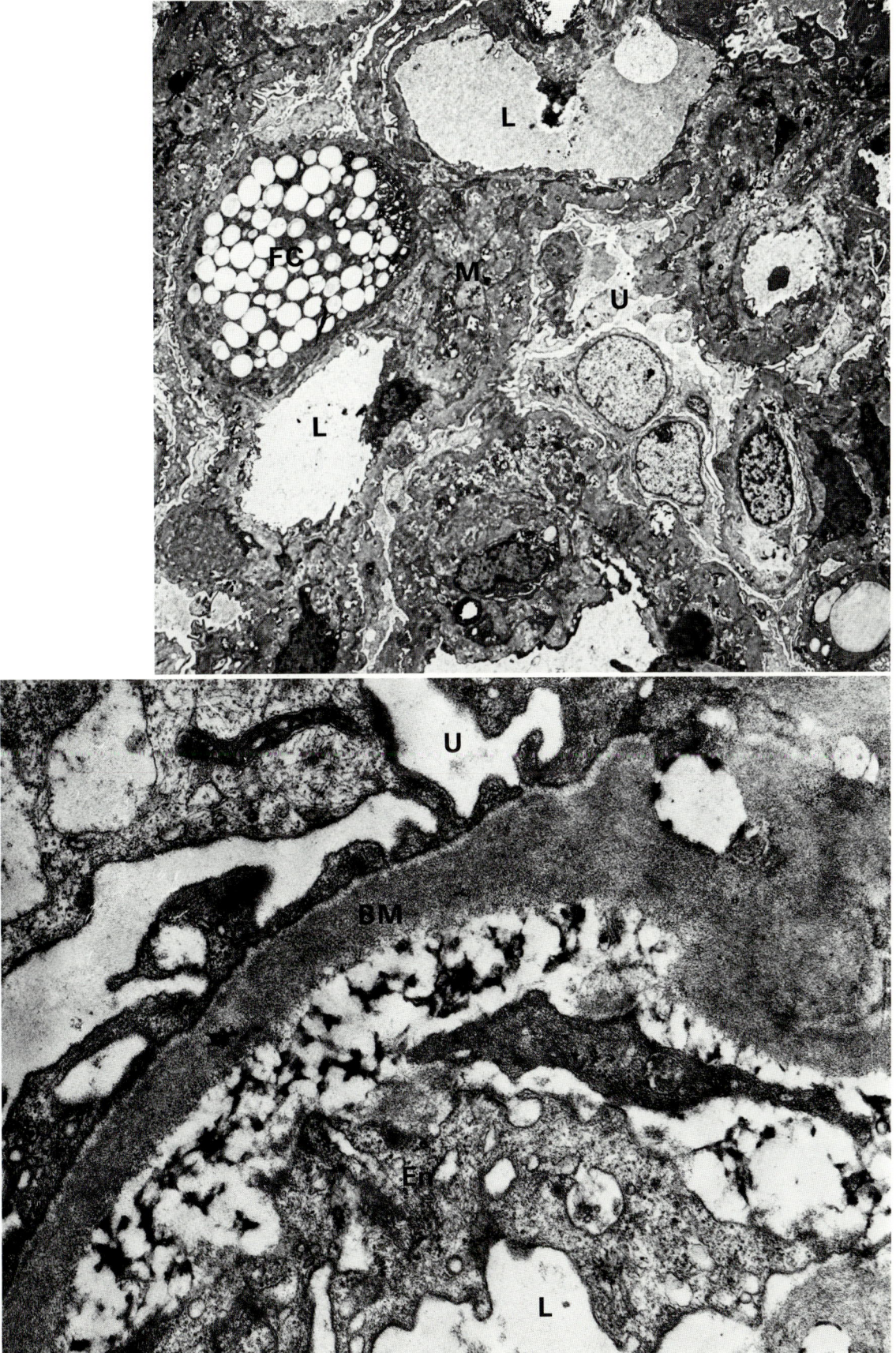

HEREDITARY NEPHROPATHIES

FAMILIAL LECITHIN-CHOLESTEROL ACYL TRANSFERASE DEFICIENCY

Fig. 18-11 Electron micrograph. Same case as Fig. 18-3. Accumulation of small membrane bound particles in the mesangial matrix (MM) and in the markedly widened subendothelial space.　　　　　　　　　　× 7,500.

Fig. 18-12 Electron micrograph. Same case as Fig. 18-3. Serpiginous fibrils in the subendothelial space.　　　　　　　　　　· × 38,000.

　　　U: urinary space, L: capillary lumen, BM: basement membrane,
　　　En: endothelial cell.

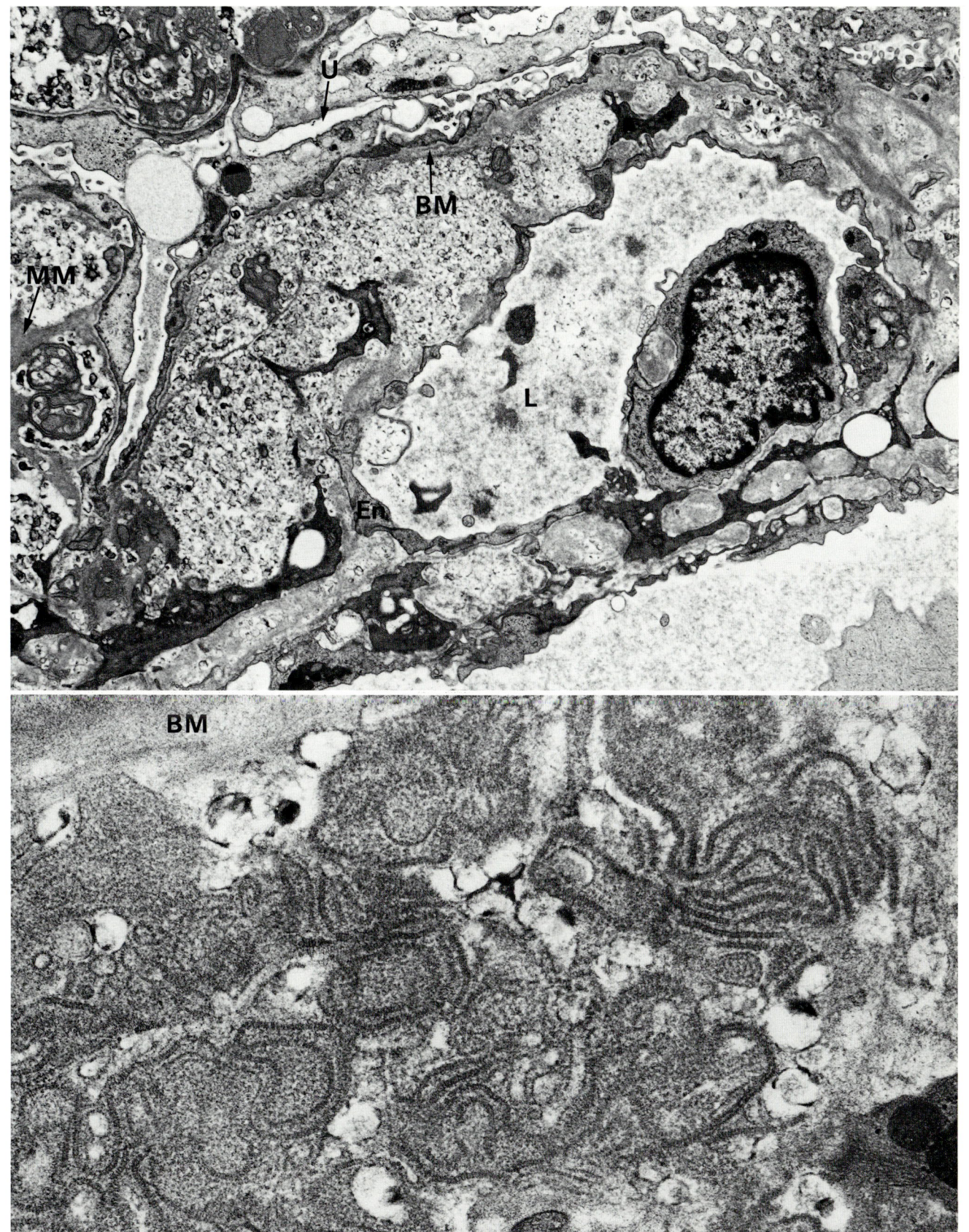

Miscellaneous Glomerular Diseases

CHAPTER 19

Nephropathy of Toxemia of Pregnancy
(Figs. 19-1 to 19-3 and Figs. 19-8 to 19-10)
Radiation Nephritis
(Figs. 19-4 to 19-7 and Fig. 19-11)

Nephropathy of Toxemia of Pregnancy
(Pre-eclamptic Nephropathy)

Definition: Glomerular changes which are specifically related to pregnancy, are accompanied by a clinical syndrome of proteinuria, edema and hypertension, and which resolve after delivery. If convulsions occur, the disease is known as eclampsia.

Clinical Manifestations: The disease occurs late in pregnancy and is more common in primigravidae than in multigravidae. Its incidence is increased in twin pregnancies, in hydramnion and in cases of hydatidiform mole. Proteinuria varies from slight to massive. Edema is frequent, but has to be distinguished from "physiologic" edema of pregnancy. Generalized edema is more significant than that limited to lower extremities. Hypertension is generally mild, but rises strikingly in eclampsia with convulsions. Glomerular filtration rate is often reduced. In severe cases, particularly in eclampsia, hemolytic-uremic syndrome may develop. The syndrome of pre-eclampsia may be superimposed upon other types of renal disease such as essential hypertension, or chronic glomerulonephritis.

Light Microscopy: The glomeruli are large and bloodless but rarely hypercellular. The capillary lumina are decreased because of enlargement of the endothelial cells and expansion of the mesangium. The endothelial cells are often vacuolated. The capillary walls may appear thickened. Capillary and arteriolar thrombi occur in eclampsia but rarely in pre-eclampsia. Eclampsia is often accompanied by hemorrhages and necrosis in the brain and in the liver. Changes of pre-eclampsia rapidly disappear from the glomeruli after delivery, but some enlargement of endothelial and mesangial cells may persist for many months.

Electron Microscopy: Swelling of endothelial and mesangial cells is the characteristic finding. In addition, electron dense deposits are found between the endothelium and the basement membrane, and in the mesangium. These deposits are finely granular and often non-homogeneous. They disappear rapidly after delivery. Rarely small amounts of fibrin can be demonstrated in the capillary wall or in the lumen. Foot processes may be focally lost but diffuse loss is rare.

Immunofluorescence Microscopy: Fibrin-related antigens are frequently seen in the endothelial and mesangial cells and under the basement membranes. Immunoglobulins (IgG, IgM) and complement (C3) are present inconstantly.

Radiation Nephritis

Definition: Renal disease following radiation injury. The kidney is moderately sensitive to radiation, and may be injured by doses exceeding 2,000 rads (less in children) administered to tumors within the kidney or in nearby tissues, especially metastatic malignancies arising from testis or ovary, and retroperitoneal lymphomas.

Clinical Manifestations: Acute radiation nephritis occurs 6–12 months after radiation and is manifested by dyspnea, anemia, fatigue and by hypertension and proteinuria. Hypertension is often of the malignant variety and may be the main clinical finding. Proteinuria will on occasion reach the nephrotic range but edema is more often due to cardiac failure. Glomerular filtration rate is decreased and more than half of patients progress to renal failure. Those who recover from the acute attack usually show persistent proteinuria and renal impairment. Chronic radiation nephritis either follows the acute phase or develops insidiously over a period of years. Its manifestations vary from isolated proteinuria or moderate hypertension to the full-blown syndrome similar to that of the acute phase, but generally milder.

Light Microscopy: A variable pattern of changes is seen depending on the dose of radiation and time interval after exposure. The earliest change at the light microscopic level is degeneration of tubular epithelium. After smaller doses, the cells regenerate, but often show nuclear abnormalities. Larger doses are followed by complete atrophy, thickening of basement membranes and interstitial fibrosis. Glomerular changes consist of segmental necrosis and cell proliferation, followed by segmental or more diffuse sclerosis and capsular adhesions. Occasionally there is thickening of capillary walls with double outlines. Arterial damage is relatively late, varying from sclerosis of the walls to fibrinoid necrosis and thrombosis. The combined effect of these changes is permanent loss of renal parenchyma.

Electron Microscopy: At electron microscopic level glomerular damage occurs early, about the same time as tubular degeneration. The glomerular endothelium becomes detached from the basement membranes with creation of clear subendothelial zones which, on the endothelial side, is limited by a newly formed thin basement membrane. Epithelial cells are also injured as evidenced by edema, foot process loss and detachment from basement membranes. The mesangium is expanded by edema, increase in cells and mesangial matrix. Mesangiolysis and collapse of capillaries lead to sclerosis.

Endothelial detachment also characterizes the early arterial changes. Necrotic zones consist of degenerated medial muscle fibers and infiltration of fibrinoid material. Degenerating tubular epithelial cells separate from the underlying basement membranes, but with partial recovery are able to form new basement membranes, creating a multilayered structure.

Immunofluorescence Microscopy: Deposits have been rarely identified. Occasionally IgM may be seen in segmental distribution.

MISCELLANEOUS GLOMERULAR DISEASES

NEPHROPATHY OF TOXEMIA OF PREGNANCY

Fig. 19-1 Pre-eclamptic toxemia of pregnancy. The glomerulus is uniformly "solid". The capillary lumina are practically invisible. There is minimal increase in cellularity.
H&E stain. × 360.

Fig. 19-2 Same case as Fig. 19-1. Part of a glomerulus under high magnification showing thickening of capillary walls, and mesangial widening without significant cellularity.
PAS stain. × 1,000.

Fig. 19-3 Immunofluorescence microscopy. Deposits of fibrinogen along the capillary walls and in the mesangium. × 260.

RADIATION NEPHRITIS

Fig. 19-4 Acute radiation injury. Large glomerulus showing congestion and focal necrosis.
H&E stain. × 260.

Fig. 19-5 Same case as Fig. 19-4. Glomerulus showing segmental cellular proliferation and an area of necrosis.
H&E stain. × 210.

Fig. 19-6 Same case as Fig. 19-4. Thickening of capillary walls with double outlines.
PAS stain. × 260.

Fig. 19-7 Chronic radiation injury in a child. Various degrees of glomerular sclerosis and tubular atrophy.
Trichrome stain. × 260.

RADIATION NEPHRITIS

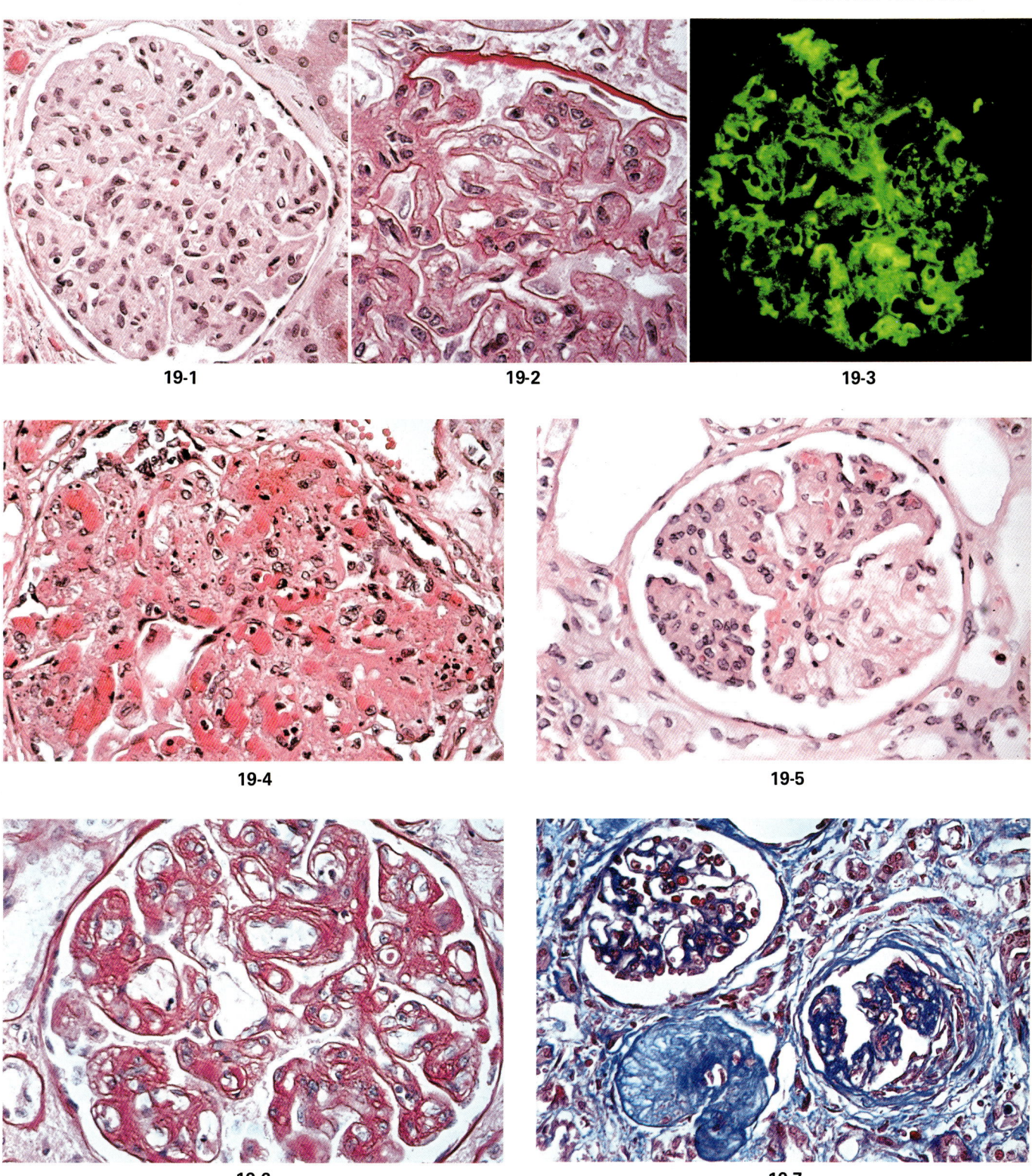

19-1

19-2

19-3

19-4

19-5

19-6

19-7

MISCELLANEOUS GLOMERULAR DISEASES

NEPHROPATHY OF TOXEMIA OF PREGNANCY

Fig. 19-8   Part of a glomerular tuft showing expansion of the mesangium, slight increase in the number of cells (MC) and the amount of matrix, swelling of the endothelial cell (En) in the capillary lumen (L) (center of the picture), and deposition (D) of light gray to dark gray material along the basement membrane of the mesangium and of the capillary wall.
PAS stain.   x 1,500.

Fig. 19-9   Electron micrograph. Glomerular capillary showing marked edema of the endothelial cells (En) with almost complete obliteration of the lumen. The capillary basement membrane (BM) and the foot processes are preserved.
x 12,000.

U: urinary space.

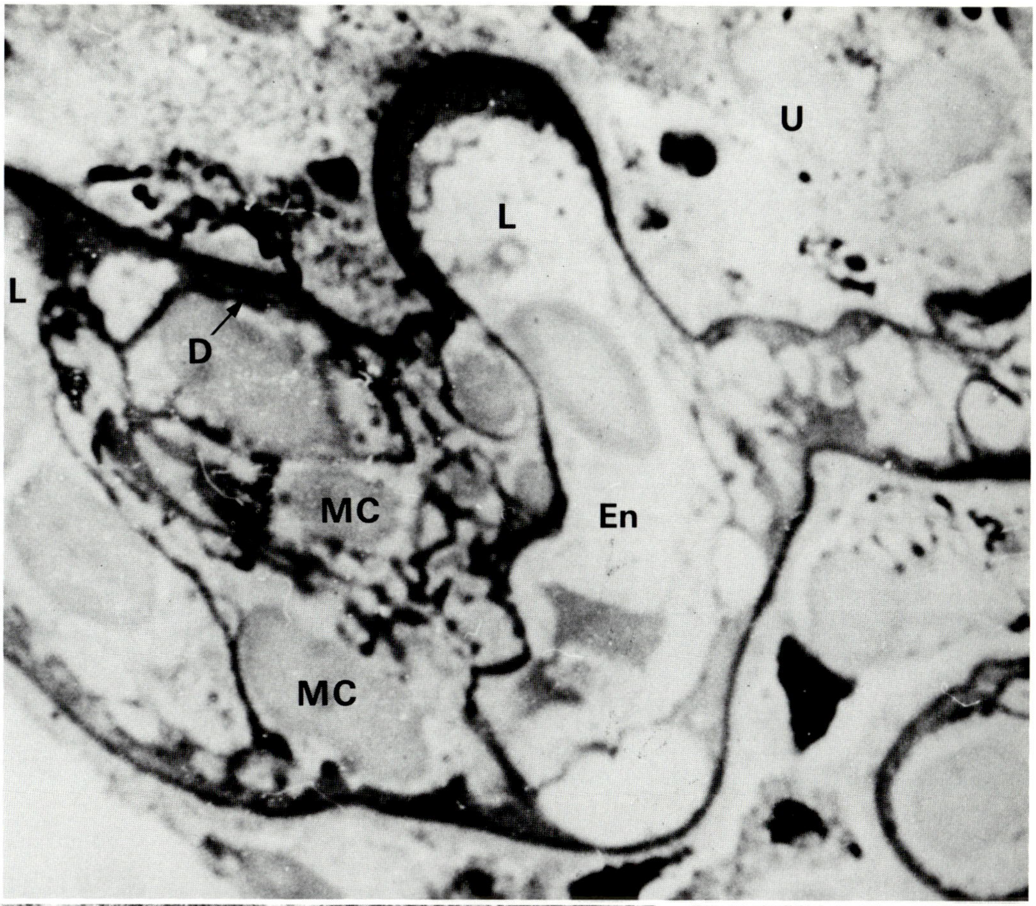

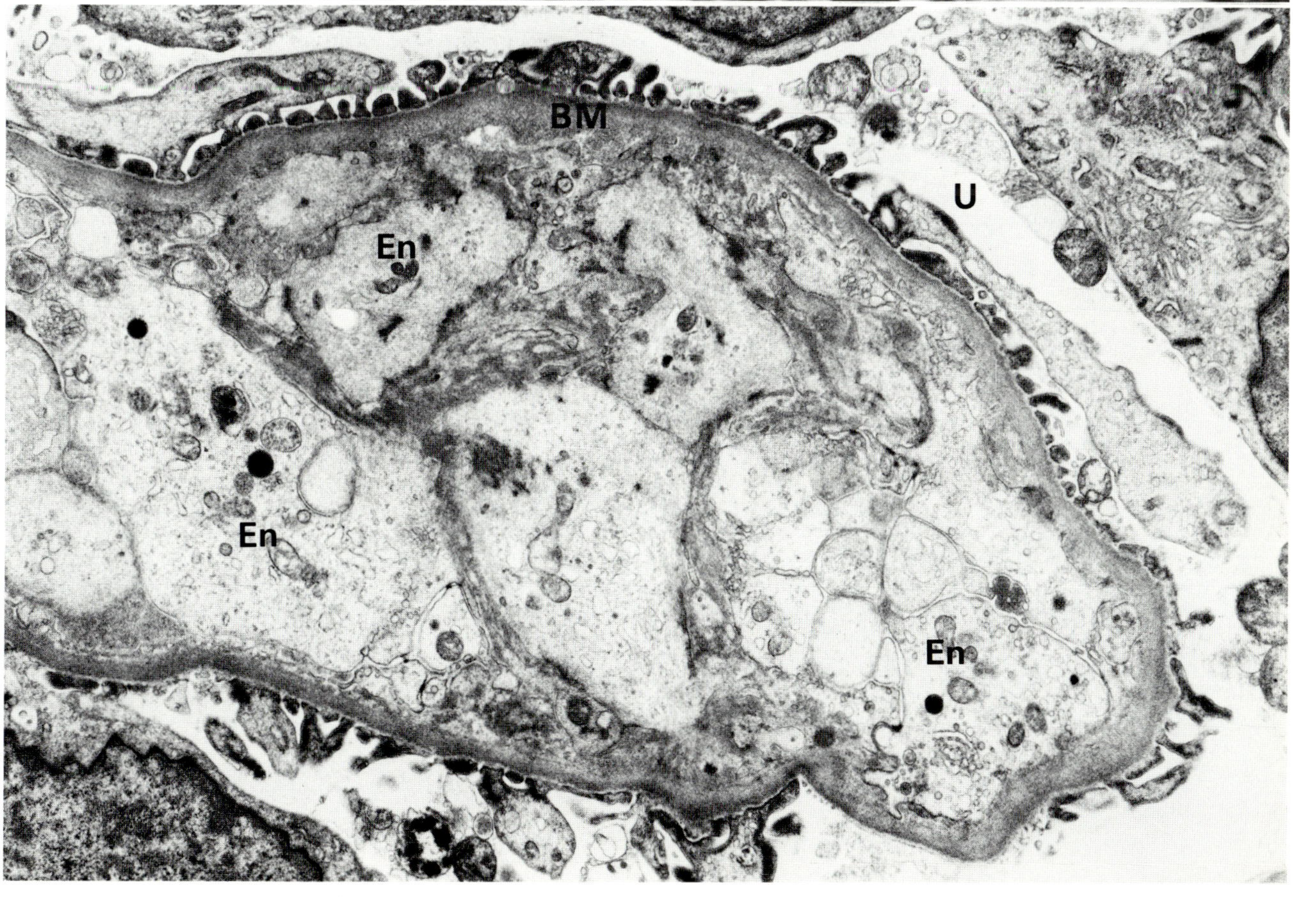

MISCELLANEOUS GLOMERULAR DISEASES

NEPHROPATHY OF TOXEMIA OF PREGNANCY

Fig. 19-10 Electron micrograph. Glomerular capillary showing subendothelial (En) (actually mesangial) deposits (D) of finely granular material.
x 11,000.

RADIATION NEPHRITIS

Fig. 19-11 Electron micrograph. Experimental acute radiation injury in a rat. Glomerular capillary showing extensive detachment of the endothelium from the basement membrane (BM). The subendothelial space contains fluffy and fibrillar material. The endothelium (En) is focally swollen; the basement membrane and the foot processes are preserved.   x 6,800.

U: urinary space, L: capillary lumen, MM: mesangial matrix, P: podocyte.

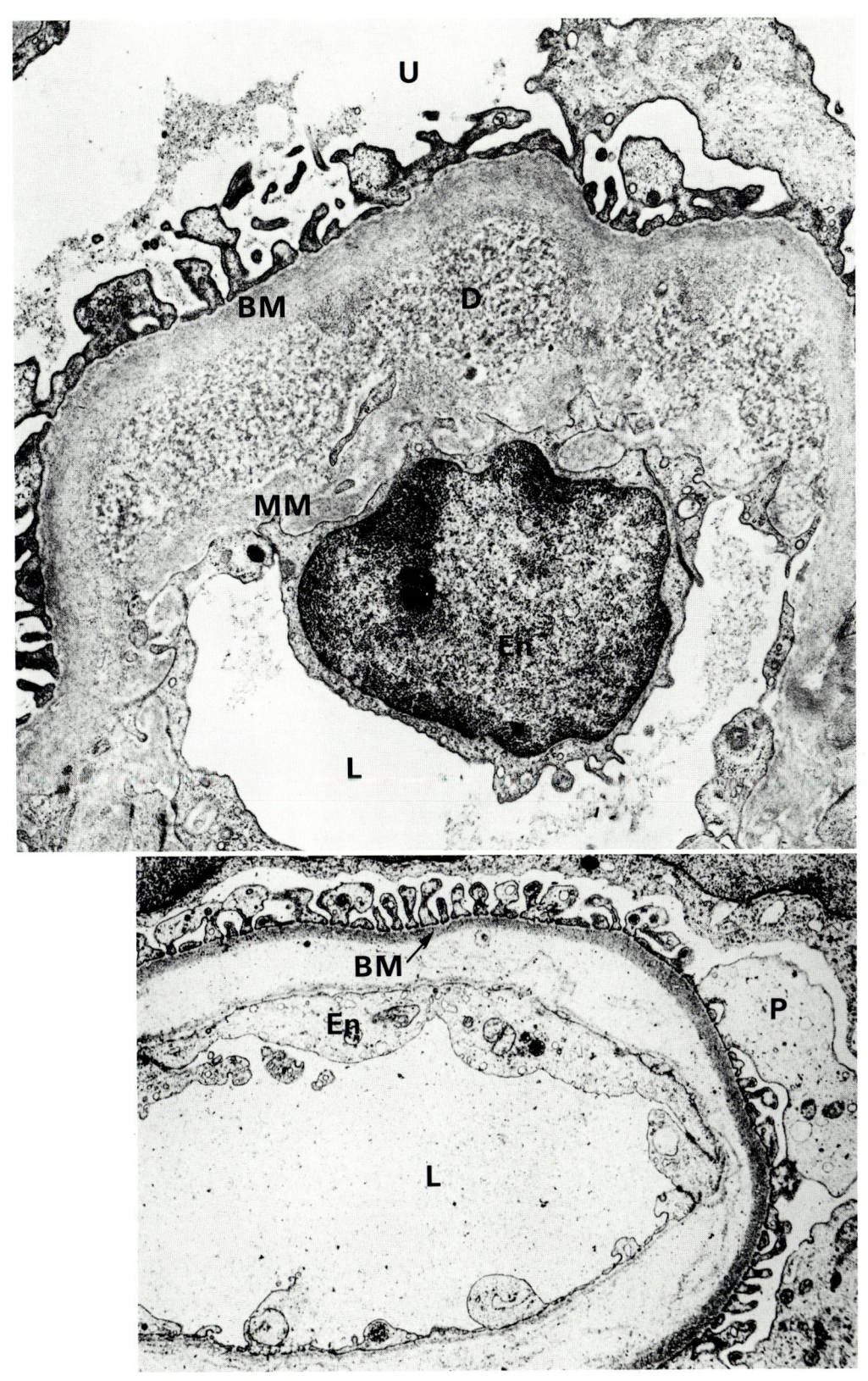

CHAPTER 20

End Stage Kidney
(Figs. 20-1 to 20-7)
Glomerular Lesions Following Transplantation
(Figs. 20-8 to 20-26)

End Stage Kidney

Definition: An extensively scarred kidney in which there is no evidence of the original process, lesion or cause. Advanced glomerular, vascular and interstitial lesions may all result in such a state. The kidney is typically shrunken, diffusely scarred and shows extensive sclerosis and fibrosis of glomeruli, blood vessels and interstitium.

Clinical Manifestations: The clinical manifestations are mainly those of advanced uremia or terminal renal failure, with accumulation in the blood of large amounts of nitrogenous waste products, severe acidosis, anemia, gastrointestinal and cerebral manifestations, hypertension and osteodystrophy. Urine formation is reduced to practically nothing, but protein and red blood cells may be present in the few cc's that are still excreted. Before the days of dialysis the survival of these patients was measured in weeks. Nowadays the patients survive much longer, often for years, allowing for progression of renal changes far beyond those seen in untreated individuals ("transstygian kidney").

Gross Appearance and Histology: The kidneys are small and shrunken often weighing less than 50 grams each. In some cases distinction can still be made between advanced primary glomerular disease with fairly uniform granular surfaces, and advanced pyelonephritis presenting large and deep scars, but these differences are by no means reliable.

Histologically, almost all glomeruli are completely sclerosed and crowded, the tubules extensively atrophied; there is prominent vascular sclerosis with luminal narrowing, and conspicuous interstitial fibrosis with some inflammatory, mostly lymphocytic infiltration. In addition, a variety of changes, rare in untreated patients, are observed in the "transstygian kidney". Among these are: acquired cystic disease due to dilatation of tubules; embryonal hyperplasia of the glomerular parietal (Bowman's) epithelium; hyperplastic smooth muscle nodules in the walls of arteries, thrombosis of veins; deposits of crystals, especially calcium oxalate, and cartilage and bone formation in the interstitium. In addition there may be adenomatous nodules, sometimes with a hint of malignant transformation, and sometimes true malignant tumors.

Electron Microscopy: The changes are non-specific and consist of capillary collapse, basement membrane wrinkling and extensive sclerosis.

Immunofluorescence Microscopy: Inconstant and variable deposits of immune globulins and C3 have been reported.

MISCELLANEOUS GLOMERULAR DISEASES

Glomerular Lesions Following Transplantation

Definition: Lesions in the glomeruli of the transplanted kidney which may be due to several different mechanisms: recurrence of the original glomerulonephritis; glomerular disease which is part of a rejection process and due to histocompatibility antigens derived from the transplanted kidney; and a new disease intercurrently acquired, e.g. poststreptococcal glomerulonephritis. The last type is very rare, while recurrence of the original glomerulonephritis is relatively uncommon in the immunosuppressed patient. However the distinction between the various types of glomerular disease is often difficult. To be acceptable as such, the recurrent glomerulonephritis must have the features of the original disease, e.g. intramembranous dense deposits in Dense Deposit Glomerulonephritis, extensive mesangial deposits of IgA in Berger's disease, or linear deposits of IgG and perhaps crescent formation in Goodpasture's syndrome.

Transplant rejection occurs in several forms: hyperacute, acute and chronic. It may also be divided into cellular and vascular types. Cellular rejection is manifested mainly by interstitial infiltration, consisting of mononuclear cells. Vascular rejection affects the arteries and the glomeruli.

Clinical Manifestations: The main manifestation is deterioration of renal function as measured by glomerular filtration rate or creatinine clearance. In hyperacute rejection, there is total absence of function, fever and systemic toxicity. In chronic rejection proteinuria is common and may reach nephrotic levels. Hematuria is seen in some patients and hypertension, occasionally of the malignant type, also occurs. Episodes of functional deterioration can be reversed by immunosuppressive therapy, but in many cases progressive loss of function develops. Nephrotic syndrome is often unresponsive to therapy.

Light Microscopy shows a great variety of lesions. All those listed in Table I and Table II occur in a variety of combinations, so that specific classification is often difficult. However, in the immunosuppressed patient, cellular proliferation is less prominent and is overshadowed by other changes. Most common of these is capillary wrinkling and collapse due to narrowing of arteries, and accompanied on occasion by fibrous crescents or fibrous thickening of Bowman's capsule. Other common lesions are thickening of the capillary walls with double outlines, mesangial expansion and sclerosis, focal and segmental sclerosis and global sclerosis. Fibrin thrombi are seen in hyperacute and acute rejection, while changes resembling those of hemolytic-uremic syndrome, including fragmented red blood cells, are not unusual in chronic rejection.

Arteries and arterioles are almost invariably affected, occasionally in diffuse, but more often, in an irregular manner. In acute rejection, there is fibrin deposition in the lumen and in the wall, "fibrinoid" necrosis with a degree of inflammation, and luminal thrombosis. In chronic rejection, marked intimal thickening develops, mucoid or fibrous in character. Numerous vacuolated cells may be present in the intima. Vascular obstruction leads to infarction and hemorrhage in the acute stage, and to parenchymal atrophy and marked interstitial fibrosis in the chronic stage. Interstitial cellular infiltrates of plasma cells and lymphocytes ("immunoblasts") occur in acute rejection episodes. Their extent and intensity is considerably modified by immunosuppression.

Electron Microscopy: The most common lesion is widening of the subendothelial space in the glomerular capillaries, which may attain striking proportions. This space is filled with pale fluffy material with a scattering of fibrils, some fibrin, platelets and occasionally red blood cells, and a few cytoplasmic processes of mesangial and endothelial cells. Rarely the presence of many cells and of electron dense deposits create the picture of mesangiocapillary glomerulonephritis (membranoproliferative Type 1). On the endothelial side the space is delimited by a thin, apparently newly formed basement membrane. The original basement membranes are often wrinkled, mostly as the result of ischemia. The foot processes are often effaced even in the absence of nephrotic syndrome. Electron dense deposits in the subendothelial space, under the epithelium or in the mesangium, are found infrequently. Intramembranous dense deposits are seen in recurrences of dense deposit glomerulonephritis.

The mesangium is expanded by edema of cells and matrix and sometimes by true mesangiolysis. Cellular proliferation is infrequent, but deposition of mesangial matrix is a frequent event. In the areas of segmental sclerosis, the expanded mesangium is surrounded by collapsed capillaries. Some of the glomerular changes correspond closely to those described under various forms of glomerulonephritis. In diabetic patients, increase of mesangial matrix and thickening of basement membranes is sometimes evident.

Immunofluorescence Microscopy: Deposits of immunoglobulins (IgM, IgG), complement (C3) and fibrinogen are frequently seen. These tend to assume interrupted linear pattern in acute rejection, granular and irregular pattern in chronic rejection. Their frequency and distribution do not correspond to the rare electron dense deposits seen by electron microscopy. Better correspondence is seen in recurrent glomerulonephritis.

MISCELLANEOUS GLOMERULAR DISEASES

END STAGE KIDNEY

Fig. 20-1 End stage kidney. Nearly complete sclerosis of the glomeruli, extensive tubular atrophy and marked thickening of the walls of arteries.
PAS stain. × 100.

Fig. 20-2 End stage kidney. Sclerosis of the glomerular tuft with adhesions to the Bowman's capsule and formation of pseudotubules. There is extensive tubular atrophy.
PAS stain. × 210.

Fig. 20-3 So-called angiomatoid obsolescence of glomeruli. The capillaries are collapsed but the lumina are still discernible. There is considerable tubular atrophy.
PAS stain. × 210.

Fig. 20-4 Glomerulus showing squamous metaplasia of the epithelium.
PASM-H&E stain. × 360.

Fig. 20-5 Sclerosed glomerulus with prominent juxta-glomerular granular cells (blue). × 360.

Fig. 20-6 Partly sclerosed glomerulus showing "glomoid" transformation of the arteriole at the hilus.
H&E stain. × 310.

Fig. 20-7 Hyperplastic arteriolar nodule. Fibrinoid necrosis (red) is noted in one lumen.
Trichrome stain. × 150.

END STAGE KIDNEY

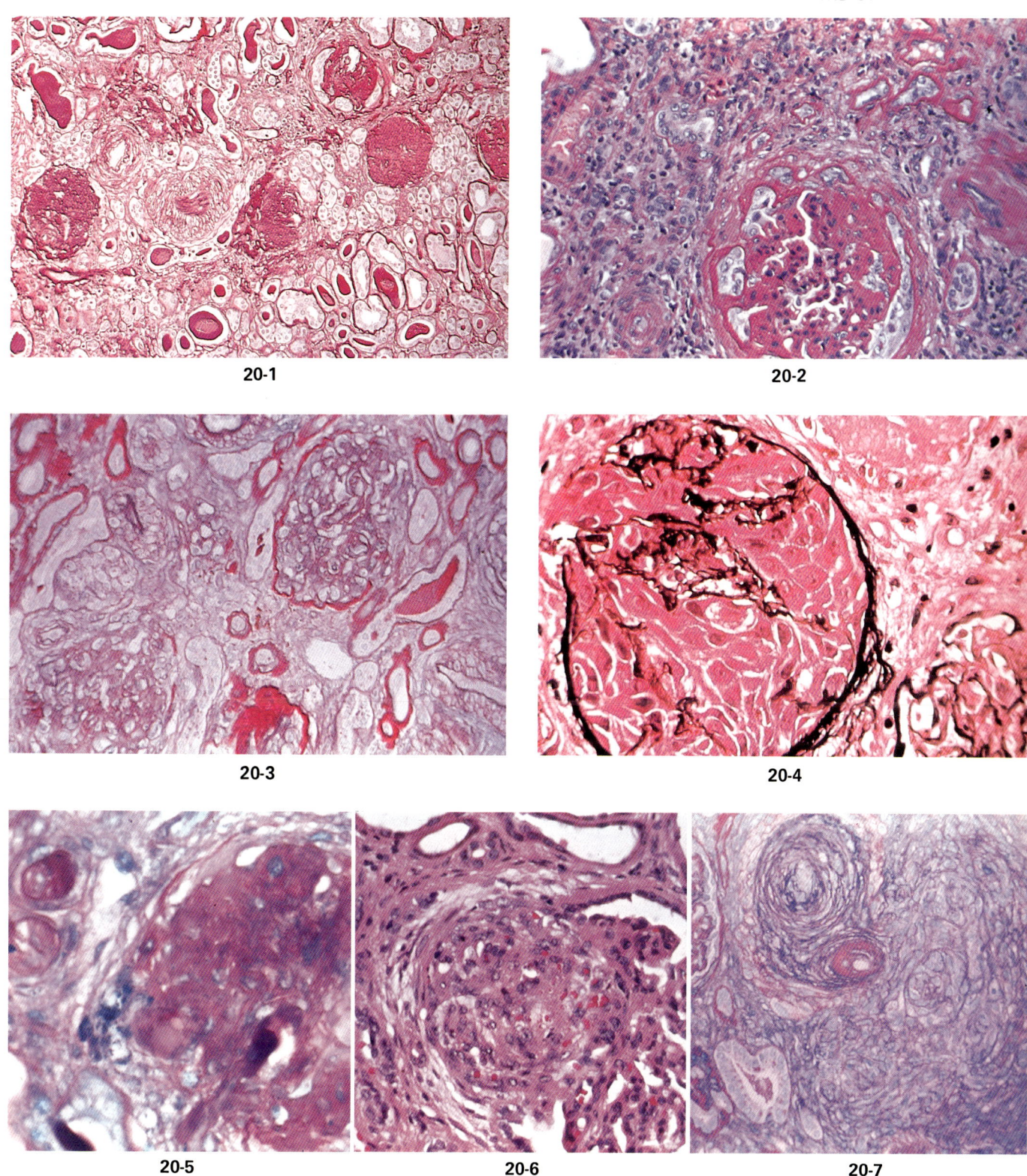

20-1

20-2

20-3

20-4

20-5

20-6

20-7

323

MISCELLANEOUS GLOMERULAR DISEASES

GLOMERULAR LESIONS FOLLOWING TRANSPLANTATION

Fig. 20-8 Kidney three months after transplantation. Acute cellular rejection. There is interstitial edema and cellular infiltration consisting mainly of small and large lymphocytes.
H&E stain.　　　　　　　　　　　　　　　　　　　　× 260.

Fig. 20-9 Renal transplant. Severe acute vascular rejection. There is necrosis in the wall of small artery and extensive polymorphonuclear infiltration.
H&E stain.　　　　　　　　　　　　　　　　　　　　× 100.

Fig. 20-10 Acute vascular rejection. Severe glomerular congestion and necrosis of renal tubules.
H&E stain.　　　　　　　　　　　　　　　　　　　　× 100.

Fig. 20-11 Chronic vascular rejection. Marked intimal proliferation in the wall of small artery with severe narrowing of the lumen.
Trichrome stain.　　　　　　　　　　　　　　　　　× 260.

Fig. 20-12 Chronic rejection. Glomerular sclerosis with almost complete collapse of glomerular capillaries. Tubular atrophy is present.
PAS stain.　　　　　　　　　　　　　　　　　　　　× 260.

Fig. 20-13 Chronic rejection. Widening and sclerosis of glomerular mesangium. The arteriole at the hilus shows only slight thickening of the wall.
PAS stain.　　　　　　　　　　　　　　　　　　　　× 260.

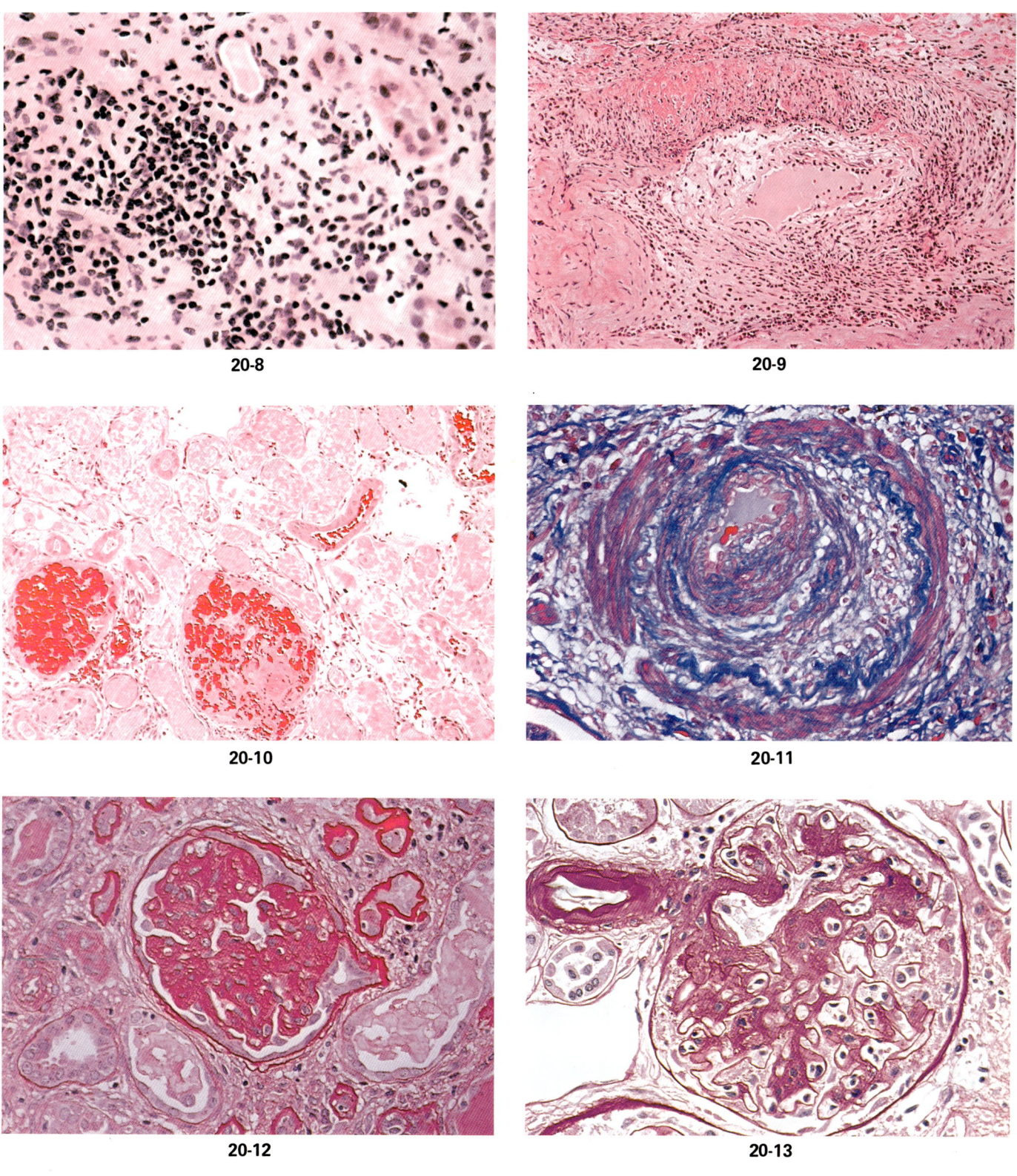

MISCELLANEOUS GLOMERULAR DISEASES

GLOMERULAR LESIONS FOLLOWING TRANSPLANTATION

Fig. 20-14 Chronic rejection. Segmental sclerosis in the glomerulus.
PAS stain. × 210.

Fig. 20-15 Hemolytic-uremic syndrome in transplant rejection. Same case as Fig. 20-8. The glomerulus is "solid" but not cellular. The capillary lumina are markedly narrowed.
H&E stain. × 260.

Fig. 20-16 Hemolytic-uremic syndrome in a transplant rejection. Fragments of red blood cells are seen in the expanded glomerular mesangium (near the top of the picture). Capillary on the left is congested.
H&E stain. × 1,000.

Fig. 20-17 Transplant rejection. Severe mesangiolysis in the upper part of the glomerular tuft. The mesangium is widened and very pale; only a few cells are seen. (Compare with the two lobules in lower part of the picture where mesangial structure is preserved.)
PAS stain. × 410.

Fig. 20-18 Transplant rejection. Diffuse but mild glomerular proliferation and narrowing of the capillary lumina.
H&E stain. × 260.

Fig. 20-19 Same case as Fig. 20-18. Mesangial proliferation and extensive mesangial interposition with double outlines in the capillary walls.
PASM stain. × 410.

GLOMERULAR LESIONS FOLLOWING TRANSPLANTATION

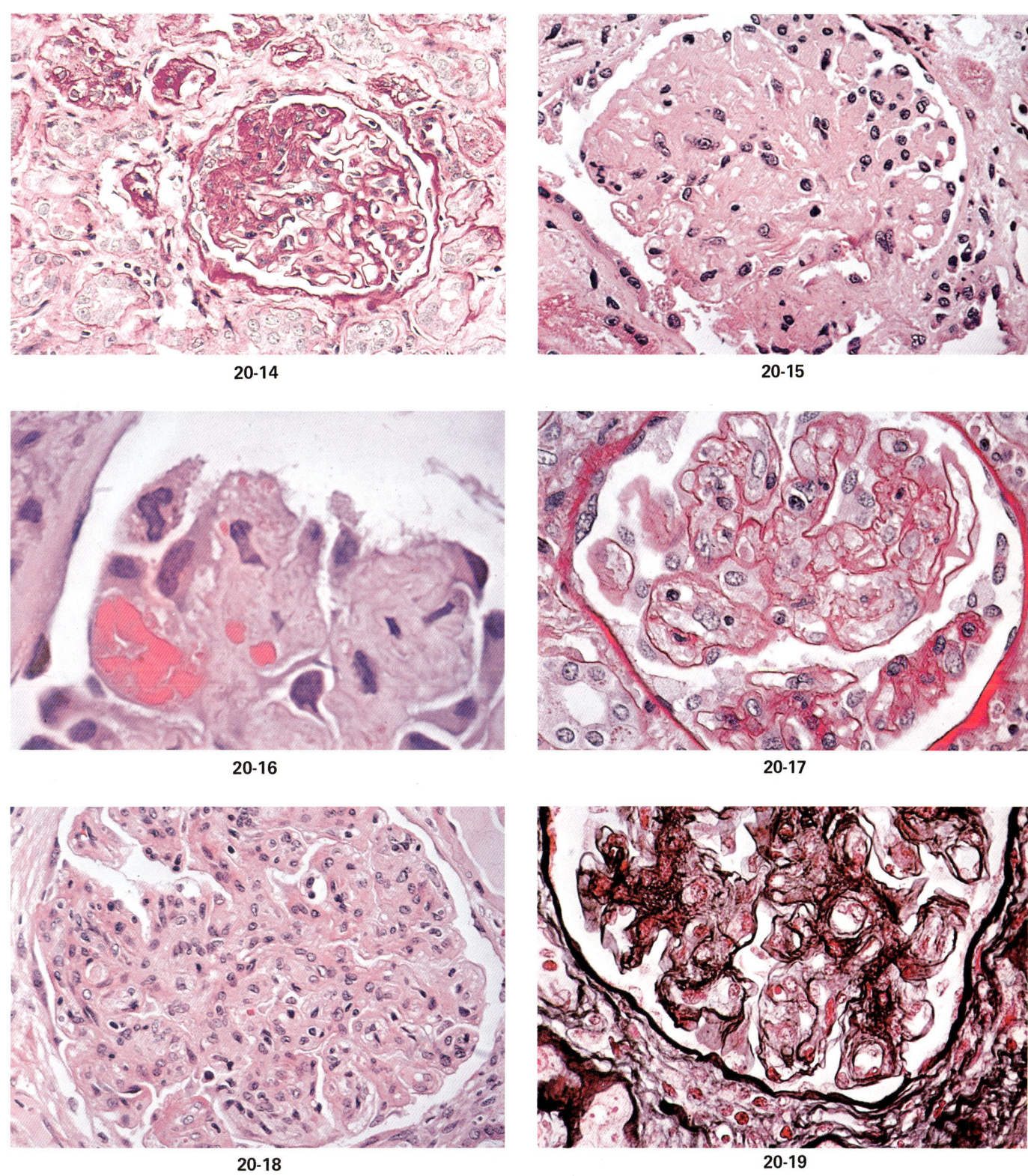

20-14

20-15

20-16

20-17

20-18

20-19

MISCELLANEOUS GLOMERULAR DISEASES

GLOMERULAR LESIONS FOLLOWING TRANSPLANTATION

Fig. 20-20 Immunofluorescence microscopy. Transplant rejection. IgM deposits in the glomerular mesangium.   x 260.

Fig. 20-21 Immunofluorescence microscopy. Transplant rejection. C3 deposits in the glomerular mesangium.   x 260.

Fig. 20-22 Immunofluorescence microscopy. Irregular deposits of fibrinogen in the glomerulus.   x 260.

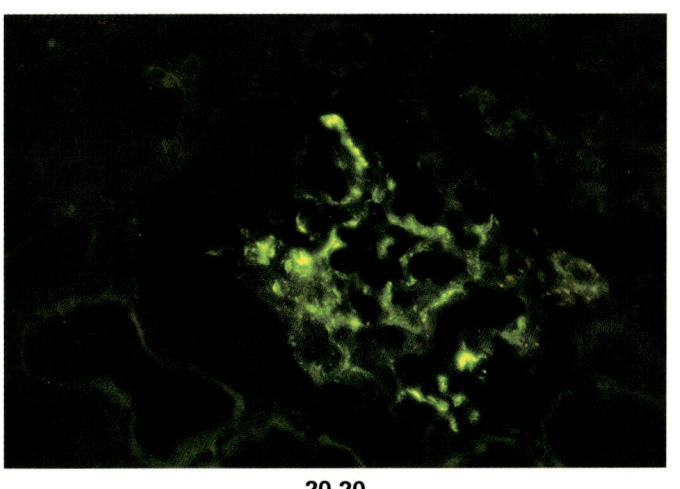

20-20

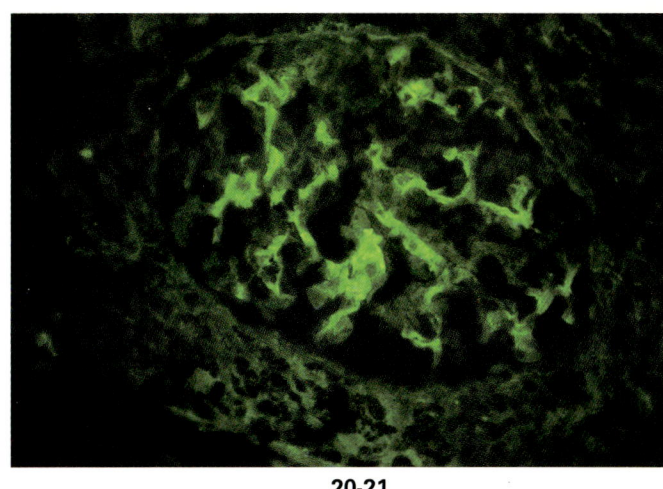

20-21

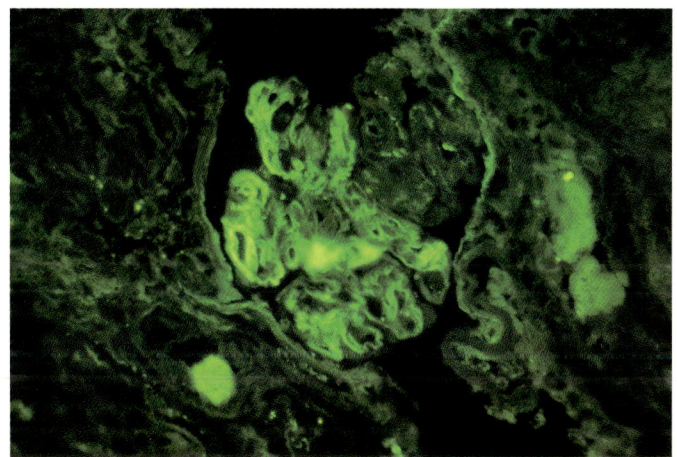

20-22

MISCELLANEOUS GLOMERULAR DISEASES

GLOMERULAR LESIONS FOLLOWING TRANSPLANTATION

Fig. 20-23 Electron micrograph. Acute rejection. Edema of the endothelial (En) and mesangial cells (MC) and accumulation of platelets in the capillary lumen (Cap). Scattered polymorphonuclear leukocytes and degenerating epithelial cells (podocytes) are visible. × 1,300.

Fig. 20-24 Electron micrograph. Same case as Fig. 20-8. Typical glomerular change consisting of separation of the endothelium (En) from the basement membrane (BM). The subendothelial space is filled with pale fluffy material. × 16,000.

P: podocyte, U: urinary space.

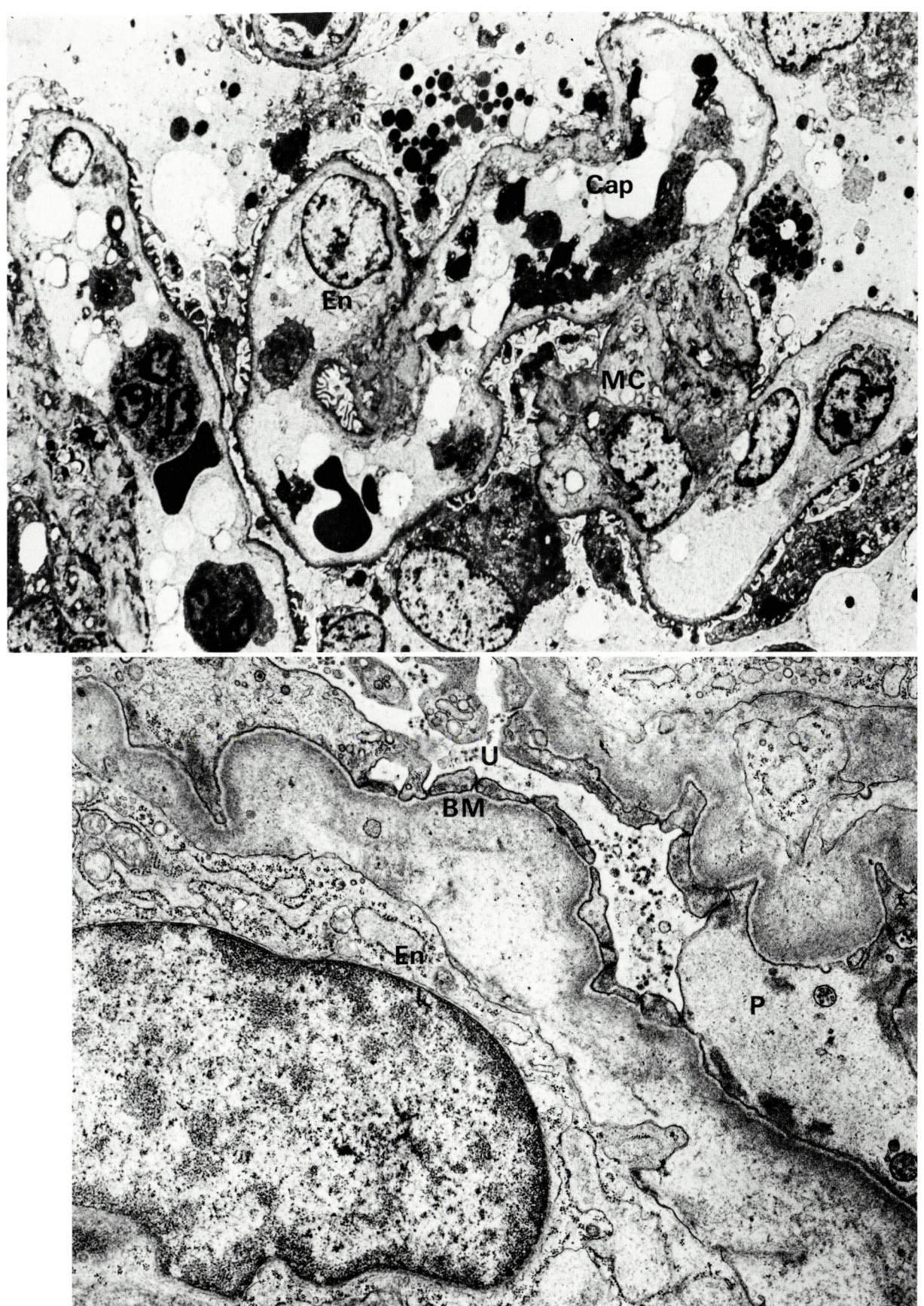

MISCELLANEOUS GLOMERULAR DISEASES

GLOMERULAR LESIONS FOLLOWING TRANSPLANTATION

Fig. 20-25 Electron micrograph. Same case as Fig. 20-18. Severe mesangiolysis with loss of capillary architecture and destruction of endothelium (En); accumulation of fluffy material, fibrils and red blood cells (RBC) is seen in the subendothelial space. × 4,400.

Fig. 20-26 Electron micrograph. Same case as Figs. 20-18 and 20-19. Circumferential mesangial interposition (MI) with marked narrowing of the capillary lumen (L). × 5,500.

BM, bm: basement membrane, U: urinary space, MM: mesangial matrix, MC: mesangial cell.

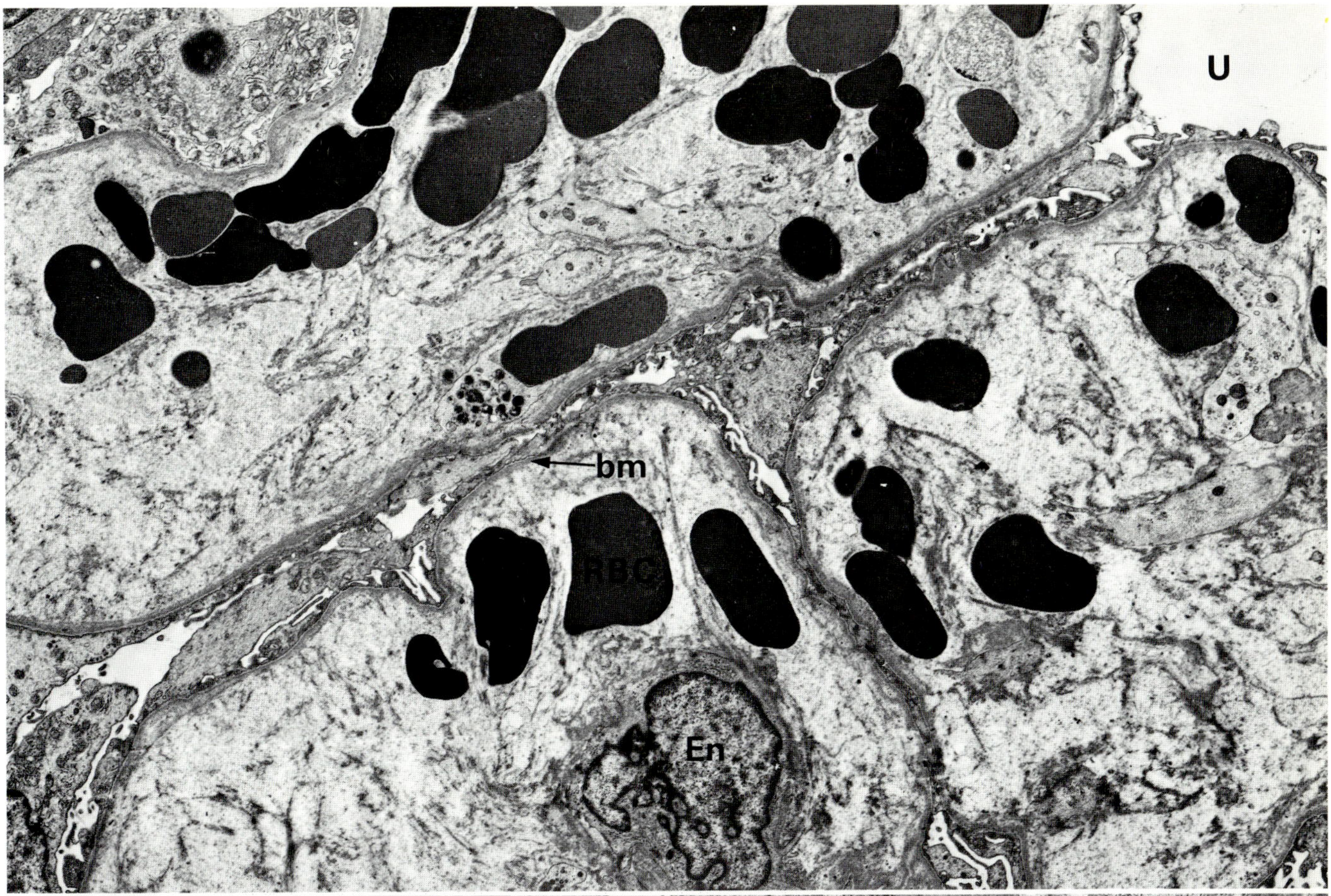

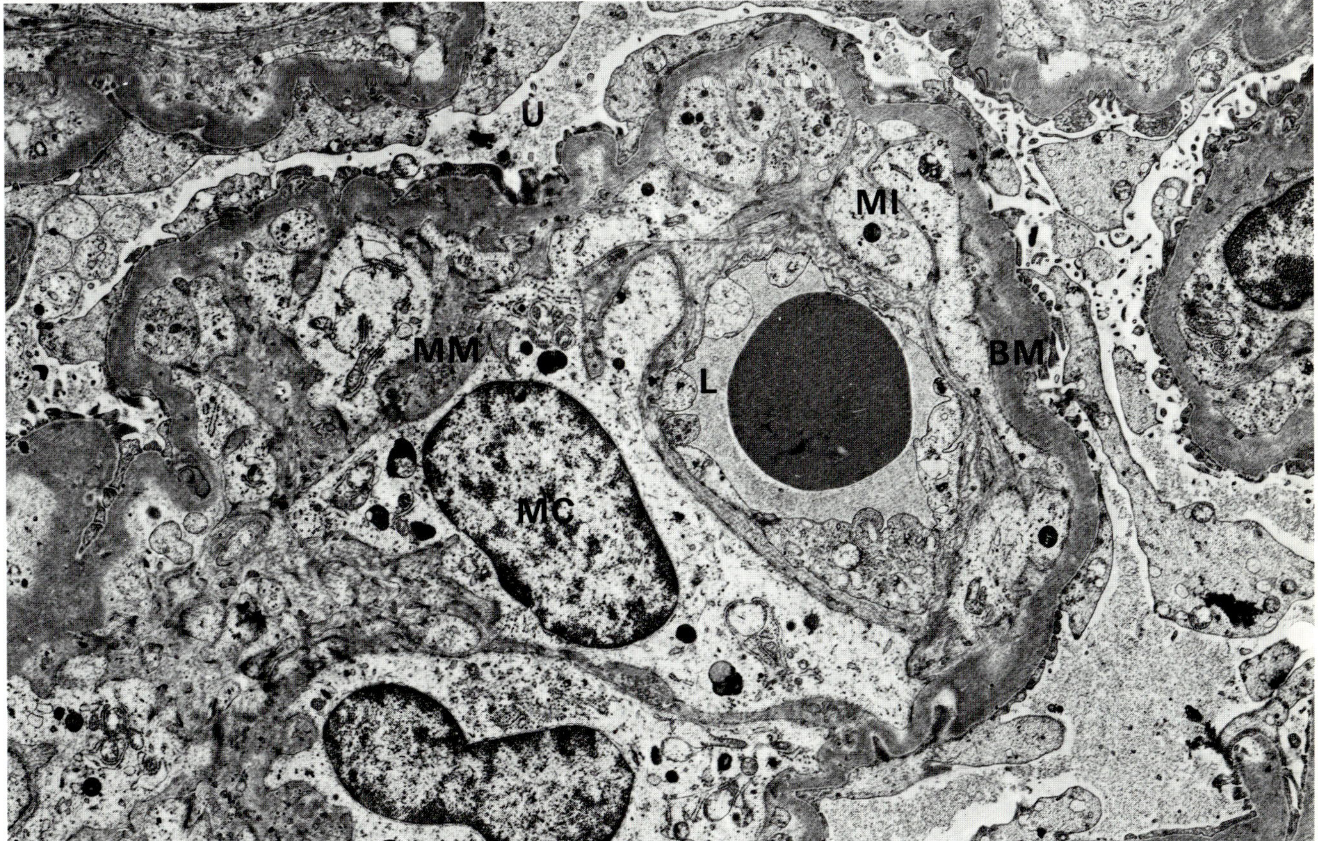

REFERENCES

Textbooks and Monographs

Included in this list are books dealing with renal pathology as well as those dealing with clinical nephrology. Most texts in the latter category have good sections on renal pathology and on normal histology.

1. Avtandilov, G.G.: Morphometry in Pathology. Meditsina, Moscow, 1973 (in Russian).
2. Becker, E.L. (Ed.): Structural Basis of Renal Disease. Hoeber Medical Division, New York, 1968.
3. Black, D.A.K. and Jones, N.F. (Eds): Renal Disease, 4th Edition. Blackwell Scientific Publications, Oxford, 1979.
4. Brenner, B.M. and Rector, F.C. Jr. (Eds): The Kidney. W.B. Saunders Co., Philadelphia, 1976.
5. Brun, C. and Olsen, S.: Atlas of Renal Biopsy. Munksgaard, Copenhagen, 1980.
6. Churg, J., Spargo, B.H., Mostofi, F.K. and Abell, M.R. (Eds): Kidney Disease: Present Status. The Williams & Wilkins Co., Baltimore, 1979.
7. Earley, L.E. and Gottschalk, C.W. (Eds): Strauss and Welt's Diseases of the Kidney, 3rd Edition. Little, Brown & Co., Boston, 1979.
8. Edelmann, C.M. (Ed): Pediatric Kidney Disease. Little, Brown & Co., Boston, 1978.
9. Hamburger, J., Crosnier, J. and Grunfeld, J-P (Eds): Nephrology. John Wiley & Sons, New York, (French Edition: Flammarion Medecine-Sciences, Paris), 1979.
10. Heptinstall, R.H.: Pathology of the Kidney, 2nd Edition. Little, Brown & Co., Boston, 1974.
11. Ignatova, M.S. and Veltishchev, Yu.E.: Diseases of the Kidneys in Children. Meditsina, Moscow, 1973 (in Russian).
12. International Committee for Nomenclature and Nosology of Renal Disease: A Handbook of Kidney Nomenclature and Nosology. Little, Brown & Co., Boston, 1975.
13. Kincaid-Smith, P., Mathew, T.H. and Becker, E.L. (Eds.): Glomerulonephritis. Morphology, Natural History and Treatment. John Wiley & Sons, New York, 1973
14. Kincaid-Smith, P., d'Apice, A.J.F. and Atkins, R.C. (Eds): Progress in Glomerulonephritis. John Wiley & Sons, New York, Brisbane, 1979.
15. Meadows, R.: Renal Histopathology, 2nd Ed., Oxford University Press, Oxford, 1978.
16. Natusch, R. and Ditscherlein, G.: Nierenbiopsien: Technik, Morphologie und Klinik. Barth, Leipzig, 1976 (in German).
17. Royer, P., Habib, R., Mathieu, H. and Broyer, M. Pediatric Nephrology. W.B. Saunders Co., Philadelphia, 1973.
18. Spargo, B.H., Seymour, A.E. and Ordonez, N.: Renal Biopsy Pathology. John Wiley & Sons, New York, 1980.
19. Tareev, E.M. (Ed): Principles of Nephrology, Vols. 1 & 2, Meditsina, Moscow, 1972 (in Russian).
20. Zollinger, H.U. and Mihatsch, M.J.: Renal Pathology in Biopsy. Springer-Verlag, Berlin, Heidelberg, New York, 1978.

ELECTRON MICROSCOPY

21. Churg, J. and Grishman, E.: Ultrastructure of Glomerular Disease: A Review. Kidney Int. 7: 254, 1975.
22. Churg, J. and Grishman, E.: Electron Microscopy of Glomerulonephritis. In: Current Topics in Pathol. Vol. 61. Springer-Verlag, Berlin, 1976. pp. 107–153.
23. Churg, J., Spargo, B.H., Sakaguchi, H. and Jones, D.B.: Diagnostic Electron Microscopy of Renal Diseases. In: Diagnostic Electron Microscopy, Vol. 3, edited by Trump, B.F. and Jones, R.T. John Wiley & Sons, New York, 1980. pp. 203–314.
24. Sakaguchi, H. and Churg, J. (Eds): Renal Disease. In: Electron Microscopy in Human Medicine, Vol. 9, edited by Johannessen, J.V. McGraw-Hill Brook Co., London, 1980. pp. 3–165.
25. Spargo, B.H. and Seymour, A.E.: The Value of Electron Microscopy in the Study of Glomerular Disease. In: Renal Disease, 4th Edition, edited by Black, D.A.K. and Jones, N.F. Blackwell, Oxford, 1979, pp. 185–218.

IMMUNOPATHOLOGY

26. Albini, B., Andres, G.A. and Brentjens, J.R.: Immunopathology of the Kidney. Arnold, London, 1979.
27. Germuth, F.G. and Rodriguez, E.: Immunopathology of the Renal Glomerulus. Little, Brown and Co., Boston, 1973.
28. Larsen, S.: Glomerular Immune Deposits in Kidneys from Patients with No Clinical or Light Microscopic Evidence of Glomerulonephritis. Acta path. microbiol. scand. Sect. A.. 87:313, 1979.
29. Serov, V.V. Morphologic Basis of Renal Immunopathology (Nephritis, Nephrosis). Meditsina, Moscow, 1973 (in Russian).
30. Wilson, C.B.: Immunologic Mechanisms of Renal Disease. Churchill-Livingstone, London, 1979.

REFERENCES

Chapter 1

NORMAL GLOMERULUS

31. Chatelanat, F.: Anatomy of the Kidney. In: Nephrology, edited by Hamburger, J., Crosnier, J. and Grunfeld, J.-P. John Wiley & Sons, New York (French Edition: Flammarion Medicine-Sciences, Paris), 1979, pp. 3–40.
32. Latta, H.: Ultrastructure of the Glomerulus and the Juxtaglomerular Apparatus. In: Handbook of Physiology, Section 8: Renal Physiology, American Physiological Society, Washington, D.C. 1973. pp. 1–29.

Chapter 2

MINOR GLOMERULAR ABNORMALITIES

33. Cameron, J.S., Turner, D.R., Ogg, C.S., Sharpstone, P. and Brown, C.B.: The Nephrotic Syndrome in Adults with "Minimal Change" Glomerular Lesions. Quart. J. Med. 43:461, 1974.
34. Habib, R. and Kleinknecht, C.: The Primary Nephrotic Syndrome of Childhood: Classification and Clinicopathologic Study of 406 Cases. Pathol. Annual 6:417, 1971.
35. Larsen, S.: Immunofluorescent Microscopy Findings in Minimal or No Change-Disease and Slight Generalized Mesangioproliferative Glomerulonephritis. Acta path. microbiol. Scand. Sect. A. 85:531, 1978.

FOCAL/SEGMENTAL LESIONS

36. Beaufils, H., Alphonse, J.C., Guedon, J. and Legrain, M.: Focal Glomerulosclerosis: Natural History and Treatment. Nephron 21: 75, 1978.
37. Bohle, A., Fischbach, H., Wehner, H., Woerz, U., Edel, H.H., Kluthe, R. and Scheler, F.: Minimal Change Lesion with Nephrotic Syndrome and Focal Glomerular Sclerosis. Clin. Nephrol. 2:52, 1974.
38. Cameron, J.S., Turner, D.R., Ogg, C.S., Chantler, C. and Williams, D.G.: The Long-term Prognosis of Patients with Focal Segmental Glomerulosclerosis. Clin. Nephrol. 10:213, 1978.
39. Grishman, E. and Churg, J.: Focal Glomerular Sclerosis in Nephrotic Patients: An Electron Microscopic Study of Glomerular Podocytes. Kidney Int. 7:111, 1975.
40. Grishman, E., Churg, J. and Porush, J.G.: Glomerular Morphology in Nephrotic Heroin Addicts. Lab. Invest. 35:415, 1976.
41. Schoeneman, M.J., Bennett, B. and Greifer, I.: The Natural History of Focal Segmental Glomerulosclerosis With and Without Mesangial Hypercellularity in Children. Clin. Nephrol. 9:45, 1978.
42. Whitworth, J.A., Turner, D.R., Leibowitz, S. and Cameron, J.S.: Focal Segmental Sclerosis or Scarred Focal Proliferative Glomerulonephritis? Clin. Nephrol. 9:229, 1978.

Chapter 3

DIFFUSE MEMBRANOUS GLOMERULONEPHRITIS (MEMBRANOUS NEPHROPATHY)

43. Collaborative Study of the Adult Idiopathic Nephrotic Syndrome: A Controlled Study of Short-Term Prednisone Treatment in Adults with Membranous Nephropathy. New Engl. J. Med. 301:1301, 1979.
44. Ehrenreich, T. and Churg, J.: Pathology of Membranous Nephropathy. Pathol. Annual 3:145, 1968.
45. Ehrenreich, T., Porush, J.G., Churg, J., Garfinkel, L., Glabman, S., Goldstein, M.H., Grishman, E. and Yunis, S.L.: Treatment of Idiopathic Membranous Nephropathy. New Engl. J. Med. 295:741, 1976.
46. Gartner, H-V, Watanabe, T., Ott, V., Adam, A., Bohle, A., Edel, H.H., Kluthe, R., Renner, E., Scheler, F., Schmulling, R.M. and Sieberth, H.G.: Correlations between Morphologic and Clinical Features in Idiopathic Perimembranous Glomerulonephritis. A Study on 403 Renal Biopsies of 367 Patients. Current Topics in Pathol. 65:1, 1977.
47. Habib, R., Kleinknecht, C. and Gubler, M.C.: Extramembranous Glomerulonephritis in Children: Report of 50 Cases. J. Pediat. 82:754, 1973.
48. Noel, L.H., Zanetti, M., Droz, D. and Barbanel, C.: Long-term Prognosis of Idiopathic Membranous Glomerulonephritis. Study of 116 Untreated Patients. Amer. J. Med. 66:82, 1979.

Chapter 4

DIFFUSE MESANGIAL PROLIFERATIVE GLOMERULONEPHRITIS

49. Bhasin, H.K., Abuelo, J.G., Nayak, R. and Esparza, A.R.: Mesangial Proliferative Glomerulonephritis. Lab. Invest. 39:21, 1978.
50. Brown, E.A., Upadhyaya, K., Hayslett, J.P., Kashgarian, M. and Siegel, N.J.: The Clinical Course of Mesangial Proliferative Glomerulonephritis. Medicine 58:295, 1979.
51. Migone, L., Olivetti, G., Allegri, L. and Dall'Aglio, P.: Mesangioproliferative Glomerulonephritis. Clin. Nephrol. 13:219, 1980.
52. Waldherr, R., Gubler, M.C., Levy, M., Broyer, M. and Habib, R.: The Significance of Pure Diffuse Mesangial Proliferation in Idiopathic Nephrotic Syndrome. Clin. Nephrol. 10:171, 1978.

DIFFUSE ENDOCAPILLARY PROLIFERATIVE GLOMERULONEPHRITIS

53. Baldwin, D.S.: Poststreptococcal Glomerulonephritis: A Progressive Disease? Amer. J. Med. 62:1, 1977.
54. Gill, D.G., Turner, D.R., Chantler, C. and Cameron, J.S.: The Progression of Acute Proliferative Poststreptococcal Glomerulonephritis to Severe Epithelial Crescent Formation. Clin. Nephrol. 8:449, 1977.
55. Hinglais, N., Garcia-Torres, R. and Kleinknecht, D.: Long-term Prognosis in Acute Glomerulonephritis. Amer. J. Med. 56:52, 1974.
56. Nissenson, A.R., Baraff, L.J., Fine, R.N. and Knutson, D.W.: Post-streptococcal Acute Glomerulonephritis: Fact and Controversy. Ann. Intern. Med. 91:76, 1979.
57. Potter, E.V., Abidh, S., Sharrett, A.R., Burt, E.G., Svartman, M., Finklea, J.F., Poon-King, T. and Earle, D.P.: Clinical Healing Two to Six Years after Poststreptococcal Glomerulonephritis in Trinidad. New Engl. J. Med. 298:767, 1978.

Chapter 5

DIFFUSE MESANGIOCAPILLARY GLOMERULONEPHRITIS (MEMBRANOPROLIFERATIVE GLOMERULONEPHRITIS TYPES 1 AND 3)

58. Anders, D., Agricola, B., Sippel, M. and Thoenes, W.: Basement Membrane Changes in Membranoproliferative Glomerulonephritis. Virchows Arch. A Path. Anat. & Histol. 376:1, 1977.
59. Bennett, W.M., Bardana, E.J., Wuepper, K., Houghtons, D., Border, W.A., Gotze, O. and Schreiber, R.: Partial Lipodystrophy, C3 Nephritic Factor and Clinically Inapparent Mesangiocapillary Glomerulonephritis. Amer. J. Med. 62:757, 1977.
60. Bohle, A., Gartner, H.V., Fischbach, H., Bock, K.D., Edel, H.H., Frotscher, U., Kluthe, R., Monninghoff, W. and Scheler, F.: The Morphological and Clinical Features of Membranoproliferative Glomerulonephritis in Adults. Virchows Arch. A Path. Anat. and Histol. 363:213, 1974.
61. Donadio, J.V. Jr., Slack, T.K., Holley, K.E. and Ilstrup, D.M.: Idiopathic Membranoproliferative (Mesangiocapillary) Glomerulonephritis. A Clinicopathologic Study. Mayo Clinic Proc. 54:141, 1979.
62. Habib, R., Kleinknecht, C., Gubler, M.C. and Levy, M.: Idiopathic Membranoproliferative Glomerulonephritis in Children. Clin. Nephrol. 1:194, 1973.
63. Jones, D.B.: Membranoproliferative Glomerulonephritis. One or Many Diseases? Arch. Pathol. Lab. Med. 101:457, 1977.
64. Strife, C.F., McEnery, P.T., McAdams, A.J. and West, C.D.: Membranoproliferative Glomerulonephritis with Disruption of the Glomerular Basement Membrane. Clin. Nephrol. 7:65, 1977.

DENSE DEPOSIT GLOMERULONEPHRITIS (DENSE DEPOSIT DISEASE)

65. Berger, J. and Galle, P.: Depots Denses au Sein des Membranes Basales du Rein. Presse Med. 49:2351, 1963. (In French)
66. Beaufils, H., Gubler, M.C., Karam, J., Gluckman, J.C., Legrain, M. and Kuss, R.: Dense Deposit Disease: Long Term Follow-up of Three Cases of Recurrence after Transplantation. Clin. Nephrol. 7:31, 1977.
67. Churg, J., Duffy, J.L. and Bernstein, J.: Identification of Dense Deposit Disease. A Report for the International Study of Kidney Diseases in Children. Arch. Pathol. Lab. Med. 103:67, 1979.
68. Droz, D., Zanetti, M., Noel, L-H and Leibowitch, J.: Dense Deposits Disease. Nephron 19:1, 1977.
69. Kim, Y., Vernier, R.L., Fish, A.J. and Michael, A.F.: Immunofluorescence Studies of Dense Deposit Disease: The Presence of Railroad Tracks and Mesangial Rings. Lab. Invest. 40:474, 1979.
70. Lamb, V., Tisher, C.C., McCoy, R.C. and Robinson, R.R.: Membranoproliferative Glomerulonephritis with Dense Intramembranous Alterations. Lab. Invest. 36:607, 1977.
71. Vargas, R.A., Thomson, K.J., Wilson, D., Cameron, J.S., Turner, D.R., Gill, D., Chantler, C. and Ogg, C.S.: Mesangiocapillary Glomerulonephritis with Dense "Deposits" in the Basement Membranes of the Kidney. Clin. Nephrol. 5:73, 1976.

Chapter 6

DIFFUSE CRESCENTIC (EXTRACAPILLARY) GLOMERULONEPHRITIS

72. Glassock, R.J.: A Clinical and Immunopathologic Dissection of Rapidly Progressive Glomerulonephritis. Nephron 22:253, 1978.
73. Morita, T., Suzuki, Y., and Churg, J.: Structure and Development of the Glomerular Crescent. Amer. J. Path. 72:349, 1973.
74. Morrin, P.A.F., Hinglais, N., Nabarra, B. and Kreis, H.: Rapidly Progressive Glomerulonephritis. A Clinical and Pathologic Study. Amer. J. Med. 65:446, 1978.
75. Olsen, S.: Extracapillary Glomerulonephritis: A Semi-quantitative Light Microscopical Study of 59 Patients. Acta pathol. Microbiol. Scand. (A) (Suppl. 249) 82:7, 1974.
76. Rosen, S.: Crescentic Glomerulonephritis: Occurrence, Mechanisms and Prognosis. Pathol. Annual 10:37, 1975.

REFERENCES

77. Spargo, B.H., Ordonez, N.G. and Ringus, J.C.: The Differential Diagnosis of Crescentic Glomerulonephritis. Human Pathol. 8:187, 1977.
78. Stilmant, M.M., Bolton, W.K., Sturgill, B.C., Schmitt, G.W. and Couser, W.G.: Crescentic Glomerulonephritis without Immune Deposits: Clinicopathologic Features. Kidney Int. 15:184, 1979.

Chapter 7

LUPUS NEPHRITIS

79. Appel, G.B., Silva, F.G., Pirani, C.L. Meltzer, J.I. and Estes, D.: Renal Involvement in Systemic Lupus Erythematosis (SLE). Medicine 57:371, 1978.
80. Baldwin, D.S., Gluck, M.C., Lowenstein, J. and Gallo, G.R.: Lupus Nephritis. Clinical Course as Related to Morphologic Forms and Their Transitions. Amer. J. Med. 62:12, 1977.
81. Cameron, J.S., Turner, D.R., Ogg, C.S., Williams, D.G., Lessof, M.H., Chantler, C. and Leibowitz, S.: Systemic Lupus with Nephritis: A Long Term Study. Quart. J. Med. 48:1, 1979.
82. Grishman, E., Porush, J.G., Lee, S.L. and Churg, J.: Renal Biopsies In Lupus Nephritis. Nephron 10:25, 1973.
83. Grishman, E., Porush, J.C., Rosen, S.M. and Churg, J.: Lupus Nephritis with Organized Deposits in the Kidneys. Lab. Invest. 16:717, 1967.
84. Hill, G.S., Hinglais, N., Tron, F. and Bach, J.-F.: Systemic Lupus Erythematosus. Morphologic Correlations with Immunologic and Clinical Data at the Time of the Biopsy. Amer. J. Med. 64:61, 1978.
85. Mahajan, S.K., Ordonez, N.G., Spargo, B.H. and Katz, A.I.: Changing Histopathology Patterns in Lupus Nephropathy. Clin. Nephrol. 10:1, 1978.
86. Sinniah, R. and Feng, P.H.: Lupus Nephritis: Correlation between Light, Electron Microscopic and Immunofluorescent Findings and Renal Function. Clin. Nephrol. 6:340, 1976.

Chapter 8

NEPHRITIS OF HENOCH SCHONLEIN PURPURA (ANAPHYLACTOID PURPURA)

87. Heaton, J.M., Turner, D.R. and Cameron, J.S.: Localization of Glomerular 'Deposits' in Henoch-Schonlein Nephritis. Histopathol. 1:93, 1977.
88. Levey, M., Broyer, M., Arson, A., Levy-Bentolila, D. and Habib, R.: Anaphylactoid Purpura Nephritis in Childhood: Natural History and Immunopathology. Adv. Nephrol. 6:183, 1976.
89. Meadow, S.R.: The Prognosis of Henoch Schonlein Nephritis. Clin. Nephrol. 9:87, 1978.
90. Sinniah, R., Feng, P.H. and Chen, B.T.M.: Henoch-Schoenlein Syndrome: A Clinical and Morphological Study of Renal Biopsies. Clin. Nephrol. 9:219, 1978.

BERGER'S DISEASE (IgA NEPHROPATHY)

91. Berger, J.: IgA Glomerular Deposits in Renal Diseases. Transpl. Proc. 1:939, 1969.
92. Clarkson, A.R., Seymour, A.E., Thompson, A.J., Haynes, W.D.G., Chan, Y-L and Jackson, B.: IgA Nephropathy: A Syndrome of Uniform Morphology, Diverse Clinical Features and Uncertain Prognosis. Clin. Nephrol. 8:459, 1977.
93. Droz, D.: Natural History of Primary Glomerulonephritis with Mesangial Deposits of IgA. Contr. Nephrol. 2:150, 1976.
94. Lamperi, S. and Carozzi, S.: Skin-Muscle Biopsy in Patients with Various Nephropathies. Nephron 24:46, 1979.
95. Sinniah, R., Pwee, H.S. and Lim, C.H.: Glomerular Lesions in Asymptomatic Microscopic Hematuria Discovered on Routine Medical Examination. Clin. Nephrol. 5:216, 1976.
96. Van der Peet, J., Arisz, L., Brentjens, J.R.H., Marrink, J. and Hoedemaeker, Ph.J.: The Clinical Course of IgA Nephropathy in Adults. Clin. Nephrol. 8:335, 1977.

GOODPASTURE'S SYNDROME

97. Andres, G., Brentjens, J., Kohli, R., Anthone, R., Anthone, S., Baliah, T., Montes, M., Mookerjee, B.K., Prezyna, A., Sepulveda, M., Venuto, R. and Elwood, C.: Histology of Human Tubulointerstitial Nephritis Associated with Antibodies to Renal Basement Membranes. Kidney Int. 13:480, 1978.
98. Briggs, W.A., Johnson, J.P., Teichman, S., Yeager, H.C. and Wilson, C.B.: Antiglomerular Basement Membrane Antibody-Mediated Glomerulonephritis in Goodpasture's Syndrome. Medicine (Baltimore) 58:348, 1979.
99. McPhaul, J.J. and Mullins, J.D.: Glomerulonephritis Mediated by Antibody to Glomerular Basement Membrane: Immunological, Clinical and Histopathological Characteristics. J. Clin. Invest. 57:351, 1976.
100. Teague, C.A., Doak, P.B., Simpson, I.J., Rainer, S.P. and Herdson, P.B.: Goodpasture's Syndrome: An Analysis of 29 Cases. Kidney Int. 13:492, 1978.

Chapter 9

GLOMERULAR LESIONS IN SYSTEMIC INFECTIONS

101. Boulton-Jones, J.M., Sissons, J.G.P., Evans, D.J. and Peters, D.K.: Renal Lesions of Subacute Infective Endocarditis. Brit. Med. J. 2:11, 1974.

102. Gutman, R.A., Striker, G.E., Gilliland, B.C. and Cutler, R.E.: The Immune Complex Glomerulonephritis of Bacterial Endocarditis. Medicine (Baltimore) 51:1, 1972.
103. Kim, Y. and Michael, A.F.: Chronic Bacteremia and Nephritis. Ann. Rev. Med. 29:319, 1978.
104. Dobrin, R.S., Day, N.K., Quie, P.G., Moore, H.L., Vernier, R.L., Michael, A.F. and Fish, A.J.: The Role of Complement, Immunoglobulin and Bacterial Antigen in Coagulase-negative Staphylococcal Shunt Nephritis. Amer. J. Med. 59:660, 1975.
105. Strife, C.F., McDonald, B.M., Ruley, E.J., McAdams, A.J. and West, C.D.: Shunt Nephritis: The Nature of the Serum Cryoglobulins and Their Relation to the Complement Profile. J. Pediat. 88:403, 1976.
106. Gamble, C. and Reardan, J.: Immunopathogenesis of Syphilitic Glomerulonephritis. Elution of Anti-treponemal Antibody from Glomerular Immune-complex Deposits. New Eng. J. Med. 292:449, 1975.
107. Hill, L.L., Singer, D.B., Falletta, J. and Stasney, R.: The Nephrotic Syndrome in Congenital Syphilis: An Immunopathy. Pediatrics 49:260, 1972.

Chapter 10

PARASITIC NEPHROPATHIES

Malarial Nephropathy

108. Hendrickse, R.G., Adeniyi, A., Edington, G.M., Glasgow, E.F., White, R.H.R. and Houba, V.: Quartan Malarial Nephrotic Syndrome. Lancet I:1143, 1972.
109. Hendrickse, R.G.: The Quartan Malarial Nephrotic Syndrome. In: Advances in Nephrology, Vol. 6, edited by Hamburger, J., Crosnier, J. and Maxwell, M.H. Year Book Medical Publishers, 1976. pp. 229–247.
110. Morel-Maroger, L., Saimot, A.G., Sloper, J.C., Woodrow, D.F., Adam, C., Niang, I. and Payet, M.: "Tropical Nephropathy" and "Tropical Extramembranous Glomerulonephritis" of Unknown Aetiology in Senegal. Brit. Med. J. 1:541, 1975.
111. White, R.H.R.: Quartan Malarial Nephrotic Syndrome. Nephron 11:147, 1973.

Schistosomal Nephropathy

112. Andrade, Z.A. and Rocha, H.: Schistosomal Glomerulopathy. Kidney Int. 16:23, 1979.

Chapter 11

PERIARTERITIS NODOSA AND WEGENER'S GRANULOMATOSIS

113. Chumbley, L.C., Harrison, E.G. and Deremee, R.A.: Allergic Granulomatosis and Angiitis (Churg-Strauss Syndrome): Report and Analysis of 30 Cases. Mayo Clin. Proc. 52:477, 1977.
114. Fauci, A.S., Haynes, B.F. and Katz, P.: The Spectrum of Vasculitis: Clinical, Pathologic, Immunologic and Therapeutic Considerations. Ann. Intern. Med. 89:660, 1978.
115. Horn, R.G., Fauci, A.S., Rosenthal, A.S. and Wolff, S.M.: Renal Biopsy Pathology in Wegener's Granulomatosis. Amer. J. Path. 74:423, 1974.
116. Saldana, M.J., Patchefsky, A.S., Israel, H.I. and Atkinson, G.W.: Pulmonary Angiitis and Granulomatosis: The Relationship Between Histological Features, Organ Involvement and Response to Treatment. Human Pathol. 8:391, 1977.

Chapter 12

THROMBOTIC MICROANGIOPATHY (HEMOLYTIC-UREMIC SYNDROME)

117. Bohle, A., Helmchen, U., Grund, K.E., Gartner, H-V, Meyer, D., Bock, K.D., Bulla, M., Bunger, P., Diekmann, L., Frotscher, U., Hayduk, K., Kosters, W., Strauch, M., Scheler, F. and Christ, H.: Malignant Nephrosclerosis in Patients with Hemolytic Uremic Syndrome (Primary Malignant Nephrosclerosis). Current Topics Pathol. 65:81, 1977.
118. Goldstein, M.H., Churg, J., Strauss, L. and Gribetz, D.: Hemolytic-uremic Syndrome. Nephron 23:263, 1979.
119. Kaplan, B.S. and Drummond, K.N.: The Hemolytic Uremic Syndrome is a Syndrome. New Engl. J. Med. 298:964, 1978.
120. Segonds, A., Louradour, N., Suc, J.M. and Orfila, C.: Postpartum Hemolytic Uremic Syndrome: A Study of Three Cases with a Review of the Literature. Clin. Nephrol. 12:229, 1979.
121. Shigematsu, H., Dikman, S.H., Churg, J., Grishman, E. and Duffy, J.L.: Mesangial Involvement in Hemolytic-Uremic Syndrome. Amer. J. Path. 85:349, 1976.

GLOMERULAR THROMBOSIS (INTRAVASCULAR COAGULATION)

122. Mant, M.J. and King, E.G.: Severe, Acute Disseminated Intravascular Coagulation. A Reappraisal of its Pathophysiology, Clinical Significance and Therapy Based on 47 Patients. Amer. J. Med. 67:557, 1979.

REFERENCES

Chapter 13

BENIGN AND MALIGNANT NEPHROSCLEROSIS

123. Hsu, H-C and Churg, J.: The Ultrastructure of Mucoid "Onionskin" Intimal Lesions in Malignant Nephrosclerosis. Amer. J. Path. 99:67, 1980.
124. Jones, D.B.: Arterial and Glomerular Lesions Associated with Severe Hypertension: Light and Electron Microscopic Studies. Lab. Invest. 31:303, 1974.
125. Pitcock, J.A., Johnson, J.G., Hatch, F.E., Acchiardo, S., Muirhead, E.E. and Brown P.S.: Malignant Hypertension in Blacks: Malignant Intrarenal Arterial Disease as Observed by Light and Electron Microscopy. Human Pathol. 7:333, 1976.
126. Shigematsu, H., Dikman, S.H., Churg, J. and Grishman, E.: Glomerular Injury in Malignant Nephrosclerosis. Nephron 22:399, 1978.

SCLERODERMA (SYSTEMIC SCLEROSIS)

127. Cannon, P.J., Hassar, M., Case, D.B., Casarella, W.J., Sommers, S.C. and Leroy, E.C.: The Relationship of Hypertension and Renal Failure in Scleroderma (Progressive Systemic Sclerosis) to Structural and Functional Abnormalities of the Renal Cortical Circulation. Medicine 53:1, 1974.
128. Kovalchik, M.T., Guggenheim, S.J., Silverman, M.H., Robertson, J.S. and Steigerwald, J.C.: The Kidney in Progressive Systemic Sclerosis: A Prospective Study. Ann. Intern. Med. 89:881, 1978.

Chapter 14

DIABETIC GLOMERULOSCLEROSIS

129. Cameron, J.S., Ireland, J.T. and Watkins, P.J.: The Kidney and Renal Tract. In: The Complications of Diabetes, edited by Keen, H. and Jarrett, R.J. Edward Arnold, London, 1975.
130. Bloodworth, J.M.B. Jr.: A Re-evaluation of Diabetic Glomerulosclerosis 50 Years after the Discovery of Insulin. Human Pathol. 9:439, 1978.
131. Dachs, S., Churg, J., Mautner, W. and Grishman, E.: Diabetic Nephropathy. Amer. J. Path. 44:155, 1964.
132. Ditscherlein, G.: Nierenveränderungen bei Diabetikern. VEB Gustav Fischer Verlag, Jena, 1969. (In German).
133. Østerby, R.: Early Phase in the Development of Diabetic Glomerulopathy. Acta Med. Scand. 197 (Suppl. 574):13, 1975.
134. Takazakara, E., Nakamoto, Y., Hayakawa, H., Kawai, K., Muramoto, S., Yoshida, K., Shimizu, M., Shinoda, A. and Takeuchi, J.: Onset and Progression of Diabetic Glomerulosclerosis: A Prospective Study Based on Renal Biopsies. Diabetes 24:1, 1975.

Chapter 15

AMYLOIDOSIS

135. Dikman, S.H., Churg, J. and Kahn, T.: Morphologic and Clinical Correlates in Renal Amyloidosis. Human Pathol. 12:160, 1981.
136. Franklin, E.C.: Some Unsolved Problems in the Amyloid Diseases. Amer. J. Med. 66:365, 1979.
137. Gise, H.v., Mikeler, E., Gruber, M., Christ, H. and Bohle, A.: Investigations on the Cause of the Nephrotic Syndrome in Renal Amyloidosis: A Discussion of Electron Microscopic Findings. Virchows Arch A. Path. Anat. Histol. 379:131, 1978.
138. Triger, D.R. and Joekes, A.M.: Renal Amyloidosis — A Fourteen Year Follow-up. Quart. J. Med. 42:15, 1973.

MULTIPLE MYELOMA AND WALDENSTROM'S MACROGLOBULINEMIA

139. Beaufils, M. and Morel-Maroger, L.: Pathogenesis of Renal Disease in Monoclonal Gammopathies: Current Concepts. Nephron 20:125, 1978.
140. Gallo, G.R., Feiner, H.D., Katz, L.A., Feldman, G.M., Correa, E.B., Chuba, J.V. and Buxbaum, J.N.: Nodular Glomerulopathy Associated with Non-amyloidotic Kappa Light Chain Deposits and Excess Immunoglobulin Light Chain Synthesis. Amer. J. Path. 99:621, 1980.
141. Lin, J.H., Orofino, D., Sherlock, J., Letteri, J. and Duffy, J.L.: Waldenstrom's Macroglobulinemia, Mesangio-capillary Glomerulonephritis, Angiitis and Myositis. Nephron 10:262, 1973.
142. Morel-Maroger, L. and Verroust, P.: Glomerular Lesions in Dysproteinemias. Kidney Int. 5:249, 1974.
143. Randall, R.E., Williamson, W.C. Jr., Mullinax, F., Tung, M.Y. and Still, W.J.S.: Manifestations of Systemic Light Chain Deposition. Amer. J. Med. 60:293, 1976.
144. Schubert, G.E., Veigel, J. and Lennert, K.: Structure and Function of the Kidney in Multiple Myeloma. Virchows Arch. Abt. A. Path. Anat. 355:135, 1972.
145. Schubert, G.E. and Adam, A.: Glomerular Nodules and Long-spacing Collagen in Kidneys of Patients with Multiple Myeloma. J. Clin. Path. 27:800, 1974.
146. Silva, F.G., Meyrier, A., Morel-Maroger, L. and Pirani, C.L.: Proliferative Glomerulonephropathy in Multiple Myeloma. J. Path. 130:229, 1980.

147. Smithline, N., Kissane, J.R. and Cohen, J.J.: Light-chain Nephropathy: Renal Tubular Dysfunction Associated with Light-chain Proteinuria. New Eng. J. Med. 294:71, 1976.
148. Solling, K., Solling, J., Jacobsen, N.O. and Thomsen, O.F.: Non-secretory Myeloma Associated with Nodular Glomerulosclerosis. Acta Med. Scand. 207:137, 1980.

CRYOGLOBULINEMIA

149. Beaufils, M. and Morel-Maroger, L.: Pathogenesis of Renal Disease in Monoclonal Gammopathies: Current Concepts. Nephron 20:125, 1978.
150. Faraggiana, T., Parolini, C., Previato, G. and Lupo, A.: Light and Electron Microscopic Findings in Five Cases of Cryoglobulinemic Glomerulonephritis. Virchows Arch. A, Path. Anat. and Histol. 384:29, 1979.
151. Feiner, H. and Gallo, G.: Ultrastructure in Glomerulonephritis Associated with Cryoglobulinemia: A Report of Six Cases and Review of the Literature. Amer. J. Path. 88:145, 1977.
152. Ogihara, T., Saruta, T., Saito, I., Abe, S., Ozawa, Y., Kato, E. and Sakaguchi, H.: Fingerprint Deposits of the Kidney in Pure Monoclonal IgG Kappa Cryoglobulinemia. Clin. Nephrol. 12:186, 1979.
153. Porush, J.G., Grishman, E., Alter, A.A., Mandelbaum, H. and Churg, J.: Paraproteinemia and Cryoglobulinemia Associated with Atypical Glomerulonephritis and the Nephrotic Syndrome. Amer. J. Med. 47:957, 1969.
154. Stoebner, P., Renversez, J.C., Groulade, J., Vialtel, P. and Cordonnier, D.: Ultrastructural Study of Human IgG and IgG-IgM Crystalcryoglobulins. Amer. J. Clin. Pathol. 71:404, 1979.

Chapter 16

NEPHROPATHY OF LIVER DISEASE

155. Berger, J., Yaneva, H. and Nabarra, B.: Glomerular Changes in Patients with Cirrhosis of the Liver. Adv. Nephrol. 7:3, 1977.
156. Nochy, D., Callard, P., Bellon, B., Bariety, J. and Druet, P.P.: Association of Overt Glomerulonephritis and Liver Disease: A Study of 34 Patients. Clin. Nephrol. 6:422, 1976.
157. Sakaguchi, H., Dachs, S., Grishman, E., Paronetto, F., Salomon, M. and Churg, J.: Hepatic Glomerulosclerosis. An Electron Microscopic Study of Renal Biopsies in Liver Diseases. Lab. Invest. 14:533, 1965.
158. Silver, M.M., Rance, P., Middleton, P.J. and Huber, J.: Hepatitis B-Associated Membranous Glomerulonephritis in a Child. Amer. J. Clin. Path. 72:1034, 1979.
159. Slusarczyk, J., Michalak, T., Nazarewicz-de Mezer, T., Krawczynski, K. and Nowoslawski, A.: Membranous Glomerulopathy Associated with Hepatitis B Core Antigen Immune Complexes in Children. Amer. J. Path. 98:29, 1980.

NEPHROPATHY OF SICKLE CELL DISEASE

160. Alleyne, G.A.O., Van Eps, L.W.S., Addae, S.K., Nicholson, G.D. and Schouten, H.: The Kidney in Sickle Cell Anemia. Kidney Int. 7:371, 1975.
160a. Elfenbein, I.B., Patchefsky, A., Schwartz, W. and Weinstein, A.G. Pathology of the Glomerulus in Sickle Cell Anemia With and Without Nephrotic Syndrome. Amer. J. Path. 77:357-376, 1974.
161. Sears, D.A.: The Morbidity of Sickle Cell Trait: A Review of the Literature. Amer. J. Med. 64:1021, 1978.

NEPHROPATHY OF CYANOTIC CONGENITAL HEART DISEASE

162. Burke, J.R., Glasgow, E.F., McCredie, D.A. and Powell, H.R.: Nephropathy in Cyanotic Congenital Heart Disease. Clin. Nephrol. 7:38, 1977.
163. Spear, G.S.: The Glomerular Lesion of Cyanotic Congenital Heart Disease. Johns Hopkins Med. J. 140:185, 1977.

Chapter 17

ALPORT'S SYNDROME

164. Churg, J. and Sherman, R.L.: Pathologic Characteristics of Hereditary Nephritis. Arch. Pathol. 95:374, 1973.
165. Hinglais, N., Grunfeld, J-P. and Bois, E.: Characteristic Ultrastructural Lesion of the Glomerular Basement Membrane in Progressive Hereditary Nephritis (Alport's Syndrome). Lab. Invest. 27:473, 1972.
166. Kohaut, E.C., Singer, D.B., Nevels, B.K. and Hill, L.L.: The Specificity of Split Renal Membranes in Hereditary Nephritis. Arch. Pathol. Lab. Med. 100:475, 1976.
167. Rumpelt, H.J., Langer, K.H., Scharer, K., Straub, E. and Thoenes, W.: Split and Extremely Thin Glomerular Basement Membranes in Hereditary Nephropathy (Alport's Syndrome). Virchows Arch A Path. Anat. Histol. 364:225, 1974.
168. Spear, G.S.: Pathology of the Kidney in Alport's Syndrome. Pathol. Annual 9:93, 1974.

BENIGN RECURRENT HEMATURIA (THIN BASEMENT MEMBRANE SYNDROME)

169. Rogers, P.W., Kurtzman, N.A., Bunn, S.M. Jr. and White, M.G.: Familial Benign Essential Hematuria. Arch. Intern Med. 131:257, 1973.

REFERENCES

NAIL-PATELLA SYNDROME (OSTEO-ONYCHODYSPLASIA)

170. Ben-Bassat, M., Cohen, L. and Rosenfeld, J.: The Glomerular Basement Membrane in the Nail-Patella Syndrome. Arch. Path. 92:350, 1971.
171. Bennett, W.M., Musgrave, J.E., Campbell, R.A., Elliot, D., Cox, R., Brooks, R.E., Lovrein, E.W., Beals, R.K. and Porter, G.A.: The Nephropathy of the Nail-Patella Syndrome. Clinicopathologic Analysis of 11 Kindred. Amer. J. Med. 54:304, 1973.
172. Morita, T., Laughlin, L.O., Kawano, K., Kimmelstiel, P., Suzuki, Y. and Churg, J.: Nail-Patella Syndrome. Light and Electron Microscopic Studies of the Kidney. Arch. Intern. Med. 131:271, 1973.

CONGENITAL NEPHROTIC SYNDROME (FINNISH TYPE) AND INFANTILE NEPHROTIC SYNDROME (FRENCH TYPE) (DIFFUSE MESANGIAL SCLEROSIS)

173. Habib, R. and Bois, E.: Congenital and Infantile Nephrotic Syndrome. In: Pediatric Nephrology, Vol. 2, edited by Strauss, J. Stratton Intercontinental Medical Book Corp., New York, 1975, p. 335.
174. Huttunen, N.-P., Rapola, J., Vilska, J. and Hallman, N.: Renal Pathology in Congenital Nephrotic Syndrome of Finnish Type: A Quantitative Light Microscopic Study on 50 Patients. International J. Pediat. Nephrol. 1:10, 1980.
175. Kaplan, B.S., Bureau, M.A. and Drummond, K.N.: The Nephrotic Syndrome in the First Year of Life: Is a Pathologic Classification Possible? J. Pediat. 85:615, 1974.
176. Rumpelt, H.J. and Bachmann, H.J.: Infantile Nephrotic Syndrome with Diffuse Mesangial Sclerosis: A Disturbance of Glomerular Basement Membrane Development? Clin. Nephrol. 13:146, 1980.

Chapter 18

FABRY'S DISEASE

177. Gubler, M-C, Lenoir, G., Grünfeld, J-P, Ulmann, A., Droz, D. and Habib, R.: Early Renal Changes in Hemizygous and Heterozygous Patients with Fabry's Disease. Kidney Int. 13:223, 1978.
178. Rosenmann, E. and Aviram, A.: Glomerular Involvement in Storage Diseases. J. Pathol. 111:61, 1973.
179. Scott, C.R., Lagunoff, D. and Pritzl, P.: A Mucopolysaccharide Storage Diseases with Involvement of the Renal Glomerular Epithelium. Amer. J. Med. 54:549, 1973.

FAMILIAL LECITHIN-CHOLESTEROL ACYL TRANSFERASE DEFICIENCY

180. Gjone, E.: Déficit Familial en Lécithine-Cholestérol Acyltransferase: Une Nouvelle Maladie Métabolique avec Atteinte Renale. Actualités Néphrologiques pp. 159–176, 1980.
181. Myhre, E., Gjone, E., Flatmark, A. and Hovig, T.: Renal Failure in Familial Lecithin-Cholesterol Acyltransferase Deficiency. Nephron 18:239, 1977.
182. Sibley, R.K.: Case of Familial Lecithin-Cholesterol Acyltransferase Deficiency, Presented at Nephropathologists Specialty Conference, Annual Meeting of the International Academy of Pathology, New Orleans, Feb. 25–29, 1980.

I-CELL DISEASE (MUCOLIPIDOSIS II)

183. Gilbert, E.F., Dawson, G., Zu Rhein, G.M., Opitz, J.M. and Spranger, J.W.: I-Cell Disease, Mucolipidosis II. Pathological, Histochemical, Ultrastructural and Biochemical Observations in Four Cases. Z. Kinderheilk. 114:259, 1973.

Chapter 19

NEPHROPATHY OF TOXEMIA OF PREGNANCY (PRE-ECLAMPTIC NEPHROPATHY)

184. Spargo, B.H., Lichtig, C., Luger, A.M., Katz, A.I. and Lindheimer, M.D.: The Renal Lesion in Pre-eclampsia. In: Hypertension in Pregnancy, edited by Lindheimer, M.D., Katz, A.I. and Zuspan, F.P. John Wiley & Sons, New York, 1976, pp. 129-137.

RADIATION NEPHRITIS

185. Churg, J. and Madrazo, A.: Radiation Nephritis. In: Seminars in Nephrology, edited by Becker, E.L. John Wiley & Sons, New York, 1977, p. 83.
186. Keane, W.F., Crosson, J.T., Staley, N.A., Anderson, W.R. and Shapiro, F.L.: Radiation-induced Renal Disease. A Clinicopathologic Study. Amer. J. Med. 60:127, 1976.
187. Madrazo, A., Suzuki, Y. and Churg, J.: Radiation Nephritis. Acute Changes Following High Dose of Radiation. Amer. J. Path. 54: 507, 1969.

Chapter 20

END STAGE KIDNEY

188. Hughson, M.D., Hennigar, G.R. and McManus, J.F.A.: Atypical Cysts, Acquired Renal Cystic Disease, and Renal Cell Tumors in End Stage Dialysis Kidneys. Lab. Invest. 42:475, 1980.

189. McManus, J.F.A. and Hughson, M.D.: New Therapies and New Pathologies. End-Stage-Dialysis Kidneys. Arch. Pathol. Lab. Med. 103:53, 1979.

GLOMERULAR LESIONS FOLLOWING TRANSPLANTATION

190. Cameron, J.S. and Turner, D.R.: Recurrent Glomerulonephritis in Allografted Kidneys. Clin. Nephrol. 7:47, 1977.
191. Hsu, H-C, Suzuki, Y., Churg, J. and Grishman, E.: Ultrastructure of Transplant Glomerulopathy. Histopathology 4:351, 1980.
192. Petersen, V.P., Olsen, T.S., Kissmeyer-Nielsen, F., Bohman, S.I., Hansen, H.E., Hansen, E.S., Skov, P.E. and Solling, K.: Late Failure of Human Renal Transplants: An Analysis of Transplant Disease and Graft Failure Among 125 Recipients Surviving from One to Eight Years. Medicine (Baltimore) 54:45, 1975.
193. Rossmann, P. and Jirka, J.: Rejection Nephropathy. Academia, Prague, 1979.
194. Rowlands, D.T. Jr., Hill, G.S. and Zmijewski, C.M.: The Pathology of Renal Homograft Rejection: A Review. Amer. J. Path. 85:774, 1976.
195. Zollinger, H.U., Moppert, J., Thiel, G. and Rohr, H.-P.: Morphology and Pathogenesis of Glomerulopathy in Cadaver Kidney Allografts Treated with Antilymphocyte Globulin. Current Topics in Pathol. 57:1, 1973.

APPENDIX

The Processing and Examination of Renal Biopsies

Introduction

The pathologist is called upon to examine two kinds of renal biopsy specimens: those obtained with a special needle (needle biopsy), and those obtained through a surgical approach (open or wedge biopsy). The pathologist also has to deal with tissue from surgically removed kidneys and with tissue obtained at autopsy.

In a needle biopsy procedure, a slender piece (core) of tissue measuring 1 mm to 2 mm in diameter and a few millimeters to 1 cm or even 2 cm in length is removed. The core generally includes both cortex and medulla, but sometimes only the medulla if the needle enters the kidney in an area of cortical-collecting tubules. Occasionally pelvic mucosa may be present. The wedge biopsy provides much more material for study, but usually consists of cortical tissue only: this, as a rule, is only a small handicap, because most diagnostic information comes from studying the cortex.

The standard methods of examination include light, electron and immunofluorescent microscopy. In many instances a diagnosis can be established by using light microscopy, but wherever possible tissue also should be set aside for the other two microscopic procedures. Thus, the person performing the biopsy should obtain more than one core of tissue, particularly when additional studies—such as culture (in cases of suspected infections), freeze-drying or freeze-substitution (for autoradiography), or enzymes (histochemistry and microchemistry)—are planned. It is best if the pathologist or a specially trained technologist is present during the biopsy to see that the tissue is handled properly and utilized to the greatest advantage. The problems caused by insufficient tissue for study are greatly reduced if a wedge biopsy instead of a needle biopsy is obtained.

The tissue is removed gently from the biopsy needle, placed in a small Petri dish containing enough cold saline to cover the tissue, and examined under a dissecting microscope, if such instrument is available. If glomeruli are present, the tissue is divided so that at least a few glomeruli are fixed for study by electron microscopy and a few are frozen for immunofluorescence; the remainder of the tissue is fixed for light microscopy. Some pathologists prefer to cut the specimen longitudinally; however, since this method introduces mechanical artifacts, *it is better to cut off small pieces from both ends of the specimen* for study by electron microscopy and immunofluorescence. The specimen should be placed on a plate of dental wax and then cut with sharp razor blades. The tissue should be covered with a drop of saline to prevent drying.

Preparation of Tissue for Light Microscopy

Fixing

The three most useful fixatives are:

1. ***Alcoholic Bouin (Dubosque-Brazil).*** The stock solution consists of 150 ml of 80% ethyl alcohol, 60 ml of concentrated formaldehyde, and 1 g of picric acid. Before use, add 1 ml of glacial acetic acid for each 14 ml of stock solution. Fix needle biopsy specimens for five to six hours and wedge biopsy specimens overnight. Transfer the tissue into neutral buffered formalin for 24 hours.

2. ***Zenker-formol.*** The stock solution is Zenker's fluid. Before use, add 1 ml of concentrated formaldehyde for each 19 ml of stock solution. Fix needle biopsy specimens for three to four hours and wedge biopsy specimens for four to six hours. Wash overnight in running water.

3. ***Formalin.*** The stock solution of neutral or slightly acid formalin consists of a 1:10 dilution of concentrated (37% to 40%) formaldehyde in phosphate or acetate buffer with a pH of between 6 and 7. Instead of an acetate buffer, one can simply add 10 g of anhydrous sodium acetate to 500 ml of a 1:10 dilution of concentrated formaldehyde in water. Formalin solutions are ready to use and keep indefinitely. Fix needle biopsy specimens in the stock solution for at least six hours and wedge biopsy specimens overnight.

Each of these fixatives has advantages and disadvantages. Alcoholic Bouin fixative produces excellent cytoplasmic preservation, but the tissue is harmed by prolonged fixation. Zenker-formol fixative requires lengthy washing to eliminate the mercury. Formaldehyde is excellent for

---

This Appendix is based on an article "The Processing and Examination of Renal Biopsies" by Jacob Churg, M.D. and Michael A. Gerber, M.D. published in Laboratory Medicine 10: 591-596, 1979 and in Technical Improvement Service, Vol. 29, 1977, American Society of Clinical Pathologists. Reproduced with permission of the Editor of Laboratory Medicine and the American Society of Clinical Pathologists.

periodic acid-Schiff (PAS) and Jones' silver methenamine stains, but tends to produce poorly differentiated trichrome stains unless sections are mordanted in mercuric bichloride or in Zenker's solution. Tissue may be left in formaldehyde for a considerable length of time without significant harm.

Recently paraformaldehyde has been used as a universal fixative for both light and electron microscopy. For that purpose, a 4% solution of paraformaldehyde is prepared in 0.1 molar phosphate buffer, pH 7.2. The solution keeps well for several weeks in the refrigerator. It penetrates the tissue quite well so that an entire needle biopsy can be dropped into the fixative and divided later into a portion for light microscopy and a portion for electron microscopy. Needle biopsies are well fixed after two to three hours. Larger pieces of tissue require several hours or overnight at room temperature.

For certain purposes special fixation is necessary. For example, to demonstrate crystals of cystine or uric acid, the tissue should be fixed in absolute alcohol. Alcohol also preserves glycogen to the best advantage, though this substance is partly preserved with formalin and other fixatives. To demonstrate lipids, use sections from the tissue that was frozen for immunofluorescence.

Embedding

The standard method of processing tissue for light microscopy is dehydration in graded alcohols and, after clearing, embedment in paraffin. Because renal biopsy specimens are very small, prolonged exposure to the dehydrating and clearing agents should be avoided. Renal biopsy tissue shoudl not be processed with other tissues but rather separately (or perhaps with other small biopsy specimens) in an automated instrument or by hand. We use the following procedure:

1. 50% ethyl alcohol – 15 minutes.
2. 95% alcohol – two changes, 15 minutes each.
3. 100% alcohol – two changes, 20 minutes each.
4. Xylene – two changes, 12 minutes each, or chloroform, 20 minutes each.

(For hand processing, place the tissue and the reagent in a tightly stoppered vial, and agitate slowly and continuously in a shaker.)

5. Xylene-paraffin (equal parts) – 10 minutes, or chloroform-paraffin (equal parts), 20 minutes.
6. Paraffin (melting point 53°C) – two changes, 20 minutes each. Agitate with a magnetic stirrer.
7. Embed in Paraplast (Sherwood Laboratories, St. Louis, MO) (melting point 56 – 57°C).

Other techniques can be used with excellent results, among them one proposed by Meadows and Shoemaker (see Ref. on page 348). Recently, embedment in plastic (glycol methacrylate) has been proposed. This material permits the cutting of very thin sections (approximately 1 um) which often produces superior images. Most stains can be used though trichrome stains are often poorly differentiated. The plastic embedded tissues can be cut with glass knives in a special microtome or in a good standard microtome equipped with a holder for glass knives. Good quality knives can be made with a special machine (such as LKB Histo Knife-maker 2078).

It is also possible to cut 1-μm sections from osmium-fixed and Epon-embedded tissue (for electron microscopy). After proper pretreatment to remove the Epon, such sections can be stained with any of the standard stains. However, the preferred method is to stain them with toluidine blue (0.5% solution in 1% borax or 2.5% sodium carbonate); in this case, the Epon does not have to be removed. The slides are stained on a hot plate at 60°C for 30 seconds, washed in running water, blotted dry, and mounted in neutral Canada balsam or in catalyzed epoxy resin mixture. Under oil immersion, these sections reveal very fine structural details. Toluidine blue tends to fade after a relatively short time, especially when exposed to light; to obtain a permanent record, the pathologist must resort to microphotography.

Cutting

Thinness is a prerequisite of good renal biopsy sections. Standard histologic sections, which generally run 6 to 8 μm in thickness, are totally unsuitable. With proper processing, a good microtome and a sharp knife, an experienced technologist can routinely obtain sections 3 μm in thickness. It is frequently stated that renal biopsy sections should be cut at 2 μm; this can be accomplished but with a fair degree of difficulty. Often the attempt to set the microtome for 2 μm sections results in skipping, compression and generally unsatisfactory preparations.

It is important that no tissue is lost by the usual method of trimming the paraffin blocks. If the biopsy specimen is properly embedded and lies flat in the block, sections can and should be taken the moment the knife reaches the level of the tissue. Because a large number of sections are needed, some laboratories cut the entire block; others are satisfied with preparing ten to 20 slides. It is advisable to place no more than two or three sections on each slide. The slides should be consecutively numbered.

Staining

Most renal pathologists routinely employ four stains: hematoxylin and eosin, PAS, trichrome, and Jones' silver methenamine. Either PAS or trichrome (depending upon the quality of the stain and individual preference) is used as the basic stain, and the others serve as special stains. We routinely stain slides 1, 4, 7 and 10 with hematoxylin and eosin; slides 2, 5, 8 and 11 with PAS; and slides 3, 6, 9 and 12 with Jones' silver methenamine. Other stains and other combinations can be used. Special stains are used as necessary. The hematoxyline and eosin stain is useful for the study of inflammatory infiltrates, tubular cytoplasm, and glomerular "fibrinoid" deposits. Trichrome is also good for these purposes and for the study of glomerular basement membranes. The PAS stain with a hematoxylin counterstain provides the greatest amount of information about the general structure of the glomerulus and the status of its basement membranes and mesangium. Silver methenamine is a superior stain for demonstrating the details of the basement membrane structure; when used with a counterstain (hematoxylin and eosin, trichrome, or chromotrope R), it also demonstrates deposits and other structural details. Whenever hematoxylin is called for, we use Mayer's formula, but other hematoxylins can be used.

For PAS stain we follow the basic procedure of Lillie. It is essential to use fresh solutions; the usual custom of keeping Schiff's reagent until a pink discoloration appears is responsible for poor results with thin sections. We prepare Schiff's reagent every week and keep it at 4°C; solutions of periodic acid are freshly prepared before staining. The thinner the section, the longer it should remain in periodic acid and in Schiff's reagent.

The trichrome stains used are Masson, Heidenhain, or chromotrope-aniline blue. If trichrome is used as a basic stain, fixation in Zenker's or in alcoholic Bouin's solution is preferred. Tissue fixed in formalin must be mordanted in acidified Zenker's solution or in an acidified saturated aqueous solution of mercuric bichloride. The mercury is removed with Lugol's solution followed by sodium thiosulfate, and the slides are washed by dipping them five to ten times in distilled water.

For best results with Jones' silver methenamine, use only double-distilled water. The staining procedure must be visually controlled. After periodic-acid oxidation, the slides are placed in a solution of silver methanamine and then in an incubator at 60°C for a predetermined period of time (in our hands, two hours or less for formalin-fixed tissue). The slides then are rinsed in distilled water and examined wet under the microscope. If the stain is too pale (as determined solely by the degree of staining of the glomerular capillary basement membranes), the slides are placed in a fresh solution of silver methenamine which has been prewarmed in the incubator, and then returned to the incubator for another half hour. The process is repeated until the desired density of stain is obtained. After washing and toning in gold, sections may be counterstained with hematoxylin and eosin, trichrome, or chromotrope R.

Examination of Renal Biopsy Specimens

Light Microscopy

As a preliminary step, the pathologist should examine all of the stained sections so that the structures are viewed at several levels. This examination compensates to some degree for the small amount of tissue available and increases the chances of finding focal lesions. Several sections are selected for detailed examination. All glomeruli in the section are counted, and each glomerulus and the intervening tissue are examined under high magnification. A high dry lens (×40) is often sufficient, but in many instances an oil immersion lens is necessary. Generally, the glomerular count establishes the adequacy of the biopsy. A minimum of 10 to 15 glomeruli are considered necessary for diagnosis. However, with a diffuse lesion a diagnosis based on the examination of even 5 glomeruli can be 95% accurate. On the other hand, focal lesions producing clinical manifestations may affect 1% or fewer glomeruli and consequently may not be found in the available renal tissue. Occasionally, as in acute interstitial inflammation or in some cases of amylodosis, a diagnosis can be made even in the absence of glomeruli.

Glomeruli are examined for the presence and the extent of abnormalities: enlargement, cellularity, mesangial expansion, thickening of capillary walls, deposits, thrombosis, necrosis, crescents, adhesions, sclerosis, and thicknening of Bowman's capsule. These lesions may affect the whole glomerulus or only a segment of it. Tubules may show epithelial changes (vacuolization, degeneration, necrosis), intraluminal casts, basement membrane thickening, and diffuse or focal atrophy. Within the *interstitial tissue,* edema, fibrosis and various types of inflammation can be noted. *Arteries and arterioles* may show sclerosis, hyalinization, narrowing of the lumen, thrombosis, necrosis and inflammation.

The pathologist should examine the sections before consulting the clinical history. After a thorough examination, the preliminary diagnosis or diagnoses can be noted and correlated with clinical and laboratory data. Each case should be discussed with the clinician in charge; a final diagnosis may be reached at the time, or further studies, including electron microscopy and immunofluorescence, may be conducted. In addition to making the specific diagnosis, evaluation should be made of the severity of the process, the degree of renal damage, and if possible the character of the disease, whether acute and self-limited or chronic and progressive.

For a complete diagnosis, special stains may be necessary. If amyloid is suspected, metachromatic stains (e.g., crystal violet), Congo red stain, and thioflavine T are useful, as is electron microscopy. Other special stains include those

APPENDIX

for hemoglobin, hemosiderin, fibrin, calcium and uric acid.

Electron Microscopy

A growing number of pathology laboratories have acquired electron microscopic facilities, along with a set of procedures for processing and examining specimens by this method. Many smaller institutions are able to establish a working relationship with an electron microscopic laboratory to which they refer the tissues and whose methods they adopt for the initial processing. The following information is addressed to those who have no immediate access to an electron microscopic facility, but who would like to preserve some tissues for future study. Once embedded in Epon or a similar medium, the tissue can be kept indefinitely.

Fixation. Preparation of tissue for electron microscopy requires fixation in osmic acid (osmium tetroxide). For a study of glomeruli, we prefer direct fixation in 1% osmic acid in a buffer solution at pH 7.2 to 7.4. Either phosphate buffer 1/15 M or collidine buffer are satisfactory. Fix for one to two hours at $4-6°C$; do not overfix.

Glutaraldehyde fixation is widely used. It preserves cytoplasmic details but tends to obscure somewhat the glomerular structure. Only purified glutaraldehyde (such as Tousimis Ultrapure Temgrade, Tousimis Research Corporation, Rockville, MD) should be used. The stock solution should be diluted with phosphate buffer (1/15 M, pH 7.2 to 7.4) to obtain a 2% working solution. Fix for two to four hours at $4-6°C$, wash in cold 0.2 M sucrose solution, and postfix in 1% osmic acid for one hour. If osmication is not carried out immediately, the tissue can be kept in sucrose overnight in the refrigerator. Overfixation in glutaraldehyde is less damaging to the tissue than overfixation in osmic acid but should be avoided whenever possible. Both osmic acid and glutaraldehyde penetrate poorly; for best results the tissue should be cut into small fragments about 0.5 mm in diameter.

Paraformaldehyde fixation has been mentioned under light microscopy. A piece of tissue to be processed for electron microscopy is cut into small fragments as mentioned above, washed in 0.1 molar phosphate buffer pH 7.2 and postfixed in 1% osmic acid for one hour.

Processing. From osmic acid, transfer the tissue into the following:

1. 0.2 M sucrose — two changes, five minutes each.
2. 70% ethyl alcohol — two changes, five minutes each.
3. 90% ethyl alcohol — two changes, five minutes each.
4. 100% ethyl alcohol — 20 minutes. (Steps 1 through 4 are carried out in a refrigerator.)
5. Second change of 100% alcohol — 20 minutes at room temperature.
6. Propylene oxide — two changes, ten minutes each.
7. Propylene oxide-Epon (equal parts) — one hour (use mixer).
8. Pure Epon — overnight in refrigerator.
9. Embed in Epon in appropriate capsules (e.g., Beem, Better Equipment for Electron Microscopy, Bronx, NY).
10. Cure for 48 to 96 hours at $55-60°C$.

If a suitable microtome (such as Porter Blum 10, Ivan Sorvall, Inc., Newtown, CT) is available, 1-μ sections can be cut with glass knives, stained with toluidine blue, and examined with the light microscope (as previously described). The same 1-μ section can be used to select the best glomeruli or other areas of interest for electron microscopic study.

Though many fine details of structure may be seen by an experienced microscopist under light microscopy, electron microscopy is extremely helpful in the examination of the individual glomerular components. Changes in the capillary wall, often crucial to the understanding of the pathologic process, can be seen clearly (e.g., endothelial detachment, ingrowth of mesangium into the subendothelial space, thickening and spitting of the basement membrane, various types of deposits, and formation of basement membrane "spikes").

Electron microscopy is also helpful in the study of the mesangium, indicating the presence and localization of deposits, from amyloid to immune complexes; the changes in the amount and character of the mesangial matrix; and the proliferation of cells. Special features that may be seen include the structure of deposits (e.g., crystals, organized patterns) or the presence of unusual constituents (e.g., myxoviruslike particles) in the cell cytoplasm.

Immunofluorescent Microscopy

Principle. The principle of immunofluorescnet microscopy is based on the specific binding of labeled antibody to antigen in tissue; identification of the label indicates the presence and localization of the particular antigen, e.g., immunoglobulin or complement as part of an immune complex.

Clinical rationale. Immunofluorescent microscopy is particularly helpful in the differential diagnosis of glomerular diseases.

Preservation of tissue. The renal tissue must be processed promptly and carefully because many antigens are labile. The specimen is surrounded by a small amount of embedding medium, such as Tissue-Tek (Ames Co., Elkhart, IN), snap-frozen in liquid nitrogen or a mixture of dry ice and isopentane, and stored at a temperature of −70°C. Paraffin-embedded tissue has been used for the labeled antibody technique; however, many antigens are destroyed during routine histologic processing.

Materials. Fluoresceinated antiserums to all known human immunoglobulin classes, light and heavy chains of immunoglobulins, and a variety of plasma proteins, including fibrinogen and several components of the complement system, are commercially available. The potency and specificity of the antiserums are of utmost importance and directly determine the reliability of the results obtained. Therefore, all antiserums should be tested by agargel double immunodiffusion, by immunoelectrophoresis, or preferably on agarose beads coated with the purified antigen. Further specificity controls include absorption of the labeled antibody with the purified antigen and blocking of the staining by the labeled antibody after prior incubation of tissue sections with unlabeled antibody.

Fluorescein isothiocyanate and rhodamine have been used most widely as labels of the anti-serums, but they require a darkfield ultraviolet microscope and fade with time, necessitating photographic documentation. Recently, products of enzyme reactions, particularly of peroxidase, have become more popular as labels because they obviate these limitations.

Methods. The snap-frozen tissue is cut in a cryostat at a thickness of 2 μm to 4 μm. The sections are mounted on slides, dried or desiccated, and fixed in acetone, ether or ethanol for ten minutes. After washing in three changes of phosphate buffered saline (pH 7.2) for 15 minutes each, the sections are incubated with the labeled antiserums for 30 to 60 minutes at room temperature or for shorter periods at 37°C. Subsequently, they are washed and coverslipped in a nonfluorescent embedding medium such as Elvanol (Du Pont Co., Wilmington, DE). If peroxidase-labeled antibodies are used, they are developed in a mixture of diaminobenzidine and hydrogen peroxide. It is advisable to include with each staining procedure a renal specimen with known staining characteristics so that technical failures can be detected. One or two sections should be set aside to be stained for examination by light microscopy; this permits a direct comparison between the histologic and immunologic findings.

Interpretation. Sections should be examined soon after staining to avoid the effects of fading. For the same reason, it is advisable to document the findings by microphotography using a high-speed film. The following points are noted:

1. Presence or absence of the antigen sought, e.g., immunoglobulin A, B_{1c} (third component of complement, C3); fibrinogen.

2. Intensity of staining (+ to ++++). The staining intensity bears some relation to the amount of antigen present, but because many other factors (e.g., thickness of section, fading, characteristics of the labeled antibody) also play a role, it is dangerous to place too much reliance on this semi-quantitative evaluation.

3. Distribution of the antigen along the glomerular capillaries, in the mesanguium, along the tubular basement membranes, and in the interstitial vessels.

4. Form of antigen deposits. Granular deposits of immunoglobulin and complement along the glomerular capillary walls are characteristic of immune complex nephritis (post-streptococcal glomerulonephritis, membranous nephropathy, systemic lupus erythematosus), whereas linear staining of the glomerular basement membrane (GBM) for IgG and complement is usually seen in anti-GBM nephritis (Goodpasture's syndrome, extracapillary glomerulonephritis) and sometimes also in diabetic glomerulosclerosis. Lipoid nephrosis or minimal change is usually free of detectable deposits. Focal glomerulonephritis often shows diffuse granular mesangial deposits with segmental accentuation (particularly IgA as in Berger nephropathy). Membranoproliferative glomerulonephritis is characterized by peripheral granular deposits of complement, usually accompanied by immunoglobulin.

References

1. Agodoa, L.C.Y., Striker, G.E. and Chi, E.: Glycol Methacrylate Embedding of Renal Biopsy Specimens for Light Microscopy. Amer. J. Clin. Path. 64:655, 1975.
2. Bancroft, J.D. and Stevens, A.: Histopathological Stains and Their Diagnostic Uses. New York, Churchill, Livingstone, Longman, 1975.
3. Churg, J. and Gerber, M.A.: Interpretation of Renal Biopsies. In: Pediatric Kidney Disease. Edited by C. M. Edelmann, Jr., Boston, Little, Brown & Co., 1978.
4. Churg, J. and Prado, A.: Rapid Mallory Trichrome Stain (Chromotrope-Aniline Blue). Arch. Pathol. 62:505, 1956.
5. Cohen, A.H.: Masson's Trichrome Stain in the Evaluation of Renal Biopsies. Amer. J. Clin. Pathol. 65:631, 1976.
6. Ehrenreich, T. and Espinosa, T.: Chromotrope Silver Methenamine Stain of Glomerular Lesions. Amer. J. Clin. Path. 56:448, 1971.
7. Hayat, M.A.: Principles and Techniques of Electron Microscopy: Biological Applications, Vol. 1, New York, Van Nostrand Reinhold Co., 1970.

APPENDIX

8. Hayat, M.A.: Basic Electron Microscopy Techniques. New York, Van Nostrand Reinhold Co., 1972.
9. Lillie, R.D.: Histopathologic Technic and Practical Histochemistry, 4th Edition, New York, McGraw-Hill Book Co., 1976.
10. Marinozzi, V. and Faraggiana, T.: Impregnazione Argentica Ed Ultramicrotomia Nella Diagnostica Delle Glomerulonefriti. Pathologica 72:1, 1980.
11. Meadows, R. and Schoemaker, H.: Improved Processing Technique for Renal Biopsies for Light Microscopy. J. Clin. Pathol. 23:548, 1970.
12. Nairn, R.C.: Fluorescent Protein Tracing, 4th Edition, New York, Churchill, Livingstone, Longman, 1976.

INDEX

Abscess, glomerular 166
Acid hydrolases deficiency, in I-cell disease 299
Acute nephritic syndrome *See* Syndrome
Adhesions, capsular 5, 6, 37, 67, 70, 118, 311
Alcohol, dehydration in 346
Alport's syndrome *See* Syndrome
Aminoaciduria, in Fabry's disease 299
Amyloidosis (Amyloid)
 –, A, 241
 –, L, 241
 –, fibril, 240
 –, primary, 240
 –, renal, 4, 13, 19, **240–241, 244, 246, 252**
 –, secondary, 240
Anaphylactoid purpura *See* Schönlein-Henoch's purpura
Angiitis, hypersensitivity, 188
 –, idiopathic necrotizing, 188
Angiokeratoma, 298
Antibodies, anti-basement membrane, 152, 153
 –, –, –, elution of 153
 –, anti-Hbs (Hepatitis B), 262
 –, anti-nuclear, 129
 –, anti-strongyloides, 177
 –, streptolysin O titer, 68
Antigen, fibrin related, 199, 212, 213, 310
 –, Hbs (Hepatitis B), 262, 266
 –, histocompatibility, 320
 –, streptococcal, 69
 –, type C virus, 131
Arteries, adventitial fibrosis, 213
 –, arcuate, in scleroderma, 213
 –, fibrin deposition, in intravascular coagulation, 204
 –, –, –, in transplant rejection, 320
 –, Fibrinoid necrosis, in periarteritis nodosa, 194
 –, –, –, in radiation nephritis, 311
 –, –, –, in transplant rejection, 320
 –, hyaline thickening, in hemolytic-uremic syndrome, 202
 –, interlobular, in scleroderma, 213
 –, intimal sclerosis (fibrosis), 199, 211, 214, 216
 –, – thickening, in transplant rejection, 320
 –, –, –, mucoid, 212, 213, 216
 –, medial hypertrophy, 211
 –, thrombosis, 204, 216, 311

Arterio-venous shunt, traumatic, 166
Arterioles, afferent, anatomy of, 23
 –, –, in benign nephrosclerosis, 211
 –, –, in diabetic glomerulosclerosis, 226, 227
 –, efferent, anatomy of, 23
 –, –, in diabetic glomerulosclerosis, 226, 227
 –, fibrin deposition, in transplanted kidney, 320
 –, fibrinoid necrosis, 190, 212, 213, 216, 320
 –, "glomeruloid" structure, in thrombotic microangiopathy, 199
 –, glomoid transformation, in end stage kidney, 322
 –, hyaline sclerosis, in benign nephrosclerosis, 211
 –, hyalinization, hyaline deposition 211, 214, 227, 238
 –, intimal thickening, 211
 –, medial hypertrophy, 199, 282
 –, subendothelial swelling, in thrombotic microangiopathy, 199
 –, thrombi, in thrombotic microangiopathy, 199
 –, –, in toxemia of pregnancy, 310
Arteriolosclerosis, hyaline, in diabetes, 227
Arteritis, fibrinoid, in scleroderma, 218
 –, in systemic lupus erythematosus, 130, 140
 –, Takayasu, 188

Bacteria, gram-negative, 166
 –, gram-positive, 166
 –, pneumococcus, 68
 –, staphylococcus, 68
 –, –, aureus, 166
 –, –, epidermidis, 167
 –, streptococcus, 68
 –, –, hemolytic, 68
 –, –, –, α, 166
 –, –, nephritogenic, 68
Basement membrane, 28, 30
 – –, "breaks", 80
 – –, disruption, 90, 120
 – –, "double contour", 83, 84
 – –, "lacunae", 177, 182, 270
 – –, membranous transformation, 175
 – –, "moth-eaten" appearance, 262
 – –, plexiform layer, 176, 182
 – –, rarefaction, 184
 – –, splitting, 83, 280

INDEX

Basement membrane (*continued*)
— —, thickening, 130, 226, 227, 242
— —, —, irregular, 176, 283
— —, —, segmental, 280
— —, thinning, segmental, 281
— —, "washed out" areas, 186
— —, wrinkled, 212, 220
Berger's disease (IgA nephropathy), 4, 10, 18, 19, 36, 39, 67, 113, **151–152, 156, 164**, 320
Biopsy
—, needle, 345
—, open, 345
—, wedge, 345
Bowman's capsule, 23, 28, 30, 85, 226
— —, adhesion   *See* Adhesion, capsular
— —, epithelium, 23
— —, —, embryonal hyperplasia, 319
— —, fibrous thickening, 211
— —, pseudotubules, 118
— —, segmental staining, 92
Bowman's space, dilatation, 283
— —, fibrous obliteration, 211
Buffer, acetate, 345
—, phosphate, 345
Burr cell   *See* Cell

Capillary (ies)
—, aneurysm (retinal), 230
—, intertubular, 146
Capillary loops, glomerular, aneurysmal dilatation, 226
— —, —, basement membrane.
  See Basement membrane
— —, —, breaks, 69, 112
— —, —, collapse, 37, 38, 48, 152, 211, 320
— —, —, —, ischemic, 212
— —, —, —, segmental, 154
— —, —, necrosis, 111, 150, 158
— —, —, —, segmental, 192, 311
— —, —, "plexiform" appearance, 274
— —, —, "plugging", by hyaline thrombi, 242
— —, —, thrombi, 5, 160, 199, 200, 310
— —, —, —, fibrin, 164, 320
— —, —, —, hyaline, 242, 248
— —, —, thrombocytes, 152
— —, —, thrombosis, 5, 6, 68, 111, 156, 158, 160
— —, —, —, segmental, 154
— —, —, wrinkling, 211, 320
—, lumina, 28
— wall, anatomy of, 23
— —, double outline, 86, 94, 96, 182, 202
— —, segmental abnormality, 5, 6
— —, thickening, 83, 84, 177, 211
— —, —, diffuse, 54
— —, —, segmental, 5, 6
Capsular drop, hyaline, 227

Casts, 68
—, multi-layered intraluminal, 241
Cell, coat, 23, 26
—, fragmented red blood, 200
—, inclusions, 299
—, red blood, "arrow", "burr", "helmet", 198, 200
Ceramide, dihexosyl, 298
—, trihexosyl, 298
—, trioxidase, 298
Chromosome, Y, in Alport's syndrome, 280
Collagen in the basement membrane, 282
Complement, deposition of, C3, 42, 88
—, depression of, 68, 69, 85
—, early components, 55, 68, 84
Complexes, DNA-anti-DNA, 129
—, non-specific trapping, 227
Congenital nephrotic syndrome   *See* Syndrome
Congo-red   *See* Stain
Crescent, 44, 68, 83, 84, 85, 92, 111, 158, 190, 192, 211, 224, 242   *See also* Glomerulonephritis, crescentic
—, beginning or early, 111
—, cellular, 5, 6
—, —, definition of, 3
—, fibro-cellular, 5, 6, 116, 120, 134
—, —, definition of, 3
—, fibrous, 116, 227
—, —, definition of, 3
—, focal, 150
—, occlusive, 152
—, segmental, 150, 212
—, small, 37, 116
Cyroglobulinemia, 4, 14, 188, 199, 240, **242–243, 248, 250, 258, 260**, 262
—, mixed, 14, 18, 19, 150, 241, 250, 262
—, monoclonal, 242
—, primary, 242
—, secondary, 242
Crystal deposition, in end-stage kidney, 319
Crystalline material in cryoglobulinemia, 250
Cystic disease, acquired, in "transstygian" kidney, 319
Cystine, demonstration of, 346
Cysts in congenital nephrotic syndrome, 282

Deafness, neurosensory, in Alport's Syndrome, 280
Dehydration of tissue, 346
Dense deposit disease   *See* Glomerulonephritis, dense deposit
Deposits, amyloid, 240, 241, 242
—, demonstration of, 347
—, electron dense, 36, 84, 104, 130, 142, 151, 160, 164, 174, 222, 263, 310
—, fibrinogen, 218
—, fine lipid, 264
—, hyaline, 37, 40, 42

INDEX

Deposits (*continued*)
—, intra-luminal, 242
—, intramembranous, 5, 6
—, linear, 55, 152, 153, 227, 320
—, lumpy, 84
—, mesangial, 5, 6, 151
—, "organized", in Cryoglobulinemia, 243
—, organized ("fingerprint"), in systemic lupus erythematosis, 130, 148
—, paramesangial, 76
—, ribbon-like granular, in light chain disease, 241
—, serpiginous fibrillar, in Lecithin-Cholesterol Acyl Transferase Deficiency, 299
—, subendothelial, 5, 6, 39, 48, 84, 96, 242
—, subepithelial, 5, 6, 76, 83, 100
—, translucent, 112, 212
—, transmembranous, 5, 6
Diabetes mellitus, 19, 226
Diabetic glomerulosclerosis *See* Glomerulosclerosis
Diffuse, definition of, 3
Disease, Fabry's, 5, 15, **298, 300, 302**
—, heart, cyanotic congenital, 263
—, I-cell, **299, 300**
—, lecithin cholesterol acyltransferase deficiency *See* Lecithin-Cholesterol Acyl Transferase (LCAT) Deficiency
—, light chain, 241, **246, 256**
—, microcystic, 282
—, nil, 35
—, pulmonary, 263
—, sickle cell, 263, 266, 268
DNA in glomeruli, in systemic lupus erythematosus, 131
Drug addicts, 166
Dysproteinemias, nephropathy in dysproteinemia, 241

Eclampsia, 310
Electron microscopy, scanning, of glomerulus, 46
Embedding, 346
—, Epon, 346
Endocarditis, acute Salmonella, 168
—, as a cause of focal glomerulonephritis, 38
—, infective, glomerular lesions in, 4, 11, 67, 68, **167, 168, 172**
—, —, as a cause of glomerulonephritis, 18, 67, 68, 166–167
—, staphylococcal, 166
Endothelium (endothelial cell), 28
—, cytoplasm, 23
—, detached (detachment), 206
—, diaphragm, 23
—, edema, 46, 314
—, enlargement, 310
—, pore, 23
—, separation (of), 199, 330
—, swelling, 68
—, vacuolated, 310
Endotoxin, 199
End stage kidney *See* Kidney
Epithelium (epithelial cell), 28
—, detachment, 38
—, parietal, 23, 30
—, squamous metaplasia, 322
—, vacuolated (vacuolization), 298, 300
Erythrocytes, fragmentation of, in hemolytic-uremic syndrome, 198
—, —, in transplanted kidney, 320
—, sludging of, 263
Extracapillary glomerulonephritis *See* Glomerulonephritis

Fabry's disease *See* Syndrome
Familial mediterranean fever, 240
Fanconi's syndrome *See* Syndrome
Fibrils, amyloid, 240
—, in subendothelial space, 320
Fibrin (Fibrinogen), 36, 52, 69, 84, 114, 132, 196, 199, 202, 213, 310, 320
Fibrosis, definition of, 3
—, interstitial, 38, 212, 282
Fixatives, alcoholic Bouin, 345, 347
—, Dubosque-Brazil *See* alcoholic Bouin
—, formalin, 345
—, glutaraldehyde, 348
—, osmic acid, 348
—, paraformaldehyde, 346, 348
—, Zenker-formol, 345, 347
Foam cells, glomerular, 280
— —, interstitial, 37, 40, 281, 284
— —, in lecithin cholesterol acyltransferase deficiency, 304
— —, lipid-laden, 299
Focal, definition of, 3
Focal/segmental lesions
  See Lesions, focal/segmental
Focal segmental hyalinosis and sclerosis, 7, **37–38**, 42 *See also* Glomerulosclerosis, focal segmental
Foot processes, 28, 30
— —, effacement (loss) of, 36, 38, 46, 84, 122, 282, 283
— —, secondary, 32
Freeze drying, 345
— substitution, 345

Generalized Shwartzman Phenomenon
  See Shwartzman phenomenon
Giant cells multinucleated, 241
Global, definition of, 3
Glomerular lesions *See* Glomerulus, lesions
Glomerulitis, alterative, 211
—, granulomatous, 189
Glomerulonephritis (GN), crescentic, 4, 9, 18, **111–112, 120, 122,** 152, 153, 166, 189, 212

353

INDEX

Glomerulonephritis, crescentic (*continued*)
–, –, early stage, 114
–, –, focal, 38, 39, 44, 52, 111
–, –, idiopathic, 111, 152
–, –, secondary, 116
–, dense deposit, 4, 9, 18
–, diffuse, 4
–, endocapillary proliferative, 4, 8, 18, **68–69, 72, 74, 78, 80, 82**
–, extracapillary *See* Glomerulonephritis, crescentic
–, focal, 8, 18, 37, **38–39, 44, 52,** 167
–, –, embolic, 167
–, –, healed, 211
–, in infective endocarditis, 11
–, lobular, 83, 102, 227
–, membranoproliferative, Type-1, 4, 9, **83–84, 86, 88, 94, 96, 98, 100, 102**
   See also mesangiocapillary
–, –, Type-2 *See* Glomerulonephritis, dense deposit
–, –, Type-3, 4, 9, **83–84, 88, 90, 102, 104**
–, membranous, 4, 7, 18, 19, 35, 37, **54–55, 56, 58, 60, 62, 64,** 69, 113, 150, 167, 177, 226, 242, 262
–, –, crescents, in, 58
–, –, early, 56
–, –, fully developed, 56
–, –, glomerular sclerosis in, 58
–, –, idiopathic, 54, 130
–, –, and proliferative, in malarial nephropathy, 177
–, –, schematic representation, 58
–, –, segmental sclerosis, 58
–, –, stage 1, 60
–, –, stage 2, 62
–, –, stage 3, 64, 234
–, –, stage 4, 64
–, mesangial proliferative, 4, 8, 18, 19, **67, 70, 72, 76**
–, –, –, in nephropathy of Cyanotic congenital heart disease, 263
–, –, –, –, of liver disease, 262
–, mesangiocapillary 4, 9, 18, 19, **83–84, 86, 88, 90, 94, 96, 98, 100, 102, 104, 134,** 150, 167, 177, 189, 242, 262, 263, 320 *See also* membranoproliferative
–, –, lobular, 86
–, necrotizing, 18
–, postinfectious, 67, 68, 188
–, poststreptococcal, 262
–, proliferative, 4
–, –, diffuse, 226
–, –, endocapillary, 4, 18, 67, **68–69, 72, 74, 78, 80, 82,** 116, 150, 154, 166, 167, 189
–, –, mesangial, 4, 8, 18, 19, 38, **67,** 69, **70, 72, 76,** 112

–, rapidly progressive, 18 *See* Glomerulonephritis, crescentic
–, recurrent, in transplanted kidney, 321
–, sclerosing, 4, 10, 18, 19, 38, 55, 68, 111, **112–113, 118,** 212, 280
–, –, chronic, 198
–, –, focal, 38
–, of systemic disease, 4, 125
–, unclassified, 4, 113
Glomerulopathy, hereditary, 280 *See also* Nephropathy
Glomerulosclerosis, diabetic 4, 13, 19, **226–227, 228, 230, 232, 234, 236, 238,** 263
–, –, diffuse, 226, 228, 232
–, –, nodular, 226, 228
–, focal segmental, 19, 36, **37–38, 40, 42, 44, 48, 50,** 211
–, hepatic, 264
Glomerulus, abnormalities of, minor, 4, 7, 35, 37
–, alterations, basic, 4
–, angiomatoid obsolescence, in Kidney, end-stage, 322
–, disease, miscellaneous, 309
–, –, primary, 3, 33
–, fibrin exudation, 190
–, hilus, 85, 211
–, immature, in congenital nephrotic syndrome, 282
–, juxtamedullary, 37
–, lesions, in infections, 4, 166
–, –, in metabolic diseases, 4, 225
–, –, in systemic disease, 4
–, –, following transplantation, 5, 17, **320–321, 324, 326, 328, 330, 332**
–, –, in vascular diseases, 4, 23, 187
–, lobule, 23, 28
–, –, accentuation of, 83, 84
–, –, collapse of, 48
–, necrosis, 150
–, –, segmental, 5, 6
–, normal, 23ff, 26, 54ff
–, sclerosis, in crescentic glomerulonephritis, 116
–, –, in nail-patella syndrome, 282
–, –, in sclerosing glomerulonephritis, 112, 118
–, "solidification", 37
–, thrombosis *See* Thrombosis, glomerular
Glycogen, preservation of, 346
Glycosaminoglycans, in I-Cell Disease, 299
Glycosphingolipids in Fabry's Disease, 298
GN. *See* Glomerulonephritis
Goodpasture's syndrome *See* Syndrome
Granules, dark irregular, in Nephropathy of liver disease, 270
Granulomatosis, allergic, 188

Heart disease, congenital cyanotic, 263

Hematoxylin bodies, 128, 130, 131, 138
Hematuria, exertional, 281
—, gross, 36, 54, 67, 68, 83, 85
—, isolated, 37
—, microscopic, 35, 36, 83
—, persistent, 18
—, "pure", 36
—, recurrent, 18, 37
—, —, benign, 5, 15, 281
Hemizygos males in Fabry's disease, 298
Hemoglobin, A, 263
—, S, 263, 274
—, SS, 266
Hemolytic uremic syndrome *See* Syndrome
Henoch-Schönlein purpura *See* Schönlein-Henoch purpura
Hepatitis, 262
—, B, 55, 176, 262
—, —, in membranous glomerulonephritis, 55
Hereditary nephropathy *See* Nephropathy
Heterozygos females in Fabry's disease, 298
Hodgkin's disease as a cause of amyloidosis, 240
"Humps" (sub-epithelial deposits), 68, 69, 78, 85, 100, 151, 166, 172
—, flame-shaped, 80
Hyaline casts, 36
—, droplets, 36
Hyalinosis, definition of, 3
—, segmental, 5, 6
Hyperprolinemia in Alport's syndrome, 280
Hypertension, 54, 83
, benign essential, 211
—, malignant, 198, 199, 212, 213
Hypotension, 240

IgA deposits, illustrations of, in Berger's disease, 156
— —, —, in nephropathy of liver disease, 264
— —, —, in Schönlein-Henoch purpura, 154
—, nephropathy *See* Berger's disease
—, in serum, 150, 151
IgG deposits, illustrations of, in lupus nephritis, 134, 136
— —, —, granular, in membranous glomerulonephritis, 56
— —, —, pseudolinear, in membranous glomerulonephritis, 56
IgM deposits, in Waldenstrom's macroglobulinemia, 242
— —, illustrations of, in focal segmental glomerulosclerosis, 42
— —, —, in mesangial proliferative glumerulonephritis, 70
Immunofluorescence findings *See* Individual Diseases, Tables III and IV and text
—, indirect, for demonstration of anti-GBM antibodies, 153

Immunoglobulin, light *See* Light chain
Infantile nephrotic syndrome *See* Syndrome
Infarcts, renal in periarteritis nodosa, 188
—, —, in scleroderma, 213
Infestation, strongyloides, 177
Infiltration, focal lymphocytic, in benign nephrosclerosis, 212
Inflammation, periglomerular, in crescentic glomerulonephritis, 112
—, purulent, of glomerulus, 166
Interstitial fibrosis, in multiple myeloma, 241
— —, in radiation nephritis, 311
— infiltration in amyloidosis, 240
— tissue, examination of, 347
Intravascular coagulation *See* Thrombosis, glomerular

Juxtaglomerular apparatus, anatomy of, 24
— —, hyperplasia (hypertrophy) of, 212, 213, 220
Juxtaglomerular granular cells, in end-stage kidney, 322

Kidney, end-stage, 5, 16, **319, 322**
—, transplanted, recurrence of dense deposits, 85
—, transstygian, 319
Knife (knives), 346
—, glass, 346

Lamina densa of basement membrane, anatomy of, 23, 30
— — —, dense deposits in, 85
— — —, —, lacunae, in Nail-Patella Syndrome, 282
— — —, "mottling" in minimal change nephrotic syndrome, 36
— — —, notching, 222
— — —, splitting, 290
— — —, thickening in LCAT deficiency, 299
— — —, thickening in Nail-Patella Syndrome, 282
— — —, thinning of, 281, 292
Lamina rara externa (subepithelial space), anatomy of, 23, 30
Lamina rara interna (subendothelial space), anatomy of, 23, 30
— — —, in LCAT deficiency, 299, 304
— — —, widening of, 36, 38, 206, 208
Latent period in progression of glomerulonephritis, 113
Lecithin-Cholesterol Acyl Transferase (LCAT) Deficiency, 15, 262, **299, 300, 304, 306**
Lesions, exudative *See* Lesions, hyaline
—, focal/segmental, 4, 35, 37
—, hyaline, 113, 226, 227, 230, 236
—, insudative *See* Lesions, hyaline

Leucocytic infiltration polymorphonuclear, 5, 6, 68, 69, 72, 84, 112, 168
Light chain, 241
– –, excretion of, 227
– –, kappa, 248
Lipid droplets (vacuoles) in endothelial cells, 37
– –, in tubular cells, 40
–, neutral, in foam cells, 299
Lipidoses, 5, 298–299
Lipodystrophy, partial, 85
Liver, cirrhosis, 262
Lupus Erythematosus, Systemic, 54, 55, 67, 68, 177, 198, 199
– –, –, acute, 129, 132
– –, –, nephritis (lupus nephritis), 4, 10, 18, 19, **127–131**, **132**, **134**, **136**, **138**, **140**, **142**, **144**, **146**, **148**
– –, –, –, diffuse, 128, 129, 131, 134, 142, 242
– –, –, –, early stage, 36, 38
– –, –, –, focal, segmental, 128, 129, 132
– –, –, –, membranous, 128, 130, 131, 136, 144
– –, –, –, mesangial, 128, 129, 131, 142
– –, –, –, mesangiocapillary, 128, 130
– –, –, –, minimal, 132
– –, –, –, morphological classification, 128

Macroglobulinemia *See* Waldenstrom's macroglobulinemia
Macrophages in crescents, 112
Malaria, nephropathy *See* Nephropathy
–, quartan, 176
Membranous, glomerulonephritis *See* Glomerulonephritis, membranous
–, nephropathy *See* Glomerulonephritis, membranous
Mesangiolysis, in hemolytic-uremic syndrome, 199
–, in malignant nephrosclerosis, 212
–, in transplant rejection, 321
Mesangium, cell, anatomy of, 23, 24
–, –, increase, in mesangial glomerulonephritis, 67
–, –, proliferation, 67, 68, 83, 85, 152, 177
–, –, vacuolization, 304
–, edema, 206
–, expansion, 310
–, interposition of, 83, 84, 85, 94, 258, 263, 276, 326
–, matrix, 23, 24, 28
–, –, disruption, 199
–, –, expansion, 37, 38, 67
–, –, increase, 67, 83, 226
–, –, sclerosis, 67, 85, 283
–, nodules, in Cyanotic congenital heart disease, 263

–, –, in diabetic glomerulosclerosis, 226, 227, 236
–, –, in dysproteinemias, 241, 242
–, reticulation of, 199
Microangiopathy, thrombotic, 4, 12
Microcysts in congenital nephrotic syndrome, 288
Microscopy, electron, 345, 348
–, –, fixation, 348
–, –, –, glutaraldehyde, 348
–, –, –, osmic acid, 348
–, –, –, paraformaldehyde, 346, 348
–, –, processing, 348
–, immunofluorescence, 345
–, –, clinical rationale, 348
–, –, interpretation, 349
–, –, materials, 349
–, –, methods, 349
–, –, preservation of tissue, 348
–, –, principle, 348
–, light, 345, 347
–, –, cutting, 346
Microthrombi, platelet, 211
Microvilli, glomerular in nephrotic syndrome, 36, 38, 46
Minimal change nephrotic syndrome *See* Syndrome
Minor glomerular abnormalities *See* Glomerulus, abnormalities of, minor
Monocyte, in crescents, 111, 112
–, in the mesangium, in diffuse proliferative glomerulonephritis, 68
Mucolipidosis, 298
–, II. *See* Disease, I-Cell
Mucopolysaccharidosis, 298
Multiple myeloma, 4, 13, 240, **241**, 242, **246**, **248**, **254**, **256**
Myelin bodies, 298
Myxovirus-like particles, in lupus nephritis, 131

Nail-Patella syndrome *See* Syndrome
Necrosis, definition of, 3
Nephritic factor C_3 (C_3NeF), 83, 85
Nephritis, hereditary, 18, 19, 36
–, lupus *See* Lupus Erythematosus, nephritis
–, radiation, 5, 16, **310–311**, **312**, **316**
–, –, acute, 311, 312
–, –, chronic, 311, 312
–, –, experimental acute, 316
–, Schönlein-Henoch's nephritis *See* Schönlein-Henoch's Purpura
–, shunt, glomerular lesions in 4, 11, **167**, **170**, **174**
Nephropathy, of cyanotic congenital heart disease, 5, 14, **263**, **268**, **276**
–, in dysproteinemia, 4
–, hereditary, 5, 279–306
–, IgA *See* Berger's disease

Nephropathy (*continued*)
 –, IgM, 18, 19
 –, of liver disease, 4, 14, **262**, **264**, **266**, **270**, **272**, **274**
 –, malarial, 4, 11, **176–177**, **178**, **182**
 –, –, advanced stage, 178
 –, –, quartan, 178
 –, membranous
  See Glomerulonephritis, membranous
 –, parasitic, 4, 176
 –, pre-eclamptic *See* Nephropathy of toxemia of pregnancy
 –, in pulmonary hypertension, 5, 263
 –, schistosomal, 4, 11, **177**, **178**, **180**, **184**
 –, of sickle cell disease, 4, 14, 19, 263, **266**, **268**, **274**, **276**
 –, strongyloides, 4, **177**, **180**, **186**
 –, of toxemia of pregnancy, 5, 16, **310**, **312**, **314**, **316**
 –, tropical, 176
Nephrosclerosis, benign, 4, 12, **211–212**, **214**, **220**
 –, malignant, 4, 12, **212**, 213, **216**, **220**
Nephrosis, lipoid *See* Syndrome, nephrotic, minimal change
Nephrotic syndrome *See* Syndrome
Nodules, adenomatous, in end-stage kidney, 319
 –, smooth muscle, in end-stage kidney, 319

Ocular abnormalities and anomalies, 280, 282
Organelles, focal increase, 36
 –, of podocytes, focal increase, 36
Osteomyelitis, as a cause of amyloidosis, 240
Osteo-onychodysplasia *See* Syndrome, nailpatella

Paraffin, 346
 –, blocks, trimming of, 346
 –, chloroform, 346
 –, xylene, 346
Paramesangial area, 24
Paraplast, 346
Parasites, as a cause of glomerulonephritis, 68
Parasitic nephropathy *See* Nephropathy
Particles, dark, irregular, in nephropathy of liver disease, 262
 –, –, membrane-bound, in LCAT Deficiency, 299
 –, virus like, in SLE, 131
Periarteritis nodosa, 4, 12, 18, 38, 68, 153, **188–189**, **190**, **194**
 –, –, classical form (Kussmaul-Maier), 188
 –, –, microscopic, 151, 188
Plasma cell dyscrasia, 227
Plasmodium, falciparum, 176
 –, malariae, 176

Plastic embedding, 346
Platelet aggregates, giant, in Alport's syndrome, 280
 –, in nephrotic syndrome, 36
Podocyte, anatomy of, 23
 –, detachment, in focal segmental hyalinosis sclerosis, 38
 –, edema, 36, 46
 –, enlargement, 36
 –, foot processes, 23
Preeclampsia, 310
Pregnancy, as a cause of hemolytic-uremic syndrome, 198
 –, toxemia, hydatidiform mole, 310
 –, toxemia of *See* Nephropathy, of toxemia of pregnancy
 –, –, hydramnion, 310
 –, –, twin pregnancy, 310
Proliferation, glomerular, segmental mesangial/endocapillary, 5, 6
 –, resolution of 74
Properdin, glomerular deposits, 90
Proteinuria, isolated, 36, 83
 –, non-selective, 37, 54
 –, orthostatic, 36
 –, selective, 35
Pseudotubules, 113
Purpura, Schönlein-Henoch *See* Schönlein-Henoch purpura
 –, thrombotic thrombocytopenic, 4, 129, **198–199**, **204**
Pyelonephritis, 37, 212, 226

Radial heads, subluxation, in nail-patella syndrome, 282
Radiation nephritis *See* Nephritis, radiation
Rapidly progressive nephritic syndrome *See* Syndrome
Raynaud's phenomenon, 213
Rejection, transplant, 19
Renal failure, acute, post partum, 198
 –, –, –, rapidly progressive, 83, 85
Rheumatic fever, as a cause of focal glomerulonephritis, 38
Rheumatoid arthritis, as a cause of amyloidosis, 240

Scar, glomerular, global, 150
 –, segmental, 55
Schistosoma, japonicum, 177
 –, mansoni, 177
Schistosomal nephropathy *See* Nephropathy
Schistosomiasis, hepatosplenic, 178
 –, nephropathy *See* Nephropathy, schistosomal
 –, as a cause of nephrotic syndrome, 54
Schönlein-Henoch purpura, 38, 67, 68, 150, 188, 199
 –, –, –, nephritis, 4, 10, 18, 19, **150–151**, **154**, **160**, **162**

INDEX

Scleroderma, 4, 13, 188, 199, **213, 216, 218, 222, 224**
Sclerosis, glomerular
–, definition of, 3
–, diffuse, 320
–, –, mesangial *See* Syndrome, nephrotic, infantile (French type)
–, focal global, 6, 8
–, global, 5, 6
–, and hyalinosis, focal segmental, 19, 36, 37, **38, 40, 42, 44, 48, 50,** 211, 298 *See also* Glomerulosclerosis, focal segmental
–, segmental, 5, 6, 54, 311
–, systemic *See* Scleroderma
–, vascular, 38
Sections, thin, 346
Segmental, definition of, 3
Sepsis, gram negative, as a cause of glomerular thrombosis, 199
Septicemia, glomerular lesions in, 4, **166, 168, 172**
–, staphylococcus aureus, **168**
Shunt, nephritis *See* Nephritis, shunt
Shwartzman phenomenon, generalized, 199
Sickle cell nephropathy *See* Nephropathy
Spicules, amyloid, 240, 246
Spikes, basement membrane, 54, 55, 56, 62, 69, 82, 100, 130, 138, 144, 186
Stain, alcian-blue, in I-Cell disease, 299
–, chromotrope R, 347
–, colloidal iron, in I-Cell disease, 26, 299
–, Congo red, 347
–, –, –, in Amyloidosis, 240, 244
–, crystal violet, in Amyloidosis, 240, 244
–, hemotoxylin and eosin, 347
–, metachromatic (crystal violet), 347
–, phosphotungstic acid, in nail-patella syndrome, 282
–, thioflavin T, 347
–, –, in amyloidosis, 240, 246
–, –, in dense deposit disease, 85, 92
–, toluidin blue, 240
–, –, in amyloidosis, 240
–, trichrome, 347
Strongyloidosis, 176, 177, 180
–, nephropathy *See* Nephropathy
Structures, dark lamellated, in Fabry's disease, 302
Subendothelial space, widening of, following transplantation, 320
Syndrome, acute nephritic, 18, 38, 83, 111, 166
–, Alport's 5, 15, 18, 19, 37, **280, 281, 284, 290**
–, chronic nephritic, 19
–, Fanconi's 241
–, Goodpasture's 4, 11, 18, 111, **152–153, 156, 158, 164,** 188, 199, 320

–, hemolytic-uremic, 4, 18, 129, **198–199, 200, 202, 204, 206, 208,** 212, 310, 320
–, Kimmelstiel-Wilson's 226
–, nail-patella, 5, 15, 19, 37, **282, 286, 294**
–, nephrotic, 19, 54
–, –, congenital (Finnish type) 5, 15, 19, **282, 288, 296**
–, –, idiopathic, 35
–, –, infantile (French type) 5, 15, 19, **283, 288**
–, –, minimal change, (Lipoid nephrosis), 19, **35–36, 40,** 46
–, –, steroid dependent, 37
–, –, steroid resistant, 35, 37
–, rapidly progressive nephritic, 18, 166
–, thin basement membrane, 5, 15, 19, **281, 286, 292**
Syphilis, 4, 55
–, acquired, 167
–, congenital, 54, 167
–, nephropathy of, **167, 170, 175**
–, secondary, 54, 167

Takayasu disease *See* Arteritis
Therapy, anti-hypertensive, 212
–, anti-syphilitic, 167
–, immunosupressive, for transplant rejection, 320
Thin basement membrane disease *See* Syndrome, thin basement membrane
Thrombocytopenia, in Alport's syndrome, 280
Thrombosis, capillary, 5, 6
–, glomerular, 4, 12, 150, 198, **199, 204**
–, renal vein, 55, 240
–, segmental, 38, 199
Thrombotic microangiopathy, 4, 12, 198
–, thrombocytopenic purpura *See* Purpura
Thrombus (thrombi) capillary, 54
–, –, fibrin, 127
–, –, hyaline, 127, 136
Toxemia of pregnancy *See* Nephropathy, of toxemia of pregnancy
Trabeculae, of podocytes, 32
Transformation, malignant (malignancy), in end-stage kidney, 319
Transplant (Transplantation) of kidney, 320
–, rejection 19, 198, 199 *See also* Glomerulus lesions following transplantation
–, –, acute, 320, 330
–, –, –, cellular, 324
–, –, –, vascular, 324
–, –, chronic, 320
–, –, –, vascular, 324
–, –, hyperacute, 320
Treatment, antimalarial, 176
–, antischistosomal, 177
Tuberculosis, as a cause of amyloidosis, 240

Tubules, atrophy, 36, 38, 212, 282
 —, basement membrane, dense deposits, 108
 —, —, —, deposits, in lupus nephritis, 146, 148
 —, —, —, thickening, in diabetes, 230
 —, calcification, 241
 —, degeneration, 112, 311
 —, examination of, 347
 —, proximal, in nephrotic syndrome, 40
 —, vacuolation, 280
Tumor, malignant, as a cause of membranous glomerulonephritis, 54
 —, protein, as antigen in membranous glomerulonephritis, 55

Uremia, 113
Uric acid, preservation of, 346
Urinary sediment, telescoped, 127, 188

Vasculitis
 —, leucocytoclastic, 151
 —, necrotizing, 152
Virus, 68, 176
 —, type C, in lupus nephritis, 131

Waldenstrom's macroglobulinemia, 4, 14, **242, 248, 258**
Wegener's granulomatosis, 4, 12, 18, 38, **188—189, 192, 196**
Wire-loop, 127, 130, 131, 134, 136, 140, 142